DISEASES OF PIGEONPEA

About the Author

Dr. S.C. Agrawal, the author of the book on "Diseases of Pigeonpea" is Principal Scientist (Plant Pathology) and Dean, JNKVV, R.A.K. College of Agriculture, Sehore, Madhya Pradesh, India. He did his M.Sc. Ag. in Plant Pathology from Vikram University Ujjain in 1963 and Ph.D. in Plant Pathology from J.N. Krishi Vishwa Vidyalaya, Jabalpur in 1985. He has put more than 38 years of experience of doing teaching, research and extension work in various capacities of which 31 years have been devoted to research on diseases of pulse crops specially pigeonpea, lentil, chickpea, mungbean and urdbean.

Dr. Agrawal has published more than 100 research papers in national and international journals, nine book chapters/review papers, three bibliographies, three technical bulletins and several extension articles. He is author of two books namely *Diseases of greengram and blackgram* and *Diseases of lentil*. He has guided several post graduate students for their thesis work and has presented more than 60 research papers in national and international symposia/seminars/workshops/conferences etc. Dr. Agrawal has contributed substantially in releasing disease resistant and high yielding varieties of pulse crops like JG 11, JG 16, JG 130, JAKI 9218 of chickpea, JL 3 of lentil and JA 4 of pigeonpea.

He is the life member of Indian Phytopathological Society, New Delhi and regular member of several scientific societies specially, Indian Society of Pulses Research and Development, Kanpur, Society of Mycology and Plant Pathology, Udaipur, Plant Protection Association of India etc. Dr. Agrawal has been honoured by the "ISPRD Recognition Award 2001" for his outstanding contribution in the field of pulses research and development. He is the member of several Committees of National level and is a well known Pulse Pathologist of the country. His work on diseases of pigeonpea and lentil is well recognized.

DISEASES OF PIGEONPEA

S.C. AGRAWAL
Principal Scientist (Plant Pathology)

CONCEPT PUBLISHING COMPANY, NEW DELHI-110059

ISBN : 81-8069-006-7

First Published 2003

Published and Printed by
Ashok Kumar Mittal
Concept Publishing Company
A/15-16, Commercial Block, Mohan Garden
New Delhi-110059 (INDIA)

Phone : 25351460, 25351794
Fax : 091-11-25357103
Email : publishing@conceptpub.com

Preface

Pigeonpea is a pulse crop highly sensitive to biotic and abiotic stresses which cause enormous losses. The research work on this aspect got momentum in the sixtees of the 20th century. Since then, lot of information has been generated and published in various journals, reports, review articles etc. There has been a long felt need by the students of higher classes, teachers, research workers and extension specialists for a comprehensive book on this aspect. The present book on "Diseases of Pigeonpea" has been written with the objective to make the scattered literature available to readers at one place. The book presents complete and up-to-date literature on the subject.

The matter of the book is dealt in 10 chapters. The introductory chapter presents the background information and the progress in relation to work done on diseases of pigeonpea. The diseases caused by fungi; bacteria; viruses, MLOs and viroides; and nematodes have been described under suitable headings in chapters 2-6. Besides the basic information on a particular disease, information on research methodologies developed specially on creation of epiphytotics and scoring plants for screening against a disease, have been described. The detailed information given on epidemiology, sources of resistance and the disease control technology are highly useful. Symptoms of different diseases have been described with original photographs which will be of great help to readers in identification and differentiation of diseases with alike symptoms.

The ecology of rhizosphere, rhizoplane, spermatosphere, seed, phyllosphere of plants play important role in development of diseases which has been covered in a chapter on Microbes in ecology of pigeonpea. Pigeonpea is highly sensitive to various meteorological parameters, soil conditions, agrochemicals etc. which result in production of typical symptoms on plants resembling to biotic diseases. This aspect has been covered in a separate chapter on abiotic diseases. This information will be of great help in avoiding misidentification of confusing biotic disorders. The integrated disease management has now been recognized as an important system for reducing the damage caused by diseases and minimizing the environmental pollution and health hazards through minimizing use of pesticides. This information covering biological, cultural and chemical control along with multiple host resistance has been dealt in the last chapter. A few packages for IDM have also been given. The concerned references have been listed in the end of each chapter. In the last, detailed Subject index has been given which will help the reader to locate the important terms and their synonyms for understanding the subject in a better way.

Literature on pigeonpea diseases published within last 3-4 decades has increased in geometrical progression. Collating this widely scattered literature and arranging it in a proper sequence is a difficult and time consuming job. In spite of my best efforts, several lapses may be noticed in the book. The readers are humbly requested to inform their views to the author for future improvement.

While preparing the manuscript of this book cooperation and help of my wife Mrs. Leela Agrawal and other family members and my colleagues Drs. H.S. Yadava, K.V.V. Prasad, A.K. Tripathi and the Dean of the College of Agriculture, Sehore, Dr. V.S. Tomar is gratefully acknowledged.

Sehore **S.C. Agrawal**

Contents

List of Tables

List of Figures

1

Introduction

Pigeonpea (*Cajanus cajan* (L.) Millsp.) is an important grain legume (Pulse) of tropics and subtropics. It is grown in the countries of Africa, Asia and Oceania and America. In Africa, it is grown in countries like Ghana, Kenya, Madagascar, Malawi, Nigeria, Senegambia, Tanzania, Uganda and Zambia while in America it is distributed to variable extents in Brazil, Colombia, Dominican Republic, Grenada, Guadeloupe, Guyana, Haiti, Jamaica, Martinique, Mexico, Panama, Peru, Puerto Rico, Trinidad, USA and Venezuela. The countries growing pigeonpea in Asia and Oceania are Australia, Bangladesh, Burma (Myanmar), India, Indonesia, Malaysia, Nepal, Pakistan, Philippines, Sri Lanka, Taiwan, Thailand and U.S.S.R. There are several other countries where pigenopea is grown in smaller areas. Pigeonpea is considered to be originated in India as 16 out of 25 species of *Atylosia* which are considered as wild prototypes of *Cajanus* exist in the western Ghats of India (Baldev 1988).

More than 350 vernacular names of pigeonpea have been recorded, however, it is commonly known as red gram, Angola pea, Congopea, No-eye pea etc. Many Sanskrit names have their modern equivalent. Adhaki or Adhuku became 'Arhar', the Dravidian Tuvarai or Tuvari used in Sanskrit since 300-4000 AD became 'Tur'. The name 'Pigeonpea' was first reported from Barbados where the seeds were once considered very useful as feed for pigeons. This name was not framed earlier than the 16th Century.

1.1 Importance

Pigeonpea is very important pulse crop which is used in various ways. Its main use is in the form of Dhal (dry, dehulled, split seed) in the Indian diet. Its green seeds are used as vegetable. It has good nutritive value although, it contains considerable amount of antinutritional polyphenolic compounds which inhibit the digestive enzymes trypsin, chymotrypsin and amylase. Faris *et al.* (1987) have tabulated the comparative nutritional values of green pigeonpeas, matured seeds and dhal of pigeonpea (Table 1.1).

Table 1.1 : Nutritive value of green, matured seeds and dhal of pigeonpea

Constituents	*Green seed*	*Matured seed*	*Dhal*
Protein (%)	21.0	18.8	24.6
Trypsin inhibitor (unit mg^{-1})	2.8	9.9	13.5
Protein digestibility (%)	66.8	58.5	60.5
Starch (%)	48.4	53.0	57.6
Amylase inhibitor (units Mg^{-1})	17.3	26.9	—
Starch digestibility (%)	36.2	—	53.0
Soluble Sugar (%)	5.1	3.1	5.2
Flatulence factors (g 100 g^{-1} soluble sugar)	10.3	53.5	—
Crude fibre (%)	8.2	6.6	1.2
Fat (%)	2.3	1.9	1.6
Minerals (mg 100 g^{-1}) :			
Calcium	94.6	120.8	16.3
Magnesium	113.7	122.0	78.9
Copper	1.4	1.3	1.3
Iron	4.6	3.9	2.9
Zinc	2.5	2.3	3.0
Cooking time (minutes)	13	53	18

Besides the human and animal diets, the green leaves of pigeonpea are used as fodder, dry stems as fuel wood and to make huts and baskets etc. The plants at various stages are also used as green manure, wind breaks, as live fence for boundaries of small farms and as substrate to culture the lac producing insects.

The pigeonpea has unique character to find important place in various intercropping systems of cereals, oilseeds, legumes, cotton etc. It is able to reduce the soil erosion on slopy lands and enrich the soil by adding the organic matter through leaf fall and about 40 kg N/ha through nitrogen fixation. This crop has good capacity to grow in poor lands and provides more stability in rainfed situations than any other crop.

Area, Production and Yield

The information on area, production and yield of pigenopea in the world is not available adequately as the substantial area under backyard crop is not included in the statistics. As per available information, it is grown in about 3974, thousand hectare of which more than 90 % lies in India

1.4 Publications Made

A critical review of published work on pigeonpea diseases (Table 1.3) shows that during first 2 decades of 20th century, only 11 references appeared which increased gradually but the increase was tremendous after 1970 reaching on peak in the last 2 decades. It coincides with the period of start of AICRP on pulses and establishment of ICRISAT. However, a large proportion of publications are on screening against diseases or the chemical control of diseases. The work on fundamental/basic research has been very limited and studies on survival of pathogens, their variability, epidemiology and forecasting, nature and extent of losses is still lacking in many diseases.

Table 1.3 : Number of research reports and publications on pigeonpea diseases during different decades

Period (Years)	*Number of publications*
Upto 1910	4
1911 to 1920	7
1921 to 1930	31
1931 to 1940	43
1941 to 1950	49
1951 to 1960	73
1961 to 1970	96
1971 to 1980	280
1981 to 1990	478
1991 to 1998	330

These references being in different reports, journals, magazines etc. are not available to all the readers at a place. The first effort for compiling the references seems to be that of Barnes (1973) who listed 184 references on pathological aspects of pigeonpea. Later, annotated bibliographies were published by Dahiya (1980) and Nene *et al.* (1985) who included 594 references with their abstracts for the period of 1906 to 1981.

The literature on diseases of pigeonpea was mostly compiled and reviewed with diseases of other pulse crops (Sen Gupta 1974, Kaiser 1976, 1981, Nene 1978, Reddy 1987, Reddy *et al.* 1986, Grewal 1988). The reviews on pigeonpea diseases alone in full were not much (Brathwaite 1981, Reddy *et al.* 1990). However, few publications have been made from extension point of view (Williams and Allen 1976, Gurha and Singh 1980, Reddy *et al.* 1993). In this book efforts have been made to review the subject *in toto*.

Lot of work on pigeonpea diseases has been done but still a lot has to be done which has been indicated for further planning in several reviews (Nene 1986, Reddy *et al.* 1992, Johansen *et al.* 1993, Kimani *et al.* 1993, Daudi 1993 and Songa and King 1994).

REFERENCES

Abrams, R., Morales, A. and Julia, P. J. 1978. Status of research on pigeonpea in Puerto Rico. *Tropical Grain Legume Bulletin* 11-12:17.

Akinola, J.P., Whiteman, P.C. ahd Wallis, E. S. 1975. The agronomy of pigeonpea (*Cajanus cajan*). Review Series, Commonwealth Bureau of Pastures and Field Crops no. 1/1975. Ferham Royal, Slough, UK: Commonwealth Agricultural Bureaux. 57 pp.

Baldev, B. 1988. Origin, distribution, taxonomy and morphology. pages 3-51, *In* Pulse Crops (Eds. B.Baldev, S. Ramanujam and H.K. Jain). Oxford & IBH Publishing Co. Pvt. Ltd., New Delhi.

Barnes, R.F. 1973. A preliminary list of literature on pigeonpea (*Cajanus cajan* (L.) Millsp). Plant Pathology Bulletin 1. St. Augustine, Trinidad, Trinidad and Tobago : University of West Indies, Department of Biological Sciences. pp 123.

Brathwaite, C.W.D. 1981. Diseases of pigeonpea in the Caribbean region. pages 129-136. *In* Proceedings of the International Workshop on Pigeonpeas, 15-19 Dec. 1980, ICRISAT Centre, Vol. 1. Patancheru, India : International Crops Research Institute for Semi Arid Tropics.

Childers, N.F., Winters, H.F., Robles, P.S. and Plank, H.K. 1950. Vegetable gardening in the tropics. Circular no. 32. Mayaguez, Puerto Rico : United States Department of Agriculture, Federal Experimental Station. 144 pp.

Dahiya, B.S. 1980. An annotated bibliography of pigeonpea 1900-1977. Patancheru, A.P., India : International Crops Research Institute for the Semi Arid Tropics. 183 pp.

Daudi, A.T. 1993. Plant protection research on pigeonpea in Malawi. pp 63-64. In improvement of pigeonpea in Eastern and Southern Africa. Annual Research Planning meeting 1993, Bulwayo, Zimbabwe, 25-27 Oct. 1993 (Eds. S.N. Slim, S. Tuwafe and L. Singh). Patancheru, India : International, Crops Research Institute for Semi Arid Tropics

Faris, D.G., Saxena, K.B., Majumdar, S. and Singh, U. 1987. Vegetable pigeonpea : A promising crop for India. Patancheru, A.P., India: ICRISAT, 13 pp.

Grewal, J.S. 1988. Diseases of pulse crops - an overview. *Indian Phytopathology* 41 : 1-14.

Gurha, S.N. and Singh, R.A. 1980. Current strategy for combating some important diseases of chickpea and pigeonpea. *Pesticides Annual* 1980-81 : 86-92.

Johansen, C., Shanower, T. G. and Reddy, M.V. 1993. ICRISAT's research on pigeonpea in a global context. In improvement of pigeonpea in eastern and southern Africa. Annual research planning meeting 1993, Bulawayo, Zimbabwe, 25-27 Oct. 1993 (Eds. S.N. Slim, S. Tuwafe and L. Singh). Patancheru, India; ICRISAT.

Kaiser, W.J. 1976. Important disease, and pests of bean (*Phaseolus vulgaris*), Lima bean (*Phaseolus lunatus*) and pigeonpea (*Cajanus cajan*) in Africa. *African Journal of Plant Protection* 1: 97-102.

Kaiser, W.J. 1981. Diseases of chickpea, lentil pigeonpea and tepary bean in continental United States and Puerto Rico. *Economic Botany* 35 : 300-321.

Kannaiyan, J., Nene, Y.L., Reddy, M.V., Ryan, J.G. and Raju, T.N. 1984. Prevalence of pigeonpea diseases and associated crop losses in Asia, Africa and the Americas. Tropical Pest Management 30:62-71

Kannaiyan, J., Reddy, M.V. and Nene, Y.L. 1981. Survey of pigeonpea diseases with special reference to wilt and sterility mosaic in India on Pages 297-303, In Proceedings of the International Workshop on pigeonpea, 15-19 Dec. 1980, ICRISAT Centre, India. vol. 2. Patancheru, A.P., India. International Crops Research Institute for Semi Arid Tropics.

Kimani, P.M., Omanga, P.A., and Slim, S.N. 1993. Status of pigeonpea research in Kenya, and future prospects. Pages 37-44. *In* Improvement of pigeonpea in eastern and southern Africa. Annual research planning meeting 1993, Bulawayo, Zimbabwe, 25-27 Oct. 1993 (Eds. S.N. Slim, S. Tuwafe and L. Singh). Patancheru, India International Crops Research Institute for Semi Arid Tropics.

Krauss, F.G. 1921. The Pigeonpea : Its culture and utilization in Hawaii. *Bulletin, Hawaii Agricultural Experiment Station* 64 : 46 : 1-23.

Krauss, F.G., 1932. The Pigeonpea (*Cajanus indicus*) : its improvement, culture and utilization in Hawaii. *Bulletin, Hawaii Agricultural Experiment Station* 64 : 46.

Morton, J.F. 1976. The Pigeonpea (*Cajanus cajan* Millsp.) : a high protein, tropical bush legume. *Horticultural Science* 11 : 11-19.

Nene, Y.L. 1978. Major disease problems of some grain legume crops in India. Pages 1-11. *In* Proceedings of the plant protection conference, 22-25 March 1978, Kuala Lumpur, Malaysia. Kuala Lumpur, Malaysia : Rubber Research Institute of Malaysia.

Nene, Y.L. 1986. Opportunities for research on diseases of pulse crops. *Indian Phytopathology* 39 : 333-342.

Nene, Y.L., Kaiser, W.J., Grewal, J.S., Kannaiyan, J. and Beniwal, S.P.S. 1985. An annotated bibliography of pigeonpea diseases, 1906-1981. Bibliography 013, Patancheru, India International Crops Research Institute for Semi Arid Tropics, 128 pp.

Nene, Y.L., Kannaiyan, J. and Reddy, M.V. 1981, "Pigeonpea Diseases, Resistance Screening Techniques". *Information Bulletin no. 9*, Patancheru, A.P., India : International Crops Research Institute for Semi Arid Tropics, 14 pp.

Nene, Y.L., Sheila, V.K. and Sharma, S.B. 1996. A world list of chickpea and pigeonpea pathogens. 5th Edn. Patancheru, A.P., India: International Crops Research Institute for Semi Arid Tropics.

Rachie, K.O. and Roberts, L.M. 1974. Grain legumes of the low land tropics. *Advances in Agronomy* 26 : 1-132.

Rachie, K.O. and Wurster, R.T. 1971. The potential of pigeonpea (*Cajanus cajan*), as a horticultural crop in east Africa. *Acta Horticulturae* 21 : 172-178.

Rathi, Y.P.S. and Nene, Y.L. 1984. "*Arhar ke Rog*". Pages 190-201 *In* "Faslon ke Rog" in Hindi (Eds. Amar Nath Mukhopadhyay and Ram Asare Singh). Directorate of Translation and Publications, G.B. Pant University of Agriculture and Technology, Pant Nagar, India.

Reddy, D.V.R., Nene, Y.L. and McDonald, D. 1986. Virus disease problems of groundnut, chickpea and pigeonpea. International Symposium on Virus diseases of rice and leguminous crops in the tropics, Yatabe, Tsukuba, Ibasaki, Japan : Tropical Agricultural Research Centre, pp. 67-75.

Reddy, M.V. 1987. Diseases of pigeonpea and chickpea and their management. Pages 175-184 *In* Plant protection in field crops (Eds. M.V. Rao and S. Sithanantham), Rajendra nagar, Hyderabad, India: Plant Protection Association of India.

Reddy, M.V., Haware, M.P., Nene, Y.L. and McDonald. D. 1992. Recent advances in fungal diseases of chickpea and pigeonpea. Pages 194-201 *In* New Frontiers of Pulses Research and Development (Eds. J.N. Sachan). Proceedings of National Symposium, 10-12 Nov. 1989, Directorate of Pulses Research, Kanpur, India.

Reddy, M.V., Sharma, S.B. and Nene, Y.L. 1990, Pigeonpea : disease management. Pages 303-347 *In* The Pigeonpea (Eds. Y.L. Nene, S.D. Hall and V.K. Sheila). Wallingford, Oxon, UK: CAB International.

Reddy, M.V., Raju, T.N., Sharma, S.B., Nene, Y.L. and McDonald, D. 1993. Handbook of pigeonpea diseases. *Information Bulletin no. 42*. Patancheru, A.P., India : International Crops Research Institute for Semi Arid Tropics.

Sen Gupta, P.K. 1974. Diseases of major pulse crops in India. *PANS* 20 : 409-415.

Songa, W. and King, S.B. 1994. Pigeonpea Pathology Research in Kenya : progress and future research strategies. Pages 45-50, *In* Improvement of pigeonpea in eastern and southern Africa. Annual research planning meeting 1993, Bulawayo, Zimbabwe, 25-27 Oct. 1993 (Eds. S.N. Slim, S. Tuwafe and L. Singh). Patancheru, A.P. India : International Crops Research Institute for Semi Arid Tropics.

Sharma, D. 1986. Breeding disease resistant varieties of pigeonpea (*Cajanus cajan* (L.) Millsp.). Pages 103-139, *In* Pigeonpea Genetics and improvement (Eds. Tikka, S.B.S.). Sharda Publishing Academy, Gujarat, India.

Viegas, A.P. 1961. Index of fungi of south America. Campinas, Brazil : Institute of Agronomica, Secao de Fitopatologia, 921 pp.

Williams, F.J. and Allen, D.J. 1976. Pigeonpea diseases. Pages 58 *In* Pathology : Grain Legume Training Course, 16 Aug. to 26 Nov. 1976 Ibadan, Nigeria : International Institute of Tropical Agriculture.

2

Fungal Diseases of Root and Stem

Large number of fungi have been reported to attack pigeonpea causing root and stem diseases but only few of them are important economically specially wilt, Phytophthora blight and dry root rot.

2.1 Damping Off

It is a minor disease of pigeonpea characterized by rotting of seedlings at soil level at pre-emergence or post-emergence stages. In pre-emergent, the young seedling is attacked at germination so that the seedling does not come out of the soil. In post-emergent, the infection of young seedlings by pathogens causes desiccation of the foliage and young shoots resulting in death. Rotting takes place at collar or stem portion of the seedling (Malik 1945). Damping off is caused mostly by species of *Pythium, Fusarium, Rhizoctonia, Phytophthora* etc.

2.1.1 Causal Organism

Pythium species : Pigeonpea has been reported to be susceptible to most species of *Pythium* isolated from various crops in U.S.A. (Sideris 1929). Out of several species, *P. splendens* var. *hawaiianum,* an aggressive isolate from pine apple, caused seedling mortality in pigeonpea (Sideris 1932). The species of *Pythium* causing damping off in pigeonpea have been reported from India (Malik 1945) and Africa (Kaiser 1976) also. So far following five species have been reported on pigeonpea.

- *Pythium aphanidermatum* (Edson) Fitzpatrik
- *Pythium splendens* Braun var. *hawaiianum* Sideris
- *Pythium arrhenomanes* Drechsler
- *Pythium debaryanum* Hesse

- *Pythium irregulare* Buisman

All these species, specially first two, are highly pathogenic to pigeonpea producing damping off symptoms. They are predominated on seed at >75% soil moisture holding capacity while *Aspergillus* species are predominated at 50 % or less.

Rhizoctonia species : Pre- and post-emergence damping off disease of pigeonpea was reported from Puerto Rico by Jehle and Wood (1926) and simultaneously by Tucker (1927). The cause was reported as *Rhizoctonia ferruginea* which was more destructive in wet weather. The host range of the pathogen includes many of the vegetable crops grown in the area. The characters of mycelium and sclerotia of *R. ferruginea* are similar to that of *Sclerotium rolfsii* which has been found to be pathogenic to pigeonpea (Kaiser 1981). Hence, it is possible that Tucker was dealing with the fungus resembling to *S. rolfsii.* The fungi *Corticium rolfsii* and *Macrophomina phaseolina (Rhizoctonia bataticola*) have been isolated from the diseased seedlings of pigeonpea (Malik 1945).

2.1.2 Control

No specific control measures have been recommended but the seed treatment with proper fungicide and reduced soil moisture may help in reducing the inoculum potential and thus the severity of the disease.

2.2 Seedling Rot

A new seedling rot of pigeonpea was reported from the areas near Allahabad caused by *Fusarium equiseti* (Bhargava *et al.* 1981). The seedlings were noticed to die between 20-30 days after sowing. The seedlings killed at early stage were necrotic and commonly covered with profuse white fungal growth. The affected seedlings showed the water-soaked spots on the radicles which later turned brown. The seedlings subsequently collapsed and toppled down due to weakening of the tissues at the collar region. The pre-emergence rot was reported as high as 65 per cent.

2.3 Fusarium Wilt

Fusarium wilt of pigeonpea was first reported from India by Butler (1906) who characterized the term wilt by gradual or rather sudden withering and drying of green parts, exactly as if they are suffering from drought, even though there may be plenty of water in the soil, with characteristic blackening of wood tissues of main root and stem. The detailed description of this disease was published later (Butler 1918). The disease being very important economically attracted attention of research workers who did substantial work which has been reviewed from time to time (Prasad 1978, Nene *et al.* 1980, Upadhyay and Rai 1989, 1992; Reddy *et al.* 1990, Haware 1993). The causal organism of pigeonpea wilt has been studied and described by various workers (Wollenweber 1931, Wollenweber and Reinking 1935, Sadasivan and Subramanian 1954 and Booth 1971). The work on this disease was initially done mostly at Imperial Agricultural Research Institute, Pusa, Bihar and later at Madras, Botany School, Madras; Indian Agricultural Research Institute, New Delhi and ICRISAT Centre, Patancheru, India.

2.3.1 Distribution and Economic Importance

The disease occurs in most of the pigeonpea growing countries of Asia, Africa, Europe and America specially Bangladesh, Germany, Ghana, Granada, India, Indonesia, Italy, Kenya, Malawi, Mauritius, Myanmar, Nepal, St. Kills & Nevis, Tanzania, Thailand, Trinidad & Tobago, Uganda, Venezuela, Vietnam and Zambia (Nene *et al.* 1996). During a systematic survey conducted in 1975-1980, the disease was found serious in Africa specially in Malawi (36.3%), Tanzania (20.4%) and Kenya (15.9%) with an annual loss of over US dollors 5 million (Kannaiyan *et al.* 1981c, 1984b). However, later surveys indicated reduced wilt incidence in Kenya (Songa *et al.* 1991) but it was high in Zambia (Kannaiyan and Sharma 1992; Mbwago 1994). The disease is not a serious problem in Bangladesh, Nepal, Malaysia and Myanmar. The disease occurs in India in almost all the pigeonpea growing states but it is comparatively less in southern states. Kannaiyan *et al.* (1981c) recorded the incidence of the wilt in Maharashtra (22.6%), Bihar (18.3%), Uttar Pradesh (8.2%), West Bengal (6.1%), Madhya Pradesh (5.4%), Andhra Pradesh (5.3%), Gujarat (5.4%), Tamil Nadu (1.4%), Karnataka (1.1%), Orissa (0.3%), and Rajasthan (0.1%). Later surveys in some areas indicated wilt to be a major problem in pigeonpea production in western Maharashtra (Podule *et al.* 1982), Gujarat (Desai *et al.* 1981), Alvar and Dholpur districts of Rajasthan (Gaur and Sharma 1989), Karnataka (Bidari 1995, Mahalinga *et al.* 1998) and lower elevations of Garhwal hills of Uttar Pradesh (Kumar *et al.* 1991).

Looking to death of plants due to wilt, one would presume total losses on per plant basis but it is not so because of partial wilting in some plants and death of plants occurring at different stages of crop growth. The losses are 100% when plants wilt at pre-pod stage but 67.1% and 29.5% at pod maturity and pre-harvest stages respectively (Kannaiyan and Nene 1981c). The wilted plants produce over 70% normal seeds and in delayed wilting, seeds are not affected adversely. Wilt percentage and yield has negative linear relationship ($r^2 = 93$) at the wilt incidence range of 69-99% in susceptible and 31-63% in moderately susceptible cultivars (Naik and Reddy 1993b). This relationship is expected to be more stable looking to the fact that soil moisture and temperature do not play major role in wilt incidence as compared to soil inoculum (Naik and Reddy 1992). The annual pigeonpea crop losses due to wilt alone have been estimated about US dollor 36 million in India (Kannaiyan *et al.* 1984b).

2.3.2 Symptoms

Symptoms of the disease were described by Butler (1906, 1910, 1918) and later by various workers (Satyanarayana and Kalyansundaram 1952, Subramanian 1963c, Amin *et al.* 1976; Nene *et al.* 1980; Upadhyay and Rai 1989) but not much has been added after Butler.

The disease appears on young seedling of 4-6 weeks age but more wilt is observed during the flowering and podding stages. The infected seedlings show loss of turgidity, interveinal clearing, chlorosis of foliage which sometimes become yellow before wilting. Under artificial inoculation, lower leaves of seedlings start yellowing within 10 days, they droop, shed within 15 days and then wilt within 20 days (Kaiser and Sen Gupta 1979). Gaur and Sharma (1989) reported yellowing of leaves, epinesty, marginal necrosis of leaves and finally complete wilting. The typical symptoms in plants are gradual or sudden withering and drying of green foliage in the way as if they are suffering from drought even in presence of sufficient soil moisture (Fig. 2.1).

The characteristic symptoms of the disease are browning of the xylem vessels from the root to the stem which can be seen as black streaks in vascular region (Fig. 2.2) and under the bark. In some cases brown or dark purple coloured bands can be seen on surface of the stem starting from base to several feet above the ground level (Fig. 2.3). The branches towards the band wilt while those on other side may remain unaffected resulting in partial wilting of plant. Browning and blackening of wood under such banded bark can be seen clearly. Such bands on the stem can be traced starting from lateral roots while the infection of tap root commonly results in complete wilting of plant. In tolerant genotypes, such bands are confined to basal part of the stem. In some cases, specially at later stages of the crop growth, the branches of affected plant may dry from top downward showing no symptoms on lower part of the stem (Reddy *et al.* 1990d). On splitting, the main stems of such plants show intensive blackening of xylem. A pinkish mycelial growth generally appears on the basal portion of diseased plants under humid condition.

The Phytophthora blight of pigeonpea has probably been mistaken for wilt disease in the past as gross symptoms of both the diseases resemble with each other (Amin *et al.* 1976). However, both can be distinguished as: (i) the leaves of plants affected by wilt turn yellow before drying while those by blight are light green with upward rolling followed by rapid drying. (ii) Leaves in case of wilt remain attached to plant while they shed in case of blight. (iii) Frequent blackening of xylem tissues occurs in wilt and not in blight.

Expression of symptoms also depend, on type of pathogen and host. Similar symptoms may be produced on a host by different species of *Fusarium* while different symptoms may be incited on the same host by the same species of *Fusarium* in different areas ranging from wilt, rots, die back, twig blight etc. (Sengupta 1974). The wilt affected plants are generally seen in patches in field and the affected area increases in size every year specially if pigeonpea is grown in the same area continuously.

2.3.3 Causal Organism

Conidial State : *Fusarium udum* Butler

Perfect state : *Gibberella indica* Rai and Upadhyay

Synonyms : *Fusarium Butleri*

F.uncinatum Wollenw.

F.lateritium Nees Var. *uncinatum* (Wollenw) Wollenw

F.oxysporum f sp. *udum* (Butler) Snyder & Hansen

F.lateritium f sp. *cajani* (Padwick) Gorden

F.udum var. *cajani* Padwick

F.vasinfectum f. *cajani*

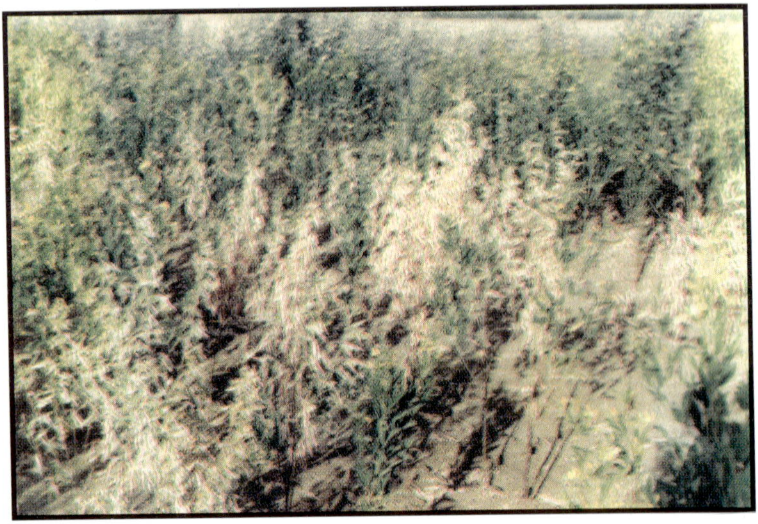

Fig. 2.1: Wilt affected plants of pigeonpea.

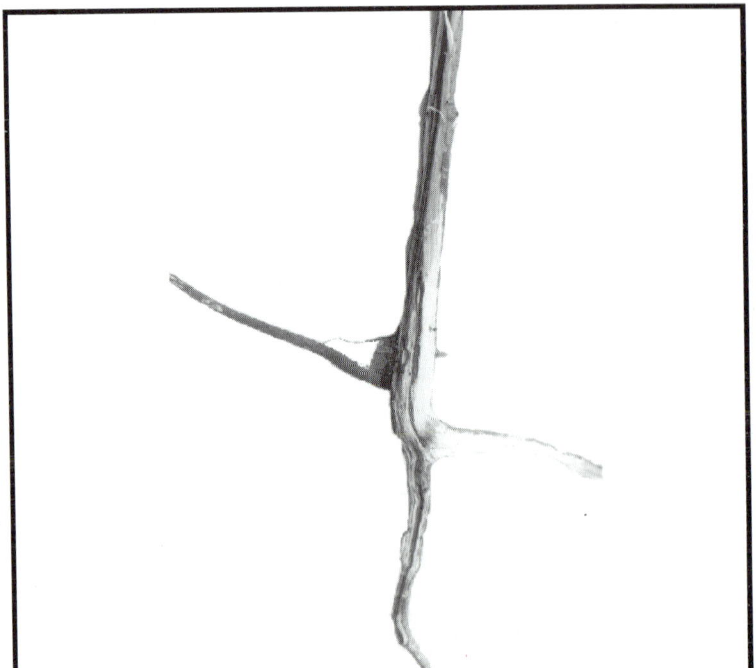

Fig. 2.2: Pigeonpea wilt: Browning of xylem.

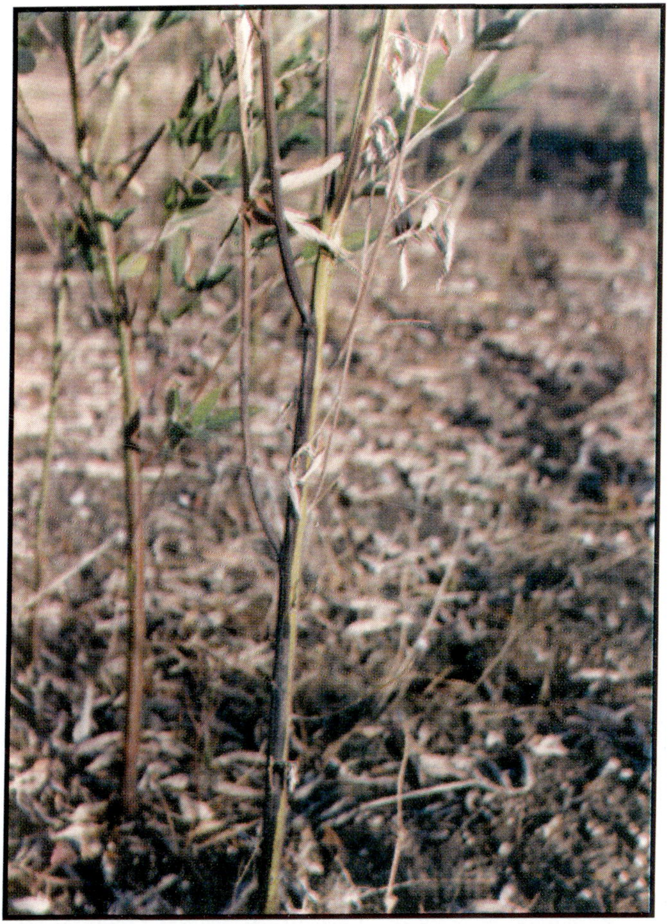

Fig. 2.3: Pigeonpea wilt: Brown band on surface of stem

The pigeonpea wilt pathogen was first described as *Fusarium udum* (Butler 1910) from India and it was later reported from Uganda (Small 1922). In Tanganyika, the causal fungus of pigeonpea seedling mortality was reported to be *F. lateritium* var. *uncinatum* (Wallace 1932) which in addition to *F. vasinfectum* caused pigeonpea diseases in India also (Mundkar 1938). Butler (1926) considered the fungi causing wilt in cotton, pigeonpea and sesamum to be the specialized isolates of *F. vasinfectum*. However, the fungus *F. udum* was found different than *F. vasinfectum* in producing prominently hooked spores in abundance in sporodochia

(Padwick 1940). He suggested the name *F.udum* var. *cajani* to pigeonpea wilt pathogen as it was morphologically and culturally identical with but pathogenically different from sunnhemp wilt pathogen. Subramanian (1955a) could not differentiate it from *F.oxysporum* var. *cubanse.* With the development of new nomenclature and reorganization of *Fusarium,* the fungus was named as *F.oxysporum* f sp. *udum* (Snyder and Hansen 1940) which was supported by Chattopadhyay and Sengupta (1967) and Kaiser and Sengupta (1976). However, the name *F.udum* is commonly accepted due to its easily distinguishable conidia with prominent hook (Booth 1971). The discovery of its perithecial stage as *Gibberella indica* (Rai and Upadhyay 1982) also suggests that it should be kept in the lateritium group of *Fusarium* and not in the Elegans group.

Morphology : According to Butler (1910), *F.udum* had *Mycelium* hyaline, slender, much branched with little aerial growth; *Microconidia Cephalosporium* type produced successively on ends of short simple or clustered conidiophores in droplets and are unicellular or with one or more septa, elliptical, hyaline singly, salmon pink in mass, occasionally developing from the surface of minute spherical stromata and then of the *Tubercularia* type, 5.15 × 2.4μ in diameter; Microconidial stage in culture usually moist and bacteria like, white to salmon pink occasionally orange red on rice agar but never green or purple. *Macroconidia* form as microconidia but on shorter conidiophores, falcate, hyaline, 3-5 septate, 15-50 × 3-5μ in size. *Chlamydospores* round or oval, thick walled, 5-10μ in diameter, may be in short chains.

According to Booth (1971) cultures of *F.udum* are often with deep purple discolouration of agar, aerial mycelium felted or absent with profuse development of pionnotes sporodochia. *Conidia* initially produced on simple verticillately branched conidiophores but later formed from pionnotes or normal sporodochia forming pinkish or salmon coloured masses. *Microconidia* are one-celled, hyaline, ovoid to fusoid or curved, 6-11 × 2-3μ in size. *Macroconidia* hyaline, typically thin walled, 1-3 and occasionally 5 septate, falcate with a distinct foot cell and an apical cell tapering towards tip which may be curved or hooked, measure 15-30 × 2.5-3.5μ in size. *Chlamydospores* are intercallary, globose, 8-10 μ in diameter. The fungus has been described by other workers also (Wollenweber 1931 and 1938, Subramanian 1955a).

The perfect state of *Fusarium udum* has been found in *Gibberella.* Hansford (1938) isolated *Gibberella* spp. from pigeonpea showing die back symptoms different from wilt. In Mauritius, outbreak of pigeonpea wilt was reported due to *Gibberella fujikuroi* var. *subglutinans* (Wiehe

1939). Singh and Edward (1978) observed abundant salmon-pink sporodochia and black, carbonaceous, apparently superficial perithecia on the diseased shoot surface of pigeonpea near the soil level. They described them as two stages of the pathogen under the names *F.butleri* and *Gibberella butleri.* Later, Singh (1980) reported perfect stage of *F.udum* as *Gibberella udum* from the same area and found that the perithecial development was favoured by cloudy weather, high humidity and a combination of low high temperature. Rai and Upadhyay (1979,1982) discovered the perfect state of *F.udum* on wilted and dead plants and named as *Gibberella indica* (Rai and Upadhyay). The fungus formed perithecia on PDA when two ascospore strains were grown together. At ICRISAT, India, dark red perithecia like bodies were observed on potato sucrose agar at 10-15°C on mating but they did not contain asci and ascospores (ICRISAT 1987).

In field, the perithecia of *G.indica* are formed on exposed roots and collar region which are superficial, commonly aggregated, globose to sub-globose, sessile and smooth walled with asci having two celled ascospores. The ascospores produce germ hyphae or conidia and are capable of inducing the disease in pigeonpea (Rai and Upadhyay 1982, Upadhyay and Rai 1983a). In addition to *F.udum*, other species like *Fusarium accuminatum, F.equiseti, F.lateritium, F.merismoides, F.moniliforme, F.oxysporum, F.vasinfectum, F.semitectum, F.solani* have also been found associated with wilt of pigeonpea (Kannaiyan and Nene 1979; Reddy *et al.* 1990d).

Physiology : The fungus grows well on Rawlin's and Richard's medium but sporulation is more on PDA and Czapek's media (Prasad and Chaudhary 1977b). The carbon and nitrogen are the major elements for growth although, several other elements are also essential in variable amount.

The fungus sporulates well at 0.2% nitrate nitrogen in standard Horne & Millers liquid medium (Sarojini and Yogeswari 1947). Amongst the carbon sources, glycerol is good for growth and lactic acid for sporulation (Subramanian 1961). For good growth as well as for sporulation of *F.udum,* the medium supplied with 3.368 and 0.03 g of carbon and nitrogen per litre in the form of sucrose and ammonium nitrate respectively, was best but production of chlamydospores was independent of nitrogen concentration (Prasad and Chaudhary 1965). The fungus can utilize nitrate, ammonical and organic nitrogen and that the source of nitrogen is more important than C : N ratio as they shift the *p*H of the medium more (Sharma 1963). The sucrose is not assimilated as such but it is hydrolysed into glucose and fructose to initiate formation of micro-and macroconidia (Prasad and Chaudhary 1973). Amino acids play important role in vegetative growth, sporulation and chlamydospore formation differently. DL-alanine and D7-valine in addition to inorganic source of nitrogen inhibit growth of the fungus at lower concentration. D7-valine initiated formation of microconidia in young culture and induced differentiation of chlamydospores in old culture. The sporulation is depressed by Di-isoleucine (Prasad and Chaudhary 1977a). The chloroethyl and trimethlyl ammonium chloride also influence sporulation of *F.udum* greatly (Prasad and Chaudhary 1978).

The micronutrients like Bo, Zn, Mn favour the growth of the fungus at 0.5 ppm but they are toxic at higher concentrations (Yogeswari 1948). The fungus does not grow on the compounds containing Al and Zn (Patel and Kulkarni 1949). Mo, Zn, Fe and Mn together stimulate growth as well as sporulation but reduce size of spores. Copper is strong inhibitor but phosphorus at 0.064% favours growth and sporulation (Prasad and Chaudhary 1966). Similarly sulphur at 0.032% is favourable but their lower concentrations enhance formation of chlamydospores (Prasad and Chaudhary 1967). Production of fusaric acid and its accumulation in the culture of *F.udum* is favoured by zinc (Prasad and Chaudhary 1974b) and in diseased tissues of pigeonpea (Prasad and Chaudhary 1974a).

Amongst the vitamins, pyridoxin and riboflavin stimulated growth and inhibited sporulation; thiamine and biotin had little effect on growth, stimulated microconidia formation but repressed macroconidia. All the vitamins stimulated chlamydospore production and influenced the size of different types of spores (Prasad and Chaudhary 1975). All of these characters and activities are influenced greatly by IAA and gibberallic acid (Prasad and Chaudhary 1976). Increased concentration of thiourea in the medium decreased dry weight of mycelium and sugar contents of *Fusarium udum* (Pandey *et al.* 1976).

Aeration of culture favours the mycelial growth of *F.udum* but inhibits sporulation (Sarojini and Yogeswari 1947). Similarly, growth and sporulation is more at *p*H 6.0 while chlamydospores are produced best at *p*H 3.5 (Prasad and Chaudhary 1977). The vegetative growth as well as sporulation are effectively induced at *p*H 5.0 and NUV irrediation but sporulation is inhibited completely in dark or NUV exposure below 3.5-4.5 and 8.5 *p*H levels (Samajpati 1973). The intermittent exposure to sunlight for 24h during 4 weeks of incubation is reported to reduce the mycelial growth and production of macroconidia but it increases formation of microconidia and chlamydospores (Chaudhary and Prasad 1975).

Variability in Pathogen : The cross inoculation experiments indicated pigeonpea and sunnhemp wilt isolates to be similar (Mitra 1934) but later, both of them were found to be highly host specific (Uppal and Kulkarni 1935; Padwick *et al.* 1940). The pathogen *F. udum* infects cotton (Venkataram 1955) and some other weed hosts also (Kannaiyan *et al.* 1985). The pathogen has been studied in detail with regard to variability in physiological, morphological and virulence to the host. It is reported that even the single spore isolates from a single strain differ from each other with regard to their growth pattern, segmentation, substrate reaction, pigmentation and secretion of metabolic products (Jeswani *et al.* 1975). Based on cultural characters, efforts have been made to distinguish 3 groups by Reddy and Chaudhary (1985), 7 groups by Gupta *et al.* (1988), 7 isolates by Shit and Sengupta (1978), 22 isolates by Rajendra and Patil (1992b) and 5 groups by Patil and Patil (1993). However, pathogenic variability is important for establishing races of a pathogen.

Sarojini (1951) isolated seven strains of *F. udum* from pigeonpea of which strain V and VI caused damping off while I, II and III were more virulent than others. Pot culture experiments on some of the isolates of the pathogen (Baldev and Amin 1974) revealed differential response of pigeonpea varieties. Pathogenic variability in pigeonpea wilt isolates collected from different locations in India has been established by several workers using different varieties of pigeonpea (Shit and Sengupta 1978, Prasad 1978, Pawar and Mayee 1983, Gupta *et al.* 1988, Singh and Pal 1990, Rajendra and Patil 1993b, Reddy and Raju 1993, Zote *et al.* 1993b, Chavan *et al.* 1995, Okirar and Kimani 1997, Das and Sengupta 1998). All these workers used different sets of pigeonpea varieties/lines for judging the pathogenic variability amongst the isolates. Some workers identified the isolates as races (Zote *et al.* 1993b) which is not justified. It is very important to standardize the technique of inoculation, differential varieties and rating scale before isolates are identified as races. The work on this aspect was started at ICRISAT centre, Patancheru, India but further work is needed.

The ultraviolet radiation of virulent strain (FU13) resulted in development of aminoacid deficient strains which became non-virulent but the virulence was restored when required aminoacid was supplemented (Purkayastha and Das 1973). These strains responded differently to aureofungin (Purkayastha and Chattopadhyay 1975).

2.3.4 Host Parasite Interaction

The pathogen *F.udum* is a soil borne facultative parasite that enters through roots and becomes systemic (Nene *et al.* 1980). The fungus produces a mass of mycelia and conidia on the surface of the host particularly on collar region and on the roots. After entry, the fungus continues to grow in xylem vessels. The fungus produces cellolase, polygalacturonase and pectin methyl esterase (Singh and Hussain 1962, 1963; Kaiser and Sengupta 1979; Shit and Sengupta 1980; Nema 1992) and Xylanase (Prasad *et al.* 1988) *in vitro* as well as *in vivo* and a toxin fusaric acid in the affected roots, stems and leaves (Singh and Hussain 1964, 1970; Prasad and Chaudhary 1974) which play important role in pathogenesis. Singh and Hussain (1968) reported that only PME was detected in root and stems of healthy plants. The sterile culture filtrate from pigeonpea wilt pathogen induces irreversible wilting, maceration of stems and browning of basal tissues of young pigeonpea cuttings (Singh and Hussain 1970). Soaking the seed in culture filtrate inhibits their germination and the radicle length if germination occurs (Reddy and Basu Chaudhary 1990). The pathogen influences host physiology and causes well marked dechlorophyllation indicating toxaemia (Satyanarayana and Kalyansundaram 1952).

The infection of pigeonpea by the pathogen causes biochemical changes in the plant. It reduces ascorbic acid and chlorophyll but increases reducing sugars (Kalyansundaram 1952, Subramanian 1963a). It also causes rapid deplition of glucose, fructose, maltose and raffinose (Chaudhary and Prasad 1974) and decrease in aminoacids (Prasad and Chaudhary 1974a). Continued presence of leucine/isoleucine in diseased tissues may stimulate fusaric acid toxin which is more in susceptible than in resistant varieties (Prasad and Chaudhary 1974a). The infection also increased the polyphenols and protein content of plants (Magdum and Nair 1988). They are known to check infection and disease development in plants. Ingham (1976) isolated four antifungal isoflavones and a isoflavonone (cajanol) from the stems of pigeonpea inoculated by *Helminthosporium carbonum.* The isoflavonone (cajanone) isolated from dried roots of pigeonpea totally inhibited the germ tube growth of *F.udum* (Preston 1977). The resistant reaction of a variety depends on the rapid synthesis of phytoalexins like hydroxygeneisein, genestein, cajanin and cajanol of which cajanol was detected more in resistant than in susceptible variety and totally inhibited conidial germination of *F.udum* (Marley and Hillocks 1993). The root knot nematodes are reported to break the resistance of pigeonpea variety ICP 9145 against *F.udum.* At least part of the mechanism of this effect is retarded cajanol accumulation due to nematodes (Marley and Hillocks 1994).

The role of extent of infection and colonization of pigeonpea by *F.udum* in causing wilting of plants has also been studied. According to Reddy *et al.* (1993), plants wilt when colonization is more than 50% and that resistance in a variety depends on the extent of colonization. However, cultivars differing in wilting may not differ in extent of infection or colonization. In different cultivars significant differences in wilt incidence were there at maturity but not at seedling stages (Reddy and Raju 1996).

2.3.5 Other Species of Fusarium

Other species of *Fusarium* reported to be associated of disease are *F.vasinfectum* (Mitra 1931, 1934; Mundkur 1938; Butler 1926), *F.lateritium* var. *uncinatum* (Wallace 1932; Mundkur 1938), *F.oxysporum* (Mukiibi 1976), *F. accuminatum, F. equiseti, F. merismoides, F.moniliforme, F.semitectum* and *F.solani* (Reddy *et al.* 1990d) some of which have been considered as synonyms to *F.udum* while others are of no significance. Padwick (1939) isolated several distinct species of *Fusarium* from wilted pigeonpea of which one differed from *F.udum* and caused severe wilt but no foot rot. The fungi *F.oxysporum* f sp. *ciceri* and *F.oxysporum* f sp. *vasinfecta* have been reported to infect pigeonpea and to cause yellowing and drooping of lower leaves but no wilting (Kaiser and Sengupta 1979; Haware and Nene 1982). In the same way. *Fusarium* species responsible for wilt of cowpea and soybean infected vascular tissues of pigeonpea (Armstrong and Armstrong 1950). Mitra (1934) reported minor wilting of pigeonpea caused by *Neocosmospora vasinfecta* which is considered as the ascigerious stage of *Fusarium* species. This fungus is responsible for root rot of pigeonpea described elsewhere. Bhargava and Singh (1978) also found *F.accuminatum, F.oxyspurum* and *F.solani* to be associated with pigeonpea soil and causing wilting in pigeonpea. Their population was high at 30% water holding capacity of soil and 20 to 30°C temperature but it declined by addition of carbohydrate specially sucrose or nitrogen as urea or ammonium sulphate (Singh and Bhargava 1981).

2.3.6 Disease Cycle and Epidemiology

Survival : The pigeonpea wilt pathogen has been reported to survive on seed and cause wilt (McRae 1924; Haware and Kannaiyan 1992;

Jeswani and Gemawat 1981). However, seed can carry only a limited amount of inculum while the bulk infection originates in soil only (Mitra 1925, McRae 1926). The seeds from general fields carry much less infection as compared to those collected from wilt sick plots (Kumar *et al.* 1998b). Some of the seeds collected from apparently healthy plants also yielded *Fusarium*. The pathogen could be traced from root, through collar region, main stems, branches to pod hulls of diseased plant but not seed of the same (Khune 1990) indicating that the infection of seed may not always be systemic. It has been reported that the pathogen is not directly transmissible from infected seeds to seedlings but it first grows over the surroundings on substrate in the soil and then infections take place through growing lateral roots (Kumar *et al.* 1998a). The seed borne inoculum plays important role in spreading the disease in new uninfected areas.

The bulk of infection of pigeonpea wilt originates in the soil where the fungus may remain alive even in absence of host up to 10 years (Butler 1918, Mitra 1925) although, its inoculum potential is reduced (McRae 1932, Zote *et al.* 1993a). According to Agnihothrudu (1954) and Subramanian (1955b), *F.udum* survives in soil on diseased plant tissues colonized by it as parasite where it has been detected alive up to 2.5 years in Vertisol and 3 years in Alfisol (Kannaiyan *et al.* 1981b) but population is detected more in Vertisol than in Alfisol (Naik *et al.* 1995). The fungus passes from decaying roots into the soil and may continue to grow and form spores under saprophytic conditions until next crop is planted (Butler 1918). Normally it forms chlamydospores entering dormant resting stage after decay of host tissues (Chakraborty 1987) or under any stress conditions. The competitive activity of the pathogen is decreased if the pigeonpea substrate is pre-colonized by other fungi like *Penicillium rubrum, P.granulatum* etc. (Upadhyay and Rai 1983b). The fungus *F.udum* is reported to be strong mycoparasite on *Rhizopus nigricans* (Rai *et al.* 1978), *Cunninghamella echinulata* (Upadhyay *et al.* 1979a, 1979b), *Mortierella subtilissima* (Upadhyay *et al.* 1981b), *Aspergillus luchuensis* and *Syncephalosporium racemosum* (Upadhyay *et al.* 1981a). It penetrates the host, mycelium, grows there, form chlamydospores and finally cause lysis of the same. Thus the mycoparasitism helps in the survival of *F.udum* in soil (Upadhyay *et al.* 1983). Maximum number of chlamydospores are detected in soil at the depth of 5-15 cm (Sharma *et al.* 1987). The fungus forms the perfect state *Gibberella indica* also on infected plants but its longevity of survival is not known.

Survival of the fungus in the soil is influenced by many factors. The optimum temperature for competitive saprophytic ability of *F.udum* in soil is 20-35°C while high soil moisture is detrimental (Mukhopadhyay and Sengupta 1991). The colonization and survival is decreased by soil amendments with Zn, Bo and Mn (Sarojini 1951); 1-2% urea, dextrose or mustard cake (Mukhopadhyay and Sengupta 1991). The pathogen survives for shorter period in the rhizosphere of resistant plant than of susceptible one (Agnihothrudu 1955). Presence of host and non-host seeds of legumes and cereals enhance the growth within 96 h, although, host seeds do not encourage sporulation (Singh 1974). Presence of certain microbes like *Bacillus subtilis* may convert the mycelium of *F.udum* into chlamydospores (Chakraborty and Sengupta 1995b).

Transmission : In the field, the infested area increases every year specially if pigeonpea crop is taken continuously. It may spread about 3cm through the soil in one season, apparently along the roots (McRae 1924). The fungus forms abundant spore masses on the infected branches at a point considerably below that which the fungus has reached in the tissues (Butler 1918, Mohanty 1946). These spore masses arise as a result of outward spread of the fungus from inside of infected branches which may cause new cases of disease at a distance from the original patch through wind late in the season. Abundant sporulation may occur at base of the infected plant causing rapid spread of the disease in irrigated plots (Sharma *et al.* 1987). The perfect state of the fungus is also observed on the collar region of the plant. Further spread of the pathogen from aerial parts in the area through the air/irrigation may be quite effective and fast. The propagules of *F.udum* have been detected on the bodies of termites from roots of the wilted plants. Such infested termites could develop the disease in plants grown in the sterilized soil (Upadhyay and Rai 1982b) and may be responsible for transmission of the pathogen.

Disease Development : The development of wilt is influenced by several factors related with the soil, host, environment and pathogen.

(i) *Inoculum Potential* : Naik *et al.* (1992) did not observe wilt at 1 : 200 dilution of wilt sick soil even in highly susceptible variety but it occurred at 1 : 100 dilution and increased with decreasing dilution. This range differs in moderately susceptible variety C 11. The ID-D curve had a slope value for susceptible and moderately susceptible genotypes as 0.93 and 0.5 respectively. The inoculum may be present in the soil up to a depth of 120 cm but that placed up to 50 cm is significant epidemiologically (Naik *et al.* 1995). Increasing levels of inoculum proportionately increase the mortality in pigeonpea (Prasad and Khan 1998) and chlamydospores have more potential than conidia (Pal *et al.* 1996). It is also observed that germination of chlamydospores is more than conidia in rhizosphere of susceptible variety of pigeonpea.

(ii) *Soils* : Heavy black soils are not favourable for pigeonpea wilt (Shukla 1975) while those slightly acidic or alkaline with 50% or more sand favour the disease incidence (Upadhyay and Rai 1989). The disease is favoured by a temperature of 12-29°C and increasing maturity (Mundkur 1935). The pathogen grows at a temperature range of 17-32°C with optimum of 28°C and 70% of soil moisture holding capacity. The infection occurs at 15-35°C but wilting occurs at 20-35°C (Naik *et al.* 1995). More pronounced effect of pathogen on plants is observed in summer than in kharif (Rajendra 1993). However, Naik and Reddy (1992) reported that the soil moisture and temperature are not the major factors for development of wilt compared to soil inoculum. The soils of southern states of India support less wilt incidence as compared to those of northern states which is correlated with higher level of soil fungistasis against the pathogen (Upadhyay and Rai 1981a). Wilt sickness of a soil may be suppressed by mixing with free soil of other field (Singh and Singh 1987).

(iii) *Crop Condition/Stage* : Wilt appears on young seedlings in August but highest mortality is caused at flowering in November-December (Butler 1906). The critical stage of infection is 6 week old plants (Naik *et al.* 1995). The physiological state of plant seems to be important in relation to infection. The wilt incidence is reduced if vegetative growth of plants is prolonged by removing flowers but it increases if defoliation occurs during the reproductive phase (Sheldrake *et al.* 1978). Thus, defoliation in the ratooned crop also aggravate the disease. There seems close relation between flowering period, wilt intensity and soil temperature that is why the early varieties suffer less due to wilt (Kotasthane and Gupta 1981, Reddy *et al.* 1988). It is probably due to lack of drought stress, efficient moisture utilization and the maturity before expression of symptoms in early maturing varieties. High wilt incidence occurs in perennial plants. In the same way higher plant biomass increases susceptibility to wilt due to increased water demand by the plant (Reddy *et al.* 1994). Hence, the factors like early sowing, well distributed rains, high fertility, freedom from weeds, good drainage, low plant density and extended maturity of plants which increase the biomass of plants increase their susceptibility to wilt. On the other hand, Chaudhary *et al.* (2000) did not find any association of flowering stage and wilt of pigeonpea. They found significant effect of sowing date on wilt. Under Kanpur condition, maximum wilt occurred in October. In soil, the germination of chlamydospores of the pathogen is supported by root exudates of susceptible variety and not by resistant one (Chakraborty and Sengupta 1991).

(iv) *Soil Biota* : Soil micro-organisms play important role in the epidemiology of soil borne diseases. The soil fungi and bacteria found antagonistic to *F.udum* are being dealt separately under biological control. The nematodes facilitate the infection of plant by injuring it and affect the growth variously (Edward and Singh 1979). The pigeonpea cyst nematode, *Heterodera cajani* increases the wilt incidence drastically (Hasan 1984). The nematode increases aggressiveness of *F.udum* on wilt susceptible varieties but not on the resistant ones (Sharma and Nene 1989). In combined inoculations, the main site of fungal entry is through the injury created by the protruding females in plants (Rai and Singh 1996). On the other hand *F.udum* is antagonistic to *H.cajani* and affects its multiplication adversely (Sharma and Nene 1989, Rai and Singh 1996). Suppression of plant growth and increase in the wilt severity of pigeonpea is caused by *M.javanica* (Salam and Khan 1986) and *M.incognita* (Dwivedi *et al.* 1992) also. Both of these species are capable of breaking resistance to wilt in variety ICP 9145 by retarding the accumulation of cajanol, a phytoalexin responsible for resistance (Marley and Hillocks 1994). This phenomenon occurs even if the nematode is present in the soil and wilt pathogen is applied on stem by puncturing, although, it does not happen in the variety ICP 8863 (Marley and Hillocks 1996). The relationship between the inoculum densities of both the organisms and plant growth parameters is inversely proportional between the final nematode population, root knot index, root colonization by the pathogen and the inoculum density (Parveen *et al.* 1998). The combined inoculation with

H.cajani, M.incognita and *F.udum* cause more effect than inoculated singly, and the combination of *F.udum* with *H.cajani* is more effective in causing wilting effect than with *Meloidogyne* spp. (Siddiqui and Mahmood 1996b).

The death of pigeonpea variety ICPL 270 due to wilt is accelerated in presence of *Rotylenchulus reniformis* (Sharma and Nene 1990 and Jain and Sharma 1996). This variety is otherwise resistant to wilt and susceptible to reniform nematode.

2.3.7 Host Resistance

Use of resistant varieties is the best and economically viable and feasible method to combat diseases like wilt. The best example on this aspect is that of Malawi in Africa where pigeonpea wilt was observed 36.3% in 1980 (Kannaiyan *et al.* 1981c) but introduction of resistant variety ICP 9145 decreased the wilt incidence to 4% by 1991 (Babu *et al.* 1992, Reddy *et al.* 1992d, 1993d, Saka *et al.* 1994 and Subramanyam *et al.* 1992). In Karnataka, India, benefit due to collaborative research on pigeonpea wilt and release of wilt resistant variety ICP 8863 as 'Maruthi' has been reported to be US dollors 62 millions representing an internal rate of return of 65%. The results, in addition to clearly quantifying the impact of fusarium wilt research also provide important lessions for research and extension policy and for formulation of future research priorities (Bantilan and Joshi 1996).

Sources of Resistance : As early as 1908, Butler tested several pigeonpea strains in wilt affected plot and selected resistant lines. There are several reports available in literature on identification of pigeonpea lines resistant to wilt with good yield, quality as well as suitability for general cultivation or as doner parents for developing suitable varieties in India (Anonymous 1931a, 1941, 1946, 1947a, 1947b, 1948, 1954a, 1954b, 1955, 1956). However, only few of them became popular amongst the farmers probably due to certain lacunae. The resistant lines identified by various workers have been compiled in Table 2.1. The oldest variety NP (WR) 15 is late maturing and small seeded and thus not preferred in central and southern India (Deshpande *et al.* 1963, Anonymous 1965). Two medium duration varieties, namely C11and C26 with resistance to wilt and fairly good seed size were released in Hyderabad (Bhaskaran 1954) of which C11 became popular in some areas including Madhya Pradesh but it does not possess high level of resistance to wilt. In Bihar,

Table 2.1: Sources of resistance to wilt of pigeonpea caused by *Fusarium udum*

Location/State	*Entries tested*	*Entries found resistant*	*Reference*
1	2	3	4
Andhra Pradesh (India)	-	C 11, C 28, C 36	Vaheeduddin (1956,1958)
	-	Yadgir, No. 3, Type 17	Anonymous (1954b)
	11000	ICP 8863	Nene & Kannaiyan (1982)
	86	ICPL 25, 108, 314	Kannaiyan *et al.* (1983b)
	92	19 lines free	Jain *et al.* (1983)
	61	ICP 4769, 8863, 9168, 11299, C11, BDN2	Nene *et al.* (1989)
	568	ICPL 37 and 16 others	Reddy *et al.* (1989b)
	2194	ICP 1641, 7118, 7120, 7198, 8858, 8859, 8860, 8863, 8864, 8865, 8868, Banda Palera, AWR 74/15, Bori 1	Nene *et al.* (1980; 1981b)
	-	*Atylosia lineata, A. Sericia*	Deodikar and Thakar (1956)
Gujarat (India)	61	GAUT 82-9, 82-23, 82-74, 82-127	Patel *et al.* (1988)
	400	BDN 2, BP 1314, 1809, 2094, 2061	Rajkule *et al.* (1989)
	35	GAUT 85-35,ICP 8863, 9175	Goyal *et al.* (1991)
	120	BDN 1, ICP 10063, 11289, 13072-1	Das & Gupta (1992)
Karnataka (India)	800	ICP 6997, 8858, 8859 8861 to 8864, 8356, 8358, 8362, 9174, 9707, 12731, 12748, 84007, 84008, 84016, 84017, 85061, 87119, 89048, 89049, 91046; BWR 23, 30, 24, 97, 105, 153, 190, 245, 301, 370; GPS 26C, 30, 33, 36, 37, 52; BSMR 198, 214, 270, 736; C 11, BDN 1, DPPA 85-5, PRG 100, Godu 1, Sharan 171-21, Sujata 1-2	Bidari *et al.* (1994)
	46	Kanpur Local	Bidari *et al.* (1995)
	522	ICP 8863 (Maruthi), GPS 3, 26C, 30, 33, 36, ICPL 87119	Bidari *et al.* (1996b)
	348	BSMR 198, PRG 100	Bidari *et al.* (1996a)
Kenya	-	ICP 9145, 9155, 10957, 10960	Reddy *et al.* (1990a)
	104	VBG 42, 52, 57	Okirar (1999)

Table 2.1 *Contd...*

1	2	3	4
Madhya Pradesh (India)	-	C11, BDN 1, Banda Palera	Kotasthane *et al.* (1981)
	-	Bori 1, ICP 8863, 9120, 9144 and 8 other lines	Sharma (1988)
	950	Ninteen lines including C 11, ICP 8863, NP (WR) 15, BDN 1, JA 3, JA 4 (AS 71-37)	Agrawal *et al.* (1991)
	-	KE 5, KE 11, KM 9, KM 18, KM 19, KM 34, KM 84, KM 112	Saxena *et al.* (1998)
Maharashtra (India)	72	No. 3 released	Plyman (1933)
	86	Type 16, 51, 80	Shaw and Kashiram (1934)
	-	EB 38	Ravi Shankar (1936)
	-	Seven selections from Bori 1, Latoor 466, DT 230, M4 X K 132	Raut & Bhombe (1971)
	-	Osmanabad, NP (WR) 15, NP 69, S 103, Balapur 10, P 1005, Jarud, Washim 4, Chandrikapur 1, Paras 5	Patil & Sable (1973)
	-	15-3-3, DT 236-63-102, Vita 1, Osmanabad 1-5, Udgir 500	Anonymous (1976)
	16	T 15-15, ICP 8860	Patel *et al.* (1981)
	-	ICP 7182, 7336, 8863, 8869, BDN 1	Zote *et al.* (1983b)
	120	Boregaon local, Yetmal	Zote *et al.* (1983a)
	13	C 11, Purple 1, BDN 44-2-7, BDN 20-6-11, ICP 7035, 7118, 7182, 7198	Zote *et al.* (1986)
	16	ICP 7336, 8862, AWR 74/15	zote *et al.* (1987a)
	-	BWR 22, 23, 24, 175, 369, BSMR 65, 146, 175, 198, 203, 294, 736	Zote *et al.* (1990)
	160	BWR 175, 369; ICP 8863	Pawar *et al.* (1992)
	31	16 cultures with BWR 369	Rajendra & Patil (1993a)
	-	Phule T 25, ICP 11290, 11296_	Pawar *et al.* (1993)
	65	BSMR 98, DA 11	Pawar & Banchod (1994)
	40	ICP 7942, 8863, 8864, 11295	Chavan *et al.* (1995)

Table 2.1 *Contd...*

1	2	3	4
	-	14 cultures including S 43, S 47, S 69 & S 122	Pandey *et al.* (1996b)
	271	BWR 175, ICPL 83924	Shrishikar *et al.* (1990)
	-	25 lines of BWR series	Zote *et al.* (1987b)
	-	ICPl 90018, 90029, 93175 to 93177, 93179, 93181, 87	Singh *et al.* (1996a)
	-	BWR 370	Shinde and Zote (1993)
Malawi	-	ICP 9134, 9142, 9145, 9156, 9177, 10960, 11299, 12738	Reddy *et al.* (1990a)
Pusa (Bihar & New Delhi)	-	Type 16, 41, 50, 51, 80, 82	McRae & Shaw (1933)
		IP 41, 80, A126-4-1, IP 51, Hybrid 5, C 38-1-2, C38-3-1, C 15, S 55 etc.	Mundkur (1946), Dastur (1946), Anonymous (1946, 1951, 1953), Vasudeva (1958a, 1958b)
	-	NP (WR) 15, 16, 42, NP 41, 51 and 80	Deshpande *et al.* (1963), Raychaudhary (1968)
	58	Nine Cultivars	Mukherjee *et al.* (1971)
	-	BDN 1, ICP 8863, Banda Palera	Pal *et al.* (1987)
	-	ICP 8863	Haque *et al.* (1987)
Rajasthan (India)	44	26 lines including BDN 1, BWR 370, ICPL 161, ICP 8863	Gaur and Sharma (1988)
Tamil Nadu (India)	168 to 218	ICPL 227, 88046, 88047, BWR 254, DPPA 84-8-3	Raguchander and Arjunan (1996)
Uttar Pradesh (India)	-	17W/2	Anoymous (1950)
	-	C 11, 28, 36, F 18, NP 41, NP (WR) 15, T17 were susceptible while Bori 192-12-5-1-2 & Bori 192-15-2-2-11-42 MR	Singh and Mishra (1976)
West Bengal (India)	21	ICP 8863, 10957, 10958, 11290, 11292 11294	Dasgupta & Sengupta (1988
Centres of AICRP	-	BWR 254, 270; ICP 8863, 8869; DPPA 82-10, 85-3, 85-5, 85-7, 85-9, 85-10, 85-11, 85-12, 85-14 and 85-15	Anonymous (1991)
	959	ICP 8863, 9174, 12745; ICPL 333, 8363, 88047; BWR 370, Banda Palera, DPPA 85-2, 85-3, 85-8, 85-13, 85-14 were resistant at 7-10 locations	Amin *et al.* (1993b)

Kanke 3 and Kanke 9 were identified with resistance to wilt, high yield and good cooking quality (Bhargava 1975). Similarly a line ICP 8863 which proved to be highly resistant to wilt in most of the states of India, performed well and thus was released in Karnataka state under the name Maruthi (Konda *et al.* 1986, Parmeswarappa *et al.* 1986). This variety possesses high yielding and medium maturity characters with good cooking quality. Another good variety identified in Karnataka was ICPL 270 (Parmeswarappa *et al.* 1987). Zaberi *et al.* (1986) recommended BDN 2 in Gujarat state owing to its wilt resistance, high yield and better agronomical characters than locally growing lines. In the state of Maharashtra, several good varieties resistant to wilt have been released specially BDN 1 (Zote *et al.* 1983a), BSMR 175 and BSMR 736 (Zote *et al.* 1995). In Madhya Pradesh, JA 4 was found to be resistant to wilt (Agrawal *et al.* 1991) and being good agronomically it was released for cultivation.

Inheritance of resistance : The study on inheritance of resistance for wilt was started at Indian Agricultural Research Institute (Anon. 1931b) and first report was published by Pal (1934) who reported that it is controlled by multiple factors and that it is not correlated with any of the important morphological characters. The resistance to wilt of pigeonpea is reported to be controlled by two complementary genes (Shaw 1936, Pathak 1970) or by a pair of duplicate genes with dominance of resistance (Joshi 1957). In a cross between TT 6 and ICP 8863 it was found monogenic symbolized as FuR 1 (Pandey *et al.* 1996a). In varieties 15-3-3 and C11 also the resistance to wilt has been reported to be dominant over susceptibility (Pawar and Mayee 1986). The dominant genes for resistance in genotypes Banda Palera, DPPA 85-7 and DPPA 85-1 are identical but different from those in DPPA 85-12 and ICPL 87119 and hence, they are symbolized as Fur 1 and Fur 2 respectively (Singh and Vishwa Dhar 1997).

On the other hand Jain and Reddy (1995) using resistant variety ICP 8863 and 2 susceptible varieties ICP 2376 and LRG 30 found resistance to be controlled by a single recessive gene designated as pwr 1. It is also reported that in some genotypes resistance to wilt is dominant while in others it is recessive (Reddy and Jain 1992). The crosses between susceptible Bahar and resistant PI 397430, PR 5149 and Banda Palera indicated that wilt resistance in pigeonpea is controlled by inhibitory gene action (Raina and Singh 1996).

Techniques of screening : Several techniques have been developed and used for screening pigeonpea genotypes for resistance against wilt caused by *Fusarium*.

(i) *Wilt Sick-Plot Technique* : As early as 1908 Butler tested a number of pigeonpea genotypes in plots severely infected by the wilt fungus. McRae and Shaw (1926) used susceptible variety as a line after every test entry for selecting wilt resistant line in wilt sick area. The pieces of diseased stems collected from the previous crop were planted between each row for creating the disease. However, they suggested to repeat the test owing to possible variation in the infection in different parts of the field. Vaheeduddin and Nanjundiha (1956) created wilt sick plot for screening the pigeonpea genotypes by spreading compost made of wilted plants. In each year, care was taken so that plot was thoroughly infested with *F.udum*. They used susceptible local varieties to serve as control. A method has been worked out for developing good wilt sick plot and recommended for efficient screening against pigeonpea wilt (Kannaiyan and Nene 1981a, Nene *et al.* 1981a) as follows :

1. Select a well drained plot of required size and isolated from other pigeonpea field so as to avoid spread of the pathogen. The plot should have had pigeonpea crop before with some wilt.
2. Collect wilted plants from other fields, chop them and incorporate in the soil of selected field.
3. Grow sole crop of pure wilt susceptible pigeonpea variety ICP 2376 or ICP 6997 or No. 1258 in this plot with normal operations.
4. By end of season, atleast 10 % wilt should appear. Chop off the tops of living plants. The fresh growth will develop and many such plants will show wilt. Wait for 30 days.
5. Chop whole crop and incorporate in the soil which will increase inoculum and make the soil sick.
6. In the next season, again plant susceptible variety and repeat steps 2 and 4 when more than 80% wilt may occur and if it is less, repeat steps 2 and 4 for one more season.
7. In the next season, screening of the material may be started. After every 2 test entries/row, one row of susceptible line is planted for monitoring and maintaining wilt sickness of the plot. The susceptible line should show 90-100 % wilt incidence.
8. From the 4th/5th year, susceptible line may be sown after every four test lines.
9. Observation on wilt incidence is recorded 2 weeks before maturity of the crop.
10. Planting of any other crop in wilt sick plot is not recommended.

For scoring against wilt, a 9-point scale has been proposed by Nene *et al.* (1981a) as follows :

Rating	*Wilt %*	*Categories*
1	No symptom on any plant	Resistant
3	10% or less mortality	Moderately resistant
5	11 - 20% mortality	Tolerant
7	21 - 50% mortality	Moderately susceptible
9	51% or more mortality	Susceptible

The test lines with rating of 1-3 are considered acceptable; the 5 is acceptable only if 1-3 are not available. This scale is best applied if total number of plants of a test line varies between 20-50. Pawar and Mayee (1983a) studied the combining ability for wilt resistance in pigeonpea and reported that there is feasibility of selection on the basis of *per se* performance of the crosses at different stages of F 1 and F 2 generations.

The wilt sick plot technique is used commonly and successfully for screening pigeonpea lines against wilt on large scale. It has been suggested that in wilt sick plot, row sowing can be replaced by hill sowing as it requires much less area and thus reduces the operation cost (Reddy *et al.* 1992a).

(ii) *Pot Culture Screening* : This technique is not adopted on large scale but it is useful for confirming the resistance in a line and for race studies. The technique was used by Patel and Kamat (1950) and later it was standardized at ICRISAT (Nene *et al.* 1981a) as follows:

1. Fill large pots (35 cm diameter) with the soil from wilt affected field and burry the pots to soil level.
2. Multiply pure culture of *F.udum* isolated locally on Sand-pigeonpea flour medium (pigeonpea flour 10 g, river sand 90 g, distilled water 20 ml in each of 250 ml flask) at 30°C for 15 days.
3. Autoclave 200 g of choped pigeonpea aerial parts in each of 1000 ml flask.
4. Mix 200 g of the fungal culture (Step 2) with 200 g of autoclaved choped plant material and incorporate the mixture in top 15 cm soil in each pot. Water the pots and wait for 2 days.
5. Plant 50 seeds of wilt susceptible variety in each pot. Remove plants after 60 days, chop wilted ones and incorporate in the soil of pot.

6. Repeat steps 4 and 5 till more that 90% wilt occurs when pots are ready for screening.
7. Use one pot of susceptible check for every 10 pots of test entries.

Screening by pot culture is completed within 2 months as completed 6-8 months required by wilt sick plot method.

(iii) *Transplanting Technique* : This technique has been developed for quick screening (Kannaiyan and Nene 1981a, Nene *et al.* 1981a). In this method the culture of *F.udum* is multiplied as described under step 2 of pot culture technique and 200 g culture is mixed with 2 kg of autoclaved soil obtained from wilt affected field. The mixture is filled in 15 cm diameter pots which are watered and kept for 2 days. Concurrently seedlings of pigeonpea test entries are grown in autoclaved river sand in 25 × 16 cm polythene bags (50 seeds/bag). When seedlings are 7-10 days old, they are removed from the sand and 2-3 cm portion of their roots are trimed. Five of such seedlings are planted in each pot. Wilt symptoms appear in 2-3 weeks and final observations are recorded 2 months after transplanting.

(iv) *Root Dip Technique* : This technique has been described by Haware and Nene (1994). It is quicker than the pot culture technique. In this method the pathogen is multiplied at 25°C for 7 days on Potato dextrose broth in flasks kept on the rotary shaker. The content is macerated in waring blender for one minute. The seedlings of test lines are grown as described under transplanting method. The seedlings are inoculated by dipping their roots in the inoculum for one minute and then they are transplanted in pot containing autoclaved sand, vertisol or alfisol soil. Uninoculated seedlings transplanted in uninoculated sand/soil are used as control.

(v) *Laboratory Technique* : It is developed for rapid screening of pigeonpea germplasm against wilt (Pandey *et al.* 1995b). In this technique, seedlings are raised on filter paper folders supported with plastic slots in a tray containing water. The trays are first kept at 28±1°C for 4 days in BOD incubator and then shifted to growth room at 25±3°C under continuous illumination. The 15 day old seedlings are used. The pure culture of the pathogen is grown on potato broth at 25±3°C for 10 days on the rotary shaker. The spores are obtained by filtration and centrifugation. The spore suspension prepared in sterile distilled water is distributed in test tubes. The tap and lateral roots of seedlings are trimmed and they are placed individually in test tubes with the support of cotton plugs so that their roots are submerged in spore suspension. The tubes are kept in BOD incubators at 28±1°C for 12h of illumination/day. Distilled water is added to tubes after every 3 days to make up the loss. Ten seedlings of each test genotype are used and seedlings of susceptible variety are used as control for comparison. The wilt appears in 28 days. The disease reaction agrees with that of pot screening method and the results are more reliable, reproducible and unaffected by weather conditions.

(vi) *Stem Inoculation Technique* : In this method the plants are inoculated by giving longitudinal cut on the stem with a sharp scalpel 10-15 cm above the ground level (Sharma *et al.* 1977). The inoculum consisting of mycelium and spores is introduced in the cut portion and absorbent cotton swab is wrapped around the inoculated portion with the help of polythene strip to avoid desiccation. Wilting symptmos appear one month after inoculation. The technique is too laborious and cumbersome and hence, not fit for large scale screening of genotypes.

Factors Governing Resistance : Inoculation studies on pigeonpea varieties ICP 8863 (Resistant) and TT 6 (Susceptible) indicated that wilt resistance is due to slow growth and localization of the pathogen (Panday *et al.* 1997).

The biochemical studies conducted by Subramanian (1963a) showed higher contents of chlorophyl l, ascorbic acid, free reducing sugars and total Mn in the resistant variety NP 15 as compared to susceptible NP 24. On the other hand, NP 24 had more total carbohydrates in roots as compared to shoot while reverse was true with NP 15. The Fe : Mn ratio increased with increasing susceptibility. Resistance to pigeonpea wilt has been observed to be associated with higher contents of total sugars, reducing sugars, amino nitrogen, amino acids, phenols, flavanols and alkaloids, xylose, cystine, tryptophane but lower amount of phenylalanine (Murthy 1975). The caffeic and chlorogenic acids and an unidentified phenolic compound present in resistant variety were inhibitory to spore germination. It is considered that Cystine counteracts the fungal infections by chelating ferric ions that activate the *Fusarium* toxin. The cystine and tryptophane were detected only in shoot of resistant variety but phenylalanine was more in susceptible one (Murthy and Bagyaraj 1978). Flavanol and alkaloid were more in resistant than in susceptible cultivar (Murthy and Bagyaraj 1980). The resistant variety had chlorogenic acid, caffeic acid and unknown phenolic acid which inhibited germination of spores of *F.udum* (Murthy and Bagyaraj 1983). The root exudates from the susceptible variety ICP 6997 allowed higher growth and spore germination of *F.udum* as compared to that from resistant varieties C11, 15-3-3, BDN 1 and Banda Palera (Kotasthane and Gupta 1983, Kotasthane *et al.* 1983). Such observations have been made on germination of chlamydospores also (Chakraborty *et al.* 1992). The resistant cultivars had higher concentration of nitrogen, total amino acids and total phenols as compared to susceptible one (Kotasthane and Gupta 1984). Differences in ascorbic acid in resistant and susceptible cultivars were not significant (Gaur and Sharma 1990). However, Kumar and Sharma (1994) reported nine amino acids in root exudates of resistant and 6 in susceptible varieties of pigeonpea. Hydroxy proline, lysine and proline were detected in resistant variety only. Total phenols were more in resistant then in susceptible variety. Concentration of each amino acid was more at seedling stage and reduced at flowering and near harvest which are the susceptible stages. Orthodihydric phenols were detected in NP 15 at seedling stage only. Total and soluble sugars decreased with the plant growth in both the varieties.

The culture filtrate of *F.udum* contained fusaric acid and thus caused mortality in resistant as well as susceptible cultivars though, extent of mortality at lower concentration was more in susceptible than in resistant varieties (Pandey *et al.* 1995a).

No spores of the pathogen are produced in least susceptible variety NP 15 due to lack of substrate in the root system or the action of some inhibitory substance in the xylem (Subramaninan 1963c). The root exudates from the susceptible plants stimulate the germination of chlamydospores greatly which is much less in exudates from resistant varieties (Dasgupta and Sengupta 1988). The xylem vessels and the vascular bundles of the resistant genotypes are wider with comparatively thinner roots than those of susceptible genotypes (Chaudhary and Kumar 2000).

Breeding for Wilt Resistance : Breeding for wilt resistance is usually done by pedegree or mass pedegree selection although, in some cases back crossing has also been successful. Dwivedi *et al.* (1989) developed several wilt resistant lines from the wilt susceptible variety LRG 30 by mutation breeding through gamma ray radiation. Interspecific crosses have also been attempted to transfer wilt resistance from *Atylosia* spp to pigeonpea (Kumar *et al.* 1958). The F2 generation is screened in wilt sick plot and resistant plants are identified. The F3 and F4 progenies are also screened in disease nursery and those with less than 10 % wilt incidence are selected for yield evaluation in a normal disease free field (Reddy and Jain 1992).

In pigeonpea, variability exists in a line with regard to wilt reaction which creates problem to select wilt free plants at early stage for use as parent. This problem can be overcome by adopting a technique (Chari *et al.* 1984) by which the pigeonea plant infected by *F.udum* can be identified before appearance of symptoms by using electric current. The prediction validity of this method is reported to be 94 per cent.

For evaluation of progenies against pigeonpea wilt, apparent infection rate ('r') values are reported to be useful compared to values of area under the disease progress curve (Naik and Reddy 1993a). It can well be adopted in studies on influence of other factors on disease development and the studies for identification of pathotypes etc.

To avoid impurities of seed due to out crossing, basic seed stock is maintained by selfing plants using muslin or nylon cloth bags. For large scale multiplications, an isolation distance of atleast 200 m is maintained.

2.3.7 Control

Chemical : Being a soil borne disease, chemical control of wilt is not much effective. However, a few reports on this aspect are available regarding *in vitro* as well as *in vivo* testing.

In Vitro Testing : The mycelial growth of *F.udum* is inhibited partly or completly by griseofulvin at 0.1 to 2.5 μg/ml (Chakrabarti and Nandi 1969), Benlate at 10 ppm (Sinha 1974), CG 450, a guazatine compound (Agrawal and Khare 1986), Bavistin, BAS 38601F (Ghosh and Sinha 1981), zineb (Gupta 1987 & 1993) and Bavistin, Topsin M 70 and thiram (Sumitha and Gaikwad 1995b). The hyphae and spores of this fungus show different degree of tolerance to fungicides (Singh and Singh 1970). The sporulation is reduced effectively by Captan (Gupta 1987 & 1993) while spore germination is inhibited by Benlate and Campogran M (Ghosh and Sinha 1981) and not by Griseofulvin even at higher concentrations (Chakrabarti and Nandi 1969).

In soil, the population of *F.udum* is reduced by thiram and ferbam at 200 ppm or more (Singh and Singh 1970), Difolatan 100 ppm (Bhargava and Singh 1978), ferbam, maneb and zineb (Gupta 1993).

Some of the plant products have also been tested against the pathogen. The extract of rhizomes of *Cyperus rotundus* in water or solvents is reported to reduce the spore germination and germ tube length of *F.udum* (Singh *et al.* 1999b). It affected the mode of germination and caused characteristic bulging of spores at high concentrations. The rhizome meal amended PDA induced sector formation and profuse sporulation by the fungus in laboratory.

In Vivo Testing : Benlate as soil drench applied at 2000-4000 ppm 10 days before to 22 days after inoculation or as foliar spray at 10000 ppm is reported to check the pigeonpea wilt although, it was ineffective as seed dresser (Sinha 1975). The disease could be checked by soil application of captan or Brassicol in rows @ 6 kg/ha (Haider *et al.* 1978) and soil drenching with thiram also (Sumitha and Gaikwad 1995b) but it is not feasible for the field crop like pigeonpea.

Seed treatment with fungicides for control of pigeonpea wilt has been found effective in case of Benlate, Bavistin and BAS 38601 F (Ghosh and Sinha 1981), Benlate + thiram (Kotasthane *et al.* 1987) or thiram alone (Sumitha and Gaikwad 1995b) or Bavistin @ 2 g/kg of seed (Pandey and Upadhyay 1999). The seed borne inoculum of *F. udum* is eliminated by seed treatment with benomyl and thiram (Haware and Kannaiyan 1992). Benlate being systemic in nature proved to be more effective but its continuous use may develop resistance in the pathogen. Hence, it is suggested to use benomyl mixed with other fungicides specially carbendazim, thiram, difolatan etc. (Kamble and Gangawane 1994). The fungicides may influence the growth of host plant also. The lower concentrations of Griseofulvin (0.1-2.5 μg/ml) is inhibitory to the growth of the pathogen but stimulatory to seedlings of pigeonpea. However, its higher concentration caused rolling and mottling of leaves and induced excessive branching, curving, stunting and hairyness in roots (Chakrabarti and Nandi 1969).

Besides fungicides, the plant extracts/products have also been tested for control of pigeonpea wilt. Leaves of *Callistimon lanceolatus* exhibited strong volatile fungi-toxic capacity inhibiting growth of the fungus completely and safe to pigeonpea plant (Pandey *et al.* 1982). Similarly essential oil from *Ageratum houstonianum* was found toxic to pathogen but not to pigeonpea plant (Pandey *et al.* 1983). *Clorodendrum fragrans* has shown inhibitory effect against *F. Oxysporum* f sp. *udum* (Verma and Singh 1997). Later, soil amendments with dry powder of leaves of *C. acuteatum* was found best for checking disease in glass house (Verma and Singh 1998).

Cultural Control : Various cultural operations exhibit great effect on disease incidence of which tillage practices are most important. Deep summer ploughing after harvest of crop exposes the soil borne pathogens to sun reducing their quantum in the soil. The efficacy of solar heat in elimination of the soil borne inoculum is increased by a technique of "Solarization" in which soil is covered with transparent polythene sheets for 6-8 weeks in April-May. This technique is highly effective against *F.udum* in presence of antagonist *A.niger* or carbendazim (Singh *et al.* 1996b).

(i) Sowing time : Most of the pathogens are restricted in their environmental requirements more as compared to their hosts. An optimum sowing time/season may thus be worked out for growing the crop so that the pathogen, although present at the site, is not able to attack the plant. However, due to meteorological and biological factors, optimum sowing time is often locally restricted in its application. It has been reported that pigeonpea suffers less due to wilt if grown in the post rainy season by sowing it in September-October as compared to that sown earlier in the rainy season (Sharma 1980, Kannaiyan and Nene 1985b).

(ii) Competition : The pigeonpea wilt is significantly decreased when plants face competition because of higher plant population or weeds possibly due to reduced development of sink under such conditions (Chauhan 1991).

(iii) Plant Nutrients : Judicious and balanced use of different plant nutrients is important for getting high yields of the crop. The manurial experiments conducted at Pusa indicated the increased incidence of pigeonpea wilt by application of superphosphate alone or high nitrogen as farm yard manure but it decreased by green manuring with *Crotalaria juncea* (McRae 1923, 1924, 1926, 1928a, 1928b, 1930, 1931). Addition of Zinc @ 80 ppm to the infested soils retards colonization of host by *F.udum* protecting seedlings from infection. It also reduces survival and persistence of the pathogen in soil exterminating it within 4-6 weeks (Sarojini 1950). Zinc is more effective in this respect compared to Bo and Mn. In the same way application of 100 to 200 ppm Mn in the soil excluded the pathogen completely. Mn when used as seed pre-soaking or foliar spray also checked the disease effectively (Subramanian 1963b). On the other hand, application of urea promotes the activity of the fungus and hence, its use should be avoided (Rai and Upadhyay 1983).

(iv) Crop Rotation : Continuous monocropping promotes harbouring and multiplication of the pathogen while crop rotation with non-host reduces the disease severity/incidence greatly. The pigeonpea wilt was not observed in large fields where it was not grown for last 8-10 years (McRae 1932). The population of the pathogen as well as disease incidence is reduced when pigeonpea is grown in rotation with Sorghum (Natrajan *et al.* 1985), cereals (Khan and Ashley 1975), tobacco or fallow (Bose 1938, Natrajan *et al.* 1985, Dasgupta *et al.* 1992). Crop

rotation has been recommended the only measure to avoid fusarium wilt of pigeonpea in Kenya (Acland 1971). On the other hand, Shirshikar and Ashtaputre (1993) could not control the disease by rotation of pigeonpea with sorghum, pearl millet, cotton or the wilt resistant pigeonpea varieties in wilt-sick plot. However, it is established fact that intelligently planned crop rotation helps in optimal utilization of nutrients with weed, insect pests and disease control surviving in the soil, although farmers show their reluctance to alternate one year economic crop with 1-3 years of low value crops.

(v) Inter and Mixed Cropping : Inter and mixed cropping of sorghum with pigeonpea reduces wilt in pigeonpea (Dey 1947, 1948, Anonymous 1949, Verma 1955, Gupta 1961, Natarajan *et al.* 1985, Sharma *et al.* 1987, Bidari *et al.* 1991, Naik *et al.* 1997, Nafde *et al.* 1998). The effect of sorghum on wilt of pigeonpea is attributed to the antifungal effect of HCN released by roots of sorghum. The quantity of the HCN depends on the stages of the crop. The effect of sorghum on pigeonpea wilt is more if the crop is grown for grain and not for fodder (Mathur 1954). It may also be attributed to deeper root system developed in inter/mixed cropping (Gupta 1961). Other crops which reduce the wilt of pigeonpea when used as inter/mixed crops are *Crotalaria medicagnea* (Upadhyay and Rai 1981b), mungbean (Chaudhary *et al.* 1998), maize and cowpea (Nafde *et al.* 1998). It has been reported that continuous inter-cropping has little effect on wilt as compared to break in the continuity by rotating sorghum alone sequenced with safflower (Naik *et al.* 1994, 1997). In fact, the production system may not have direct beneficial effects in field with high pathogen population but by reducing the population of the pathogen it helps in reducing the wilt incidence.

(vi) Irrigation : The wilt of pigeonpea is reported to be more at IW/CPE ratio of 1.0 and 0.8 than at 0.6 or no irrigation (Sharma *et al.* 1987). The spread of the inoculum of the wilt pathogen may be reduced by avoiding flow of the water from infested areas to uninfested one. The growth of the pathogen on surface of the soil ceases at 7% MHC (Dasgupta and Sengupta 1993) and the optimum temperature for growth is 28°C.

(vii) Sanitation : Roguing of diseased plants with roots and their destruction by burning is partially helpful in reducing the diseased area (Mathur 1954).

Biological Control : The bacterium *Bacillus subtilis* has been reported to be antagonistic against *F.udum* (Vasudeva 1949, Vasudeva and Govindaswami 1953). Less pigeonpea wilt observed in unsterilized soil as compared to sterilized soil has been attributed to antagonism of *B.subtilis* (Vasudeva and Roy 1950). It has been reported that the *B.subtilis* produces an antibiotic and that the production is more on the medium developed by Vasudeva *et al.* (1952) specially in presence of $MgSO_4$, Mn and Fe. The active principle is absorved by soil and kaolin. It is thermostable and active at 4.5-9.8 *p*H even at 1 : 10000 concentration (Anonymous 1954a). Another thermostable antibiotic produced by *B.subtilis* has been named as 'Bulbiformin' because it induces formation of characteristic bulbs in the spores and hyphae of *F.udum* (Vasudeva *et al.* 1958). Production of bulbiformin is favoured by sterile soil enriched with asparatic acid or asparagine and dextrose or root residues of sweet clover, molasses and groundnut cake (Vasudeva *et al.* 1962, 1963, Mahmood 1964). Addition of bulbiformin in soil directly reduces the severity of *F.udum* (Vasudeva 1958b). The production of bulbiformin is maximum on seed coat, spermatosphere and rhizosphere of pigeonpea treated with *B.subtilis* mixed with molasses and ground nut cake (Singh *et al.* 1965). The antibiotic becomes systemic in plant tissues forming protective zone round the root reducing the wilt incidence. Most of the cultures of *B.subtilis* and *B.cereus* tested by Singh and Singh (1980a) inhibited growth and caused lysis of the mycelium and germ tubes of *F.udum* and enhanced formation of chlamydospores in culture of the same (Singh and Singh 1983c). The culture of *B.subtilis* did not have any adverse effect on pigeonpea seed germination and growth of seedlings (Sumitha and Gaikwad 1995a). The lytic action of *B.subtilis* on mycelium of *F.udum* is favoured by soil amendments with cakes of neem, and castor, rice husk and other organic matter (Singh and Singh 1980b, 1981). Bapat and Shah (2000) isolated several bacterial cultures antagonistic to *F. udum*. *Bacillus brevis* (*Brevibacillus brevis*) produced extra cellular substances which induced swellings of hyphal tips and cells with shrunken and granulated cytoplasm. It reduced wilt in pots and field when used on seed. Its formulation with vermiculite has shelf life of 6 months. A few isolates of *Pseudomonas fluorescens* have also been found antagonistic to *F.udum* controlling the wilt of pigeonpea when used as seed treatment + root zone application specially in combination with *Trichoderma viride* although, bacterium inhibited *T.viride* also *in vitro* (Sethuraman and Vidyasekaran 1994). The talc formulation of *P. fluorescens* has been found effective even after 6 months of storage and peat formulations up to 60 days. The unformulated bacteria could not be stored even for 10 days (Vidhyasekaran *et al.* 1997).

Amongst the fungi, *Trichoderma viride, T.harzianum, T. koningii* and *T. hamatum* are strong antagonists against *F.udum* (Sumitha and Gaikwad 1995a, Bhatnagar 1996, Somasekhara *et al.* 1996) and in few cases their application on seed/soil reduced the disease considerably. Seed treatment with *T.viride* is reported to reduce the pigeonpea wilt by 28% in wilt sick plot (Bidari and Gundappagol 1997). According to Biswas and Das (1999) *T.harzianum* is most effective against *F.udum* followed by *T.hamatum, T.longikonis* and *T.koningii* while *T.viride* is not effective. In pot cultures, none of them were effective when used on seed but *T.harzianum* reduced the wilt by 89% when used in soil as maize-meal-sand culture @ 40 to 60 g/kg soil. On the other hand, Pandey and Upadhyay (1999) found *T.viride* as well as *T.harzianum* best for checking pigeonpea wilt by seed application. In combination with *Verticillium chlamydosporum* the antagonist *T.harzianum* was found highly effective against wilt complex of pigeonpea involving *F.udum* and *Heterodera cajani* (Siddiqui and Mahmood 1996a). In the integrated treatment *T. harzianum* + thiram was best with 68% disease control (Pandey and Upadhyay 1999).

The wilt of pigeonpea or its pathogen is reported to be suppressed in the presence of *Rhizopus nigricans* and *Cunninghamella elegans* (Anonymous 1952) and *Aspergillus nidulans* (Upadhyay 1987) in the root region of pigeonpea. The ecology of *F.udum* in root region of pigeonpea in relation to antagonism and control of wilt has been studied in detail by Upadhyay and Rai (1982a, 1985, 1987). In the dual cultures, *Micromonospora globosa* was found to parasitize hyphae of *F.udum* by coiling and penetration resulting in granulation, coagulation and vacuolation of cytoplast ultimately causing lysis. Chlamydospores of the wilt pathogen were also attacked resulting in disintegration of their outer walls (Upadhyaya and Rai 1978, Rai and Upadhyay 1979a).

The growth as well as other activities of the bilogical agents, the pathogen as well as host plant are directly or indirectly influenced by the soil amendments. Thus soil amendments are important in biological control of a disease. The population of *F.udum* in the soil is reduced greatly by soil amendment with cakes of groundnut, mustard, Neem or Mahua (Singh and Singh 1980b, 1983a, Rai and Singh 1995). On the other hand, soil amendments, with cakes of margosa and castor (Singh and Singh 1982b), saw dust with or without urea (Singh and Singh 1982a) and rice husk (Singh and Singh 1983d) increases the acitivity of the pathogen for first 2-3 weeks but later the activity declines with the decomposition process. The soil amendments with leaves of

Crotalaria medicagnea (Upadhyay and Rai 1981b), Neem cake (Singh and Singh 1983d, Rai and Singh 1995) and oat crop residues (Kotasthane *et al.* 1987) have been found effective in controlling the disease. The soil amendments with neem cake and compost are reported to control the disease under pot culture conditions (Goudar and Kulkarni 1998). The amendments may reduce the pathogenic ability of the pathogen also (Dasgupta and Sengupta 1989).

The vesicular-arbuscular mycorrhyzae like *Glomus mosseae, G.constrictum* and *G.monosporum* did not show any influence on the wilt of pigeonpea specially under high inoculum conditions (Reddy *et al.* 1989a).

Fungicides carbendazim and captan were non injurious to antagonists *T. viride* and *T. harzianum* and their use with antagonists increased the efficacy of treatment for control of wilt (Goudar and Kulkarni 1999).

The wilt incidence was reduced with increased yields by simultaneous inoculations with *Rhizobium* strain JCC/C3 (Bhattacharya 1998).

Cross Protection : The pigeonpea plants infected by sterility virus become protected from wilt pathogen and the sap from virus infected plant does not contain glutamic acid or alanine and exhibit inhibition of spore germination of *F.udum* (Anonymous 1964, Chadha and Raychaudhuri 1965).

Inoculation of pigeonpea with non-pathogenic *Fusarium oxysporum* f sp. *ciceri* and *F. oxysporum* f sp. *vasinfectum* controlled the wilt caused by *F.udum* (Kaiser and Sengupta 1969, Maitra and Sinha 1973). This effect is more if inoculation with non-pathogenic fungus is done 6-3 days before inoculation with pathogen. In the combined infection the hyphae of all the three species could be detected in host tissues in similar manner except that the *F.udum* was concentrated more in vascular. bundles and produced conidia (Kaiser and Sengupta 1975). Seedlings infected with non-pathogenic species induced wilt symptoms initially but later they recovered. The extracts of seedlings inoculated with *F.oxysporum* from other hosts showed antifungal properties against *F.oxysporum* f sp. *udum* (Kaiser and Sengupta 1977). Cross protection of pigeonpea seedlings from *F.udum* has been obsevered by using non-pathogenic *F.oxysporum niveum, F. oxysporum ciceri, F.solani* f sp. *pisi* and *Cephalosporium sacchari* also (Chakrabarty and Sengupta 1995a). Injury to plant roots, however, decreased the effect of cross protection while exposure of seedlings at 20-30°C before inoculation increased the effect. Pigeonpea, lentil and pea have been found symptomless carriers of chickpea wilt pathogen (Haware and Nene 1982).

The true phenomenon of cross protection against *F.udum* has been reported by Rajendra and Patil (1992a) who identified some strains of *F.udum* antagonistic to pathogenic strains of the same.

2.4 Phytophthora Blight

The occurrence of Phytophthora blight of pigeonpea caused by some Phycomycetous fungus was first suspected in New Delhi in the form of typical cankers on stems near the ground level which resulted in rapid wilting of plants (Williams *et al.* 1968). The detailed description of the disease was given for the first time under the name Stem rot caused by *Phytophthora drechsleri* var. *cajani* (Pal *et al.* 1970). The disease was reported to cause serious losses to pigeonpea crop at certain places in northern parts of India. Five years later, Williams *et al.* (1975) described the disease as Phytophthora stem blight but the cause of the disease could not be identified up to the level of species. The same group of workers (Amin *et al.* 1978) later identified the cause of the disease as *Phytophthora cajani*. The disease was studied in detail at ICRISAT, India where Kannaiyan *et al.* (1980c) named the disease as Stem blight but finally name phytophthora blight caused by *P.drechsleri* f sp. *cajani* has been accepted (Nene *et al.* 1996). The literature on Phytophthora blight of pigeonpea has been reviewed by Nene *et al.* (1980), Singh and Chauhan (1992), Mehrotra (1992), Reddy and Sheila (1994) and Bajpai and Tripathi (1999).

The disease has so far been reported from Dominican Republic, India, Kenya, Panama, Puerto Rico (Nene *et al.* 1996) and Sri Lanka (Reddy *et al.* 1992c). In India, the disease occurs in most of the pigeonpea growing states specially West Bengal, Uttar Pradesh, Bihar, Andhra Pradesh (Kannaiyan *et al.* 1981c) and Madhya Pradesh (Agrawal 1985). The disease incidence in West Bengal was as high as 26.3 % while in Madhya Pradesh it was estimated to be 0.97 % on over all basis with an yield loss of 416.14 tonnes (Agrawal & Khare 1988b). Kumar *et al.* (1991) reported the disease to occur at most of the elevations of Garhwal hills in U.P. In the past, the disease has probably been confused with the wilt.

2.4.1 Symptoms

According to Pal *et al.* (1970), the symptoms of Phytophthora blight appear as brown to dark brown distinctly marked lesions on base of the stem or above it (Fig. 2.4). These lesions increase in size and girdle the stem causing drying and death of affected part above the girdled portion (Fig. 2.5). The lesion generally starts from the point of leaf scar and extends several centimetres in each direction.

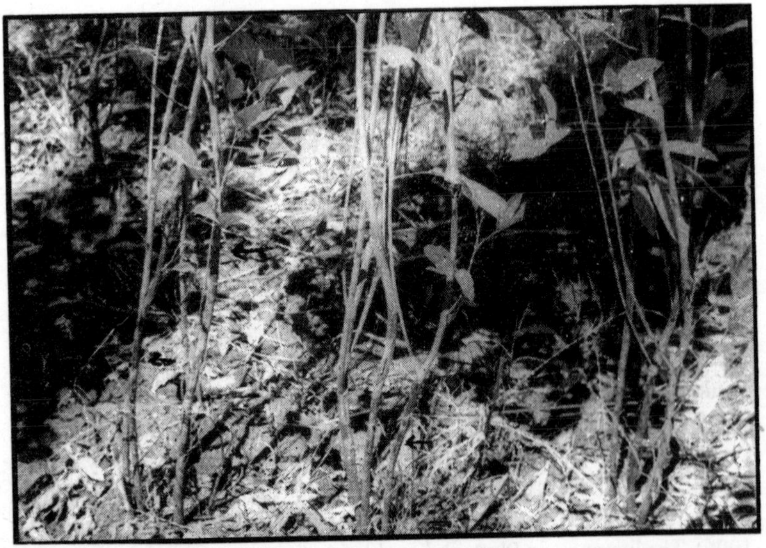

Fig. 2.4: Phytophthora blight of pigeonpea: Lesions on stems/branchs

The disease is characterized by rapid wilting of plants above the invasion site; dessication and upward rolling or leaflets usually without chlorosis; withering of petioles and small stems (Williams *et al.* 1975). The lesions on base of stem often extend 15-20 cm or even more. On the upper part of the plant, lesions may be formed on main stem, branches or petioles. They usually have definite margins and plain surface but later become slightly depressed. Longitudinal cuts into newly formed lesions show brown to black discolouration of the bark and cambium but older xylems are discoloured late. The stem or branches may break at lesion site with strong wind or other force. The stems infected late in the season may escape the death. In such cases, the stem at the edge of lesion swells into cankerous structure (Agrawal 1985). White to pinkish fungal growth may appear on the blighted area under congineal weather conditions (Pandey *et al.* 1987). The foliage of plant may also be infected showing brown water soaked circular to irregular lesions up to 1 cm diameter on leaves which may result in blighting of whole foliage within a week

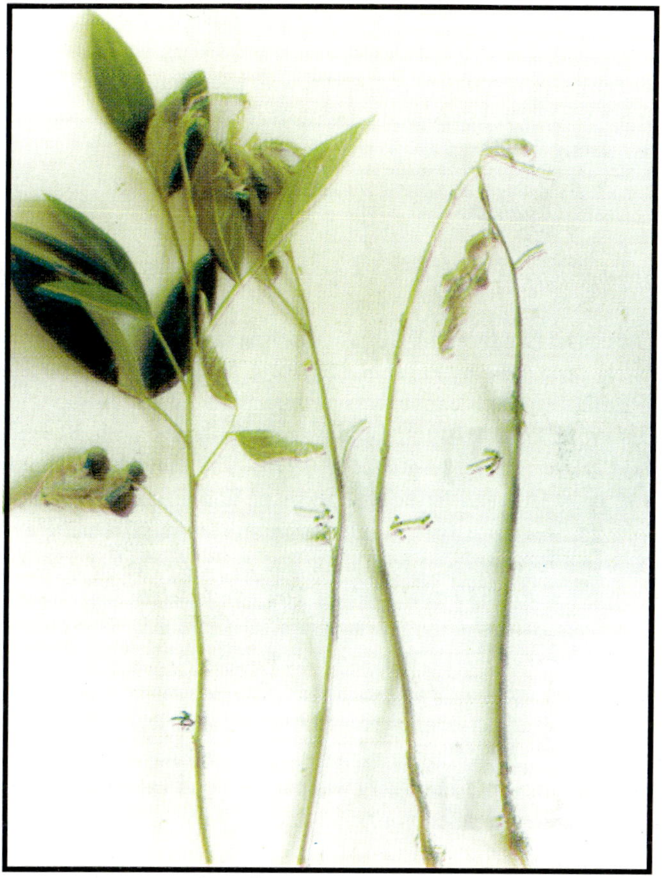

Fig. 2.5: Phytophthora blight of pigeonpea: Lesion girdling stem.

(None) *et al.* 1980). The seedlings may also be infected as soon as they emerge. Such seedlings are killed within 3 days and hence may go unnoticed (Reddy *et al.*, 1990d).

The gross symptoms of Phytophthora blight resemble with wilt and it is possible that it has been confused with wilt in the past. However, both the diseases can easily be differentiated on the basis of their field symptoms. The roots of the blight affected plants remain healthy whereas they are internally rotten and discoloured in case of wilt. The plants affected by wilt exhibit purple to dark brown streaks extending upward from soil level while those affected by blight show girdling with necrotic lesion extending several centimetres from soil level up to the stem. The lesions can be found on upper part also. In case of wilt, the older xylem is discoloured but not in case of blight (Amin *et al.* 1976). The plants affected by wilt can be pulled out from the soil with roots but those affected by Phytophthora blight break at the point of infection during pulling and even by strong wind.

2.4.2 Causal Organism

Phytophthora drechsleri Tucker f sp. *cajani* (Pal *et al.*) Kannaiyan *et al*

The causal fungus of this disease was first identified as *Phytophthora drechsleri* var. *cajani* by Pal *et al.* (1970). A few years later, the disease was studied and the cause was reported to be a new species as *Phytophthora cajani* Amin, Baldev and Williams without refering *P.drechsleri* var. *cajani* (Amin *et al.* 1978). The fungus was studied in detail at ICRISAT and based on the shape and size of the sporangia, oogonia and oospore formation; temperature requirement and its specificity to pigeonpea, it was identified as *P. drechsleri* f sp. *cajani* (Kannaiyan *et al.* 1979 and 1980c). The comparative morphology of these isolates of the pathogen is given in Table 2.2. The characters described by Pal *et al.* (1970) resembled to those of *P.drechsleri* except size of zoosporangium and presence of the evanescent vesicle with a minute papilla and hence, they named it as a new variety of *P. drechsleri*. The *mycelium* is intracellular, branched, hyaline, filamentous to slender; aerial mycelium white and fluffy when grown on PDA or oat meal agar medium, coenocytic when young but later septate with thick plugs and abundant hyphal swellings of 13-15 μ in diameter with tube like projections.

The culture of *Phytophthora cajani* could not be available and hence, Mehrotra (1992) was not sure that it is the same as *Phytophthora drechsleri* f sp. *cajani*.

Physiology : The fungus grew best on Mehrotra's medium and the optimum levels for good growth of the fungus were incubation period of 3 weeks, *p*H 6.5 and temperature 30°C (Pal and Grewal 1975c). Out of 14 carbon sources used, hexoses specially D-glucose, D-fructose, D-mannose and D-galactose were good while raffinose, insulin, sorbitol, manitol, D-xylose and lactose were poor growth supporters. The nitrogen was best utilized from ammonium salts specially ammonium nitrate (Pal and Grewal 1975a). The fungus showed partial deficiency for thiamine. The growth was supported by biotin, ascorbic acid and pyridoxine also (Pal and Grewal 1978).

Table 2.2: Comparative morphological characters of isolates of *Phytophthora* from pigeonpea

Characters	*P.drechsleri var. cajani (Pal et al. 1970)*	*P.cajani (Amin et al. 1978)*	*P.drechsleri f sp. cajani (Kannaiyan et al. 1980c)*
(1)	(2)	(3)	(4)
1. Mycelium	Variable in width (3-6 μ), devoid of granular content	Fluffy at 30°C, 4-9μ wide, vacuolate,	—
2. Hyphal swellings	Not mentioned.	Abundent at 15-20°C but not at 30°C	Present at 9-18°C.
3. Sporangiophore	—	Simple, 400 μ long, proliferated from base of sporangium, internally or externally in aged culture.	—
4. Sporangia	Ovate to pyriform and few spherical, 9.33 × 4.7-13.9 μ (av. 17.4-22 × 8-11.6 μ) with minute papilla.	Ovoid to obpyriform, non-pedicillate, terminal, persistent and with slightly conspicuous papilla, germinate directly or form new sporangium. First formed 49-82 × 19-44 μ (av. 60×32μ), later formed 16-23 × 9-14 μ in size.	Ovate to pyriform, proliferating with stalk narrowly tapered and widened at the base of sporangium. Sporangia 42-83 × 29-48 μ (av. 61.8 × 37.3 μ) in size.
5. Zoospores	Some time liberating with an evanescent vesicle or proliferation of zoosporangium, 8-20 per sporangium.	Zoospores differentiated within sporangium 2-25, released one by one through exit pore of 6.6-11 μ in diameter, 10-25 μ (14 μ) in size; germinate after encystment forming 1-4 germ tubes.	—
6. Sex organs	Oogonia spherical, 23.4-37 μ (Most 25.5-28 μ); antheridia amphigynous basal, persistent, nearly spherical, 8.1-15 ×	Oogonia with amphigynous antheridia, persistent, 15-16 μ, hyaline. Oospores single, spherical, smooth, light	Oogonia with amphigynous antheridia. Oospores spherical, 27.5-47.5 μ (37.3μ) in diameter.

Table 2.1 *Contd...*

(1)	(2)	(3)	(4)
	spherical, 8.1-15 × 8-14 μ (11.6 × 12.7 μ). Oospores spherical, to globose, 23.4-37μ (30 μ) in diameter, thick-walled and 2.4-4.8μ in size.	smooth, light brown, pleurotic, 20-37 μ in size.	
7. Optimum temperature for growth	30 – 32°C	30°C	27-33°C
8. Chlamydospores	Intercallary or terminal, 11.2-20.8 μ (14.4 μ) in size.	Not present.	Not present.
9. Host range	Not tested	Pigeonpea only (host specific).	*Cajanus cajan* and *Atylosia* spp. only which are wild relatives of pigeonpea.

The fungus grows well on V 8 juice agar medium: V 8 juice 100 ml, calcium carbonate 2 g, agar 20 g, distilled water 900 ml (Nene *et al.* 1981a); pigeonpea infusion agar medium made of infusion from 40 g pigeonpea seed meal, agar 20 g and distilled water to make 1000 ml (Sheila *et al.* 1983). A selective medium for *P. drechsleri* f sp. *cajani* has also been developed by Bisht and Nene (1988) which is prepared using V 8 juice agar, Benlate 20 ppm, hymexazol 20 ppm, mycostatin 10 ppm, PCNB 20 ppm, pimaricin 5 ppm, vanomycin 200 ppm and rifamycin 10 ppm.

Studies have been conducted on formation of sporangia and germination of zoospores of *P. drechsleri* f sp. *cajani*. Abundant sporangia are formed by the fungus adopting the technique developed by Kannaiyan *et al.* (1994) in which fungus is grown for 5 days at 30°C on V 8 juice agar medium. The fungal discs of 5 mm diameter are obtained from perifery of the colony and floated in clear V 8 juice and sterile distilled water (1 : 5) for a further 24 h at 30°C under fluorescent light. The discs are rinsed twice in sterile distilled water after 16 h of which abundant sporangia are formed. The fungus is very sensitive to plant growth regulators and indole 3-butyric acid (IBA) results in least sporangia formation (Rai 1994). According to Singh and Chauhan (1988b), the zoospores encyst within 2 h at 5-10°C or 35-50°C. They germinate forming 1-5 germ tubes and some produce microsporangia after germination. The optimum temperature, *p*H and light for zoospore germination are 30°C, 7.5 *p*H and complete darkness (Chauhan and Singh 1991c).

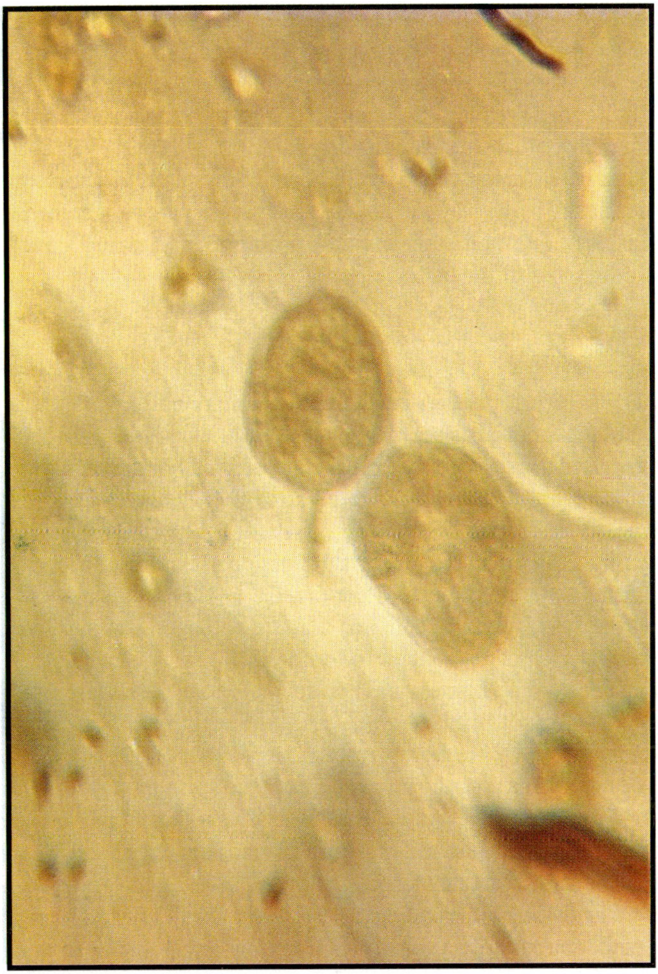

Fig. 2.6 : Sporangia of *Phytophthora drechsleri f sp. cajani*

The oospores are formed well on pigeonpea leaves floated in 5% sucrose solution incubated in dark at 25°C (Singh and Chauhan 1988a). The host is not essential for oospore formation but temperture is the critical factor. They are formed by transferring the mycelium in distilled water on glass slide and kept at 25°C for 36 h.

Pathogenic Races : The pathogen *P. drechsleri* f sp. *cajani* has been found variable pathogenically. Sarkar (1988) differentiated 8 isolates collected from different parts of India on the basis of reaction of 13 pigeonpea genotypes. They were P2, P3, P4, BHU, KPR, HIS, and P2 BF. These isolates have shown variability with regard to their pathogenicity (Nene *et al.* 1991) as well as growth and morphology (Nene *et al.* 1992). Variability in physiological parameters like nutritional and temperature requirements of isolates from Hyderabad (P2), Varanasi (VP) and Delhi (DP) has been demonstrated by Singh and Singh (1994) also. However, inconsistency in the reaction and loss in aggressiveness of some isolates on frequent sub-culturing created problem in drawing conclusion regarding races of the pathogen.

2.4.3 Disease Cycle and Epidemiology

(i) *Survival* : Information on the epidemiology of Phytophthora stem blight of pigeonpea has been reviewed by Agrawal (1987b). The fungus was reported to survive only for 133 days under laboratory conditions on V 8 juice agar medium when stored at 15°C (Kannaiyan *et al.* 1980b). Kannaiyan *et al.* (1983) reported survival of the pathogen on infected bits of pigeonpea in the field for a short period of time and hence, they did not attribute the recurrence of the disease to survival of the pathogen. However, it was later established that the pathogen can survive in the infected stems of pigeonpea in the field till commencement of rains when the next crop is sown and that such diseased stems left in the field are the sources of primary inoculum (Agrawal 1985, Bisht and Nene 1986, Agrawal 1987b, Agrawal and Khare 1988a). The survival period is favoured by burying the infected bits in the soil and may vary from 3-7 months (Sharma and Singh 1996) to one year (Bisht and Nene 1990) depending on depth and soil moisture levels. The fungus survives in the field in the form of chlamydospores (Sarkar 1988). There is no evidence of seed transmission of the pathogen (Agrawal 1985, Bisht and Nene 1990). The pathogen can infect *Atylosia scarabaeoides* (Kannaiyan and Nene 1985a), *Cajanus goensis* and *C. platycarpus* (Sarkar *et al.* 1991) which are mostly the perennial weeds and may play the role as alternate hosts for survival of the pathogen.

(ii) *Dispersal* : The splashing rain and the wind contribute to short distance dispersal of the pathogen in the field while water flowing from an infested field may carry the inoculum to uninfested field (Agrawal 1985, Bisht and Nene 1990).

(iii) *Disease Development*: The disease severity is influenced by several factors related to host pathogen and environment as described below:

Host Injury : The infection of pigeonpea stem by *P.drechsleri* f sp. *cajani* oftenly takes place on a leaf scar (Williams *et al.* 1975) and the injury to the host facilitate the infection.

Environment : The meteorological parameters specially rainfall, RH and temperature play important role in development of this disease. High humidity helps in rapid development of disease (Pal *et al.* 1970). Inoculation of plants early in the season when the RH was high with 30-35°C temperature resulted in blighting of plants (Williams *et al.* 1975) while inoculation at decreasing temperature caused only marginal kill of plants. Role of meteorological parameters in the development of Phytophthora blight and spread of the pathogen has been worked out and documented well (Agrawal 1985, 1987b, Agrawal and Khare 1987b, Chauhan and Saha 1999). Number of rainy days, rainfall and RH are positively correlated with the infection index/disease incidence while it was negative with the temperature levels. More number of rainy days are more favourable to the disease as compared to heavy rains which probably do not allow the inoculum to settle on the host surface. The death of plants due to blight is favoured by more rainfall, rainy days, RH and less difference between the maximum and minimum temperatures. The high daily temperature (33°C) during July and August may impede the growth of the pathogen (Singh and Chauhan 1985a). The spread of the disease depends on formation and dispersal of sporangia and release and germination of zoospores which are favoured by the temperature levels of 25-30°C and 25-27°C respectively (Pal and Grewal 1984). The zoospores encyst rapidly at 5-10 or 35-50°C. The cyst germinates best at 30°C but not below 10°C or above 45°C. The germination is favoured by darkness (Chauhan and Singh 1991c) and the disease develops more fast at night (Singh and Chauhan 1985a). The infection and subsequent disease develops well at day temperature of 28°C prevailing after a rain for 5-7 consecutive days (Reddy *et al.* 1992b). The soil inoculum increases with decrease in the day temperature, more rainfall and cloudy weather.

Drainage : Poor drainage causes temporary water stagnation in the field which favours the disease causing heavy losses (Agrawal 1985, Singh and Chauhan 1985a, Pandey *et al.* 1987). During a survery of the disease in the state of Madhya Pradesh, higher incidence was observed in poorly drained fields than in well drained ones. Even on slopy land with good drainage, the disease occurs more severely on low-land as compared to mid-land and up-land areas (Agrawal 1989a). Such differences are apparent specially when susceptible variety is used.

Plant Nutrients : The plant nutrients influence the growth and strength of tissues and thus affect the disease incidence and severity. High doses of nitrogen increase the incidence of Phytophthora blight in absence of potassium (Pal and Grewal 1976a). On the other hand, addition of K decrease the disease regardless of presence or absence of N or P in the soil. The P had little effect on the disease.

Cultural Practices : The soybean as intercorp with pigeonpea in blight sick plot could not check the dispersal of inoculum of pathogen through rain splashes from soil to pigeonpea foliage (Agrawal 1985). It did not work due to the fact that both the crops were sown simultaneously and hence soybean could not form the crop canopy sufficiently thick to check the rain splashes. However, Chauhan and Singh (1991a) reported less disease in the weed-infested pigeonpea plots as compared to weed free plots.

General observations revealed the reduced disease incidence in pigeonpea crop grown in rotation with other crops as compared to the area where pigeonpea is grown repeatedly (Mishra and Shukla 1987). Date of sowing also influences the disease greatly. It is reported less in early and pre-monsoon sown crop as compared to late sown crop (Agrawal 1985). On the other hand, delayed sowing is reported to reduce the disease greatly at ICRISAT.

Host : The plants are infected more at the age of 15 days and the susceptibility of plants decreases with the advancing age (Mishra and Shukla 1986a). Agrawal and Khare (1987a) studied the comparative epidemic growth of the disease on four genotypes having different degrees of resistance. The epidemic curves of all the genotypes showed the sigmoid pattern but rate of the disease progress ('r') varied in all the cases. Thus it was suggested that the 'r' values should be supported by areas under curve ('A') for better interpretation. The disease causes heavy losses to short duration varieties as compared to medium and long duration ones. It is probably due to the close spacing used for short duration and also due to the fact that they do not have time and plasticity to compensate the lost plants as is the case with medium and long duration types (Reddy *et al.* 1990d).

2.4.4 Host Resistance

Screening of pigeonpea genotypes for resistance to Phytophthora blight was first done by Pal *et al.* (1970) by leaf scar inoculation method and AS

3, 2357 and 4419 were found as moderately resistant. The systematic screening work against this disease was, however, started at ICRISAT centre, Patancheru, India in 1976-77 where large number of resistant genotypes were identified as summarized in Table 2.3. None of the line of pigeonpea was found resistant to P3 isolate of the pathogen (ICRISAT 1986). Later, screening was taken up at various centres under All India Coordinated Pulses Improvement Programme and several entries have been identified with multilocation resistance (Reddy *et al.* 1990c, Amin *et al.* 1993). Screening was also done to identify multiple disease resistance specially against wilt, Phytophthora blight and sterility mosaic (Anon. 1992). Reddy *et al.* (1991) reported that out of 6873 germplasm of pigeonpea, none was resistant to P3 isolate of *P.drechsleri* f sp. *cajani.*

Table 2.3: Pigeonpea entries resistant to Phytophthora blight

Number of test entries	*Entries found resistant*	*Reference*
268	AS 3, 2357 and 4419	Pal *et al.* (1970)
1543	ICP 28, 113, 214, 231, 339, 580, 752, 913, 914, 934, 1088, 1090, 1120, 1123, 1149, 1150, 1151, 1258, 1321, 1529, 1535, 1570, 1950, 2376, 3753, 6974, 7065, 7182, *Atylosia sericia* and *A. platycarpa.*	Nene *et al.* (1980)
6488	122 lines including those with multiple disease resistance	Nene *et al.* (1981b)
2842	77 germplasm, 3 cultivars and 2 species of *Atylosia.*	Kannaiyan *et al.* (1981a)
46	BDO 3, ICPL 6, S 80, S 197, ICPL 150 from early; ICPL 5, ICPL 6, ICPL 234, No. 148, AS 71-37, BDN 2, ICPL 270, PDA 5 from medium and late group.	Bhargava and Gupta (1983)
7I	ICPL 161, METH 12, COMP 1, ESR 6, Pant A 3, Pant A 83-14.	Singh *et al.* (1985)
250	KPBR 79-1, S 786-1, KPBR 80-1, KPBR 80-2.	Mishra and Shukla (1986b)
—	GAUT 82-53-1, GAUT 82-55-1, ICP 28, KPBR 80, KPBR 80-1-4 DA 13 and Pant A 1-1	Pal *et al.* (1987, 1989a, 1989b)
322	13 lines were resistant	Reddy *et al.* (1989b)
6873	10 were promising to P2 & P3 isolates and KPBR 80-2-1	Reddy *et al.* (1990c)
—	ICPL 8564, 8610, 8692, 9046, 9252	Anonymous (1992)
1010	KPBR 80—2-1, 80-2-2 & ICP 9252	Amin *et al.* (1993a)
—	*Atylosia platycarpa* to P2 & P3	Reddy *et al.* (1996)
13	Accessions of *C.platycarpa* ICPW 61, 65, 69, and 70	Saxena *et al.* (1996)
300	Exn 7, ICPL 90039, 92042, 91047, DTOTSP, AL 601, ICPL 87119	Kant *et al.* (1998)
—	KE 11 and KM 10	Saxena *et al.* (1998)

Khare and Lakpale (1997) screened several entries of pigeonpea belonging to five maturity groups but none was resistant although, 14 were moderately resistant. A line KPBR 80-2 was found to possess resistance to P2 and P3 isolates of Phytophthora, wilt and sterility mosaic (Anonymous 1990).

Perfect screening with reproducible results depends on the technique used for screening, i.e. for creation of the disease and scoring procedure. Pal *et al.* (1970) used leaf scar method of inoculation for developing the disease in the test population in which 1-2 month old plants were inoculated at leaf scar after removal of leaf. The techniques for screening have been developed at ICRISAT and standardized for screening the pigeonpea population on large scale (Kannaiyan and Nene 1978 and 1981b). The techniques so developed with the standard grading scales have been described in detail by Nene *et al.* (1981a) as follows :

(i) *Stem Inoculation Method* : This method is recommended for large scale screening. The test entries are sown in a well levelled plot. A line of susceptible check (ICP 7119) is sown after every 10 lines of test entries for monitoring. Culture of *P.drechsleri* f sp. *cajani* is grown on V8 juice agar (V8 juice 100ml, calcium carbonate 2 g, agar 20 g, distilled water 900 ml) or pigeonpea infusion agar (Infusion from 40 g pigeonpea seed, agar 20 g, distilled water to make 1000 ml) at 28-30°C. One week old culture is macerated after adding 0.2% of 600 mesh carborundum. The stems of one month old plants are inoculated at base by rubbing small amount of mycelial mass with fingers. The field is then flooded with water immediately after inoculation. Blight symptoms appear in about 10 days. There should be atleast 20-50 plants in each line. The following rating scale is recommended for observation.

Rating	*Description*	*Interpretation*
1	No symptoms on any plant	Resistant
3	Symptons on 10% or fewer plants	Moderately resistant
5	Symptoms on 11-20% plants	Tolerant
7	Symptoms on 21-50% plants	Moderately susceptible
9	Symptoms on 51% or more plants	Susceptible

The test lines with ratings of 1-3 are acceptable, 5 is acceptable if 1-3 is not available, 7-9 is not acceptable.

Rating against Phytophthora blight of pigeonpea and other root diseases is done on the basis of per cent mortality as Resistant (0-10%), Moderately resistant (11-20%), Moderately susceptible (21-50%), Susceptible (51-80%) and Highly susceptible (81-100%). However, based on the type of symptoms, Reddy and Jain (1992) proposed a nine-point scale as follows:

Rating	*Plant mortality(%)*	*Stem lesion type*
1	0	No symptoms.
2	1-5	Less than 5 mm long smooth lesions.
3	6-10	6-10 mm long smooth lesions.
4	11-20	10 mm long smooth lesions with girdle.
5	21-30	10 mm long lesion with cracking.
6	31-50	Smooth galls without cracking.
7	51-75	Large galls with cracking and girdling.
8	76-100	Galls with cracking, girdling and breaking of branches.
9	Plants killed	Plants killed completely.

Singh and Chauhan (1985b) suggested only three categories of host reaction for identifying resistnace in pigeopea against Phytophthora blight as 1 = No symptoms (Highly resistant), 2 = Formation of galls (Moderately resistant) and 3 = Appearance of brown lesions resulting in collapse and death of plants (Susceptible).

(ii) *Pot Culture Screening Method*: It is done by soil drench method in which culture of *P.drechsleri* f sp. *cajani* is multiplied on V8 juice broth or pigeonpea infusion broth as described before. Test entries are sown in plastic pots (20 cm diameter & filled with red alfisol) @ 25-30 seeds per pot. The mycelial mats are washed and mashed with water in waring blender for 1-2 minutes. The suspension is diluted and 5-10 day old seedlings are inoculated by pouring 100 ml mycelial suspension around base of seedlings in each pot. Pots with susceptible (ICP 7119) and resistant (BDN 1) checks are maintained for monitoring. Plants are watered liberally atleast 3 times a day. Symptoms start appearing in 48 h. Final observations are recorded 10 days after inoculation.

The spray inoculation method is practiced in pots as described above but inoculation is done by spraying 15-30 days old seedlings with 50 ml suspension per pot. The inoculated plants are covered with polythene bags for 48 h after which bags are removed and plants are sprayed with tap water every 2-3 h during day until 96 h after inoculation. Afterward these are sprayed 3 times a day until final recording after ten days of inoculation.

(iii) *Diseased Debris Field Inoculation Technique* : This technique has been developed for large scale screening of pigeonpea lines for resistance to Phytophthora blight in the field (Reddy *et al.* 1990b). In this technique, the test entries are sown in field using ICP 2376 and ICP 7119 (resistant and susceptible checks respectively) alternately after every 4 rows of test entries. The infected plant debris from last season crop are scattered in the field. Irrigation is not required and 250 kg debris are required per hectare. The field inoculated with diseased debris in beginning and incorporation of deseased crop in soil at end result in development of good blight sick plot. Observations on disease are recorded at frequent interval.

Biotechnological Approach : Asthana *et al.* (1998) adopted tissue culture method for selecting pigeonpea lines resistant to Phytophthora blight *in vitro.* The calli were initiated from 10-15 days old immature embryo explant on MS medium supplemented with BAP (2 mg/1 + 2,4-D 1.5 mg/1). Three weeks old calli were cut into pieces and sub-cultured on callusing medium containing 0.1-1.5 per cent of culture filtrate of the pathogen. The concentration 1.5 % proved lethal to calli but 8-15% calli from 1% culture filtrate treatment survived after 4 cycles selection. They were selected and transferred on filtrate free medium for multiplication. Some of the calli turned green and showed shoot differentiation when transferred to regeneration medium.

Inheritence of Resistance : The resistance in pigeonpea genotypes to isolates P2 of *P. drechsleri* f sp. *cajani* has been found to be governed by a single dominant gene named as Pd1 (Sharma *et al.* 1982). Similarly in case of P3 isolate also resistance is reported to be monogenic and dominant but presence of some minor genes has also been reported which are involved in expression of resistance (Gupta *et al.* 1996). It is suggested to fully utilize this durable source of resistance (Pd3) in pigeonpea breeding programmes.

Mechanism of Resistance : Several factors have been studied in relation to resistance in pigeonpea plants against Phytophthora blight.

(i) *Chemical contents* : The biochemical analysis of resistant and susceptible varieties revealed total phenols to be more in susceptible than in resistant varieties (Pal and Grewal 1975b, Agrawal 1989b). However, stem inoculation caused increase of phenoles in resistant varieties while in susceptible ones phenoles decreased in leaves but increased in stem indicating their mobilization from leaves to infection site (Agrawal 1989b). All the 9 phenolic acids were detected in resistant as well susceptible varieties except ferulic acid which was absent in resistant variety Pant A 3. Gallic acid, protocatechuic acid and chlorogenic acid were high in resistant than in susceptible genotypes. It is not very conclusive that phenolic acids have some correlation with resistance. In fact, resistance may be due to cumulative effect of other chemical constituents of plants (Chaurasia *et al.* 1993).

The non-reducing sugars increase with time but after infection by *P.drechsleri* f sp. *cajani* they decrease and more so in susceptible than in resistant varieties (Pal and Grewal 1976b). According to Agrawal (1991), total sugar contents did not differ in resistant and susceptible varieties but after stem inoculation, they increased in leaves as well as in stems of resistant variety while in susceptible variety they decreased in leaves and increased in stems indicating transport of sugars from leaves to stem.

The resistant varieties contain less amino acids than the susceptible ones but after inoculation, they increase in resistant variety and decrease in susceptible ones. The protein did not show any correlation with resistance or susceptibility of pigeonpea plants (Agrawal 1990).

(ii) *Age of Plant* : The plants are highly susceptible at the age of 15 days and the susceptibility decreases with the increasing age resulting in minimum infection at the age of 120 days (Mishra and Shukla 1986a). However, this phenomenon may differ from genotype to genotype and isolate to isolate (Sarkar *et al.* 1992).

(iii) *Phytoalexines* : The chemicals—phytoalexin-84 and inducer are claimed to act as elicitor and to help plants to increase their phytoalexin level. These chemicals when sprayed or soil drenched before inoculation reduced blight incidence greatly. The effect was more pronounced in case of soil drenching as compared to foliar spray (Sheila and Nene 1987).

2.4.5 Control

Chemical Control : Fungicides and plant extracts have been evaluated against *P.drechsleri* f sp. *cajani in vitro* as well as *in vivo.*

In vitro Evaluation : The growth of the pathogen is inhibited completely by zineb, copper oxychloride, metalaxyl, thiram and captan at 250 ppm each and by mancozeb at 1000 ppm (Agrawal 1987a); Blue copper -50, Brestan 60, Ceresan wet, Cuman, Daconil, Difolatan, Miltox, Plantvax, Thiram and Vitavax (Mishra and Shukla 1989). As soil drench, Blue copper-50 and Ceresan wet controlled the fungus completely. Some of the herbicides like fluchloralin and pendimethalin at more than 50 μ/1 reduced growth and sporangia formation by *P.drechsleri* f sp. *cajani* completely (Singh *et al.* 1999a).

Some of the plant products have also been found effective against the pathogen. Ajoene, a compound derived from garlic (*Allium sativum)* inhibited growth, sporangia formation and germination of sporangia and zoospores of the pathogen effectively (Singh *et al.* 1992). However, at low concentrations it enhanced all these activities of the pathogen.

In vivo testing : Effective disease control could be obtained by pre-inoculation spray with some conventional fungicides like Brestan-60 (Pal and Grewal 1983), Difolatan chlorothalonil and Brestan-60 (Mishra and Shukla 1989).

The disease could be controlled in greenhouse experiments up to initial stage only by seed treatment with metalaxyl @ 4g/kg (Sinha 1983 and Kannaiyan and Nene 1984) but it was not effective in field. Similar observations have been made by Pandey *et al.* (1987). Rajdan (1985) detected sufficient amount of metalaxyl in seedlings raised from treated seeds. However, later metalaxyl as seed treatment was found ineffective in controlling the disease even up to 5g/kg of seed. It could be controlled by 0.3% spray of metalaxyl at 40, 55 and 70 DAS alone or in combination with seed treatment (Kannaiyan *et al.* 1984; Pandey *et al.* 1987 and Bisht *et al.* 1988). Effective control of the disease could be achieved even by two sprays of metalaxyl at 30 and 45 DAS (Agrawal 1987a). According to Chauhan and Singh (1991b) the disease is controlled by metalaxyl spray even at 125 ppm in greenhouse experiments but in field complete control is not possible due to interference of rains. Control of disease by metalaxyl spray was achieved by Singh and Sharma also

(1996). High rates of Apron (4 & 8 g/kg) were phytotoxic and 2-4 g/kg could be recommended as cost effective (Singh *et al.* 1999). Ridomil NZ 72 (8% metalaxyl +64% mancozeb) was as effective as Apron 35 WS.

The translocation and persistence studies on metalaxyl in pigeonpea have clearly explained that why seed treatment alone is not effective in controlling Phytophthora blight of pigeonpea. The metalaxyl is absorbed by seed, root and leaves and becomes ambimobile within seedling/plant (Kotwal *et al.* 1981; Chaube *et al.* 1984), although, some workers have reported that it moves upward only (Vyas *et al.* 1983). It persists in seed coat and cotyledons for 11 days after seed treatment and for 20 and 15 days in leaves and roots respectively after root treatment (Vyas *et al.* 1983). In case of seed treatment, the quantity of fungicide translocated to susceptible parts of seedlings is insufficient to check the infection (Chaube *et al.* 1987b) as major part is retained with seed. In case of root treatments, most part is translocated to leaves where it is distributed uniformly in the lamina and later it accumulates at tips and margins of leaf. The translocation is enhanced by adding sugar. In case of seed treatment, only 14.4, 6.3 and 3.3 % of the metalaxyl applied to seed could be recovered from seedlings of 15, 30 and 45 days age respectively (Chaube *et al.* 1987a). The herbicides like fluchloralin and pendimethalin are reported to increase the toxicity of Apron and Ridomil but reduced that of captafol (Singh *et al.* 1999a). The fungicide does not affect the nodulation adversely (Vyas *et al.* 1983).

Among the plant products, 2% aquous extract of *Aegle marmelos* proved to be highly effective against Phytophthora blight when used for seed treatment (Dayaram 1994). Upadhyay *et al.* (1998) reported Neem oil and Neem soap to be effective for disease control in field when used as seed treatment.

Resistance to Fungicides : The isolates P2 and P3 from ICRISAT are reported to develop resistance to benomyl (Gangawane *et al.* 1988) and the resistance was not reduced by use of Captan, thiram or Difolatan alternately or as mixture. The resistant mutants could be developed by various chemical and physical treatments. The virulence of resistant isolates was, however, reduced on pigeonpea variety HY 3C. The resistance increased with successive passes of fungus on benomyl individually or in mixture with mancozeb, tridemorph and thiophanate methyl but PCNB reduced it even in mixture (Gangawane *et al.* 1989). Alternate use of these fungicides may prove beneficial in managing resistance in fungi to fungicides. The fungus *P.drechsleri* f sp. *cajani* has exhibited resistance to metalaxyl also (Chauhan and Singh 1987,

Gangawane 1995). It emphasizes need of careful use of chemicals for control of plant diseases, although, their use becomes very necessary under certain conditions.

Biological Control : In pot experiments, *Gigaspora calospora,* a vesicular-arbuscular mycorrhiza has been reported to inhibit the development of Phytophthora blight of pigeonpea (Bisht *et al.* 1985). In the same way, isolates of *Bacillus subtilis* or its cell free culture filtrate inhibited growth of the pathogen *in vitro* (Podile and Dube 1987). The disease is reported to be reduced in presence of VAM (ICRISAT 1986).

Integrated Management : Phytophthora blight of pigeonpea could be controlled best by integrated treatment involving resistant variety (KPBR 80-2 or ICP 8564), seed treatment with metalaxyl followed by 1-2 sprays of metalaxyl at 15 days interval (Raju and Reddy 1993). Chaurasia and Rathi (1993) evaluated several combinations of various management practices of which seed treatment with metalaxyl @ 5g/kg with ridge planting and no weeding for two months provided maximum protection. Seed treatment + 3 sprays of ridomil + No weeding + ridge planting was also effective. Agrawal and Prasad (Unpublished data) reported that the integrated treatment had highly significant effect when susceptible variety was used as compared to tolerant or resistant varieties and that no weeding treatment can be replaced by using soybean as cover crop in between the rows of pigeonpea.

2.5 Phoma Stem Canker

The pathogen of this disease *Phoma cajani* was first reported to occur on pigeonpea in Brazil (Rangel 1915) followed by Trinidad (Leach and Wright 1930) and the Antilles region of Caribbean (Cook 1939). However, the disease was first reported in its epidemic form from Puerto Rico by Garcia (1960) who described it in detail. The disease has also been reported from India (Somani *et al.* 1981), Malawi and Zambia (Kannaiyan *et al.* 1981c) and West Indies (Goodling 1962). In India, the disease occurs in the states of Gujarat (Kannaiyan *et al.* 1981c), Madhya Pradesh (Agrawal and Nema 1985) and Maharashtra (Somani *et al.* 1981). In Trinidad, the disease appears late and hence, it may not become a major problem if single crop is taken (Leach and Wright 1930). However, the disease may cause heavy losses under favourable agroclimatic conditions. It is reported to occur in epiphytotic proportions in Puerto Rico periodically on commercial plantings of pigeonpea (Garcia 1962, Lopez 1969). The disease occurs widely in Zambia also causing economic losses. In some experimental crop of pigeonpea, Agrawal and Nema (1985) observed practically 100% plants infected by the disease. The disease affects seedlings as well as old plants and may cause death (Aponte and Aponte 1963). Thus, the importance of the disease cannot be disregarded specially in dense stands of pigeonpea in row crop system.

2.5.1 Symptoms

According to Leach and Wright (1930), the primary symptoms of the disease are the formation of gray, scutiform dark edged lesions averaging 5 cm long on stem and branches (Fig 2.7). Many lesions turn dark brown

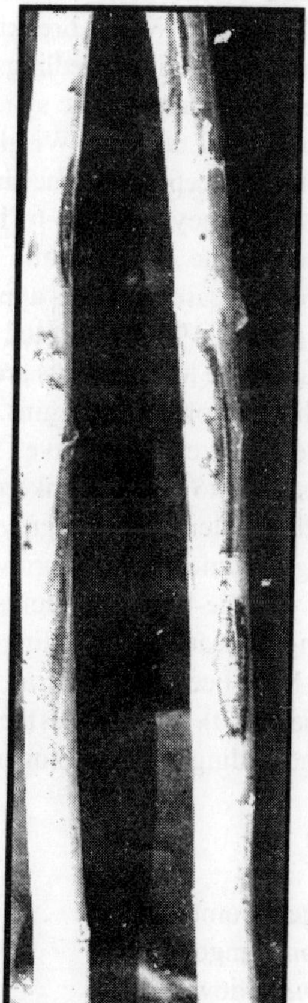

Fig. 2.7: Phoma stem canker of pigeonpea.

and at the collar they change into large deep cankers with a verrucose, carbonaceous surface. The canker usually girdles the collar region killing the affected plant. The diagnostic character is unequal development of the wood near the lesions giving twisted appearance to the stem. In later stages, discolouration of internal tissues extends from a canker for a distance of many centimetres along the stem. Similar symptoms of collar and stem canker of pigeonpea have been reported due to *Physalospora cajani* (Goodling 1962) which is considered to be the perfect stage of *Phoma* and *Macrophoma* species.

According to Garcia (1960), the Phoma stem canker of pigeonpea is characterized by the presence of swollen, cankerous areas of 2-3 cm length on branches and stems. The lesions generally enlarge longitudinally. The affected site swells breaking open the bark and becoming more cankerous with the age. Seedlings are attacked early with sooty spots which is the most characteristic symptom of the disease.

The symptoms reported by Leach and Wright (1930) and by Garcia (1960) are more or less similar except that former authors reported presence of *Diplodia* sp. also which they thought to be responsible for the carbonaceous appearance of the canker while Garcia mentioned that *Phoma* sp. alone can produce carbonaceous appearance of cankers.

Khune and Kapoor (1981a, 1981b) reported the symptoms on stems as well as leaves. On leaves, the lesions/spots are circular, tan coloured, circular to irregular with dark coloured margins. The necrotic tissues of spots become brittle and detached from leaves forming the shot holes. On the stem, numerous grey to brown cankerous lesions are formed which coalesce and girdle the stem showing grey centre with dark brown margin at advanced stage. Numerous dark brown pycnidia can be seen embeded in the spot area. Die-back symptoms are seen but no stem deformities like twisting appearance, swellings of affected parts and breaking open of bark have been observed as reported by Leach and Wright (1930) and Garcia (1960). It seems that the symptoms of pigeonpea stem canker may vary according to the pathogens involved.

2.5.2 Causal Organism

Phoma cajani (Rangel) Comb. Nov.
= *Phyllosticta cajani* Rangel
= *Phyllosticta cajani* Sydow
= *Phyllosticta cajanicola* (Syd.) Trotter

Phyllosticta cajani and *Phoma cajani* were first described by Rangel (1915) on pigeonpea from Brazil. Leach and Wright (1930) observed *Phoma* and *Macrophoma* type pycnidia associated with the canker of pigeonpea and showed them to be the stages of *Physalospora* in culture. The *Phoma* sp. has *pycnidia* papillate, variable in size and structure, united as stroma in culture but separate in plant tissues. Whole of their inner surface contain the *conidiophores* bearing hyaline, obtuse *conidia* from 3.1 to 6.2 μ (4 × 1.6 μ) in size. *Macrophoma* Type *Pycnidia* are not papillate, with *conidia* elongate, subellipsoid to sub-rhomboid, obtuse, 18.5-35μ in length and averaged 24.5 × 7 μ. They are hyaline with non-vacuolated granular contents.

The *perithecia* of *Physalospora* are corriaceous, globose and short beaked, 164-226 μ in diameter. They contain basally born clavate-cylindrical, apically thickened *asci* 126-134.8 μ long by 25-35 μ broad. The *ascospores* extrude in a gelatinous matrix through a pore formed by the splitting off of an apical cap and are fusoid, elliptical with thick walls, hyaline with 1-3 central vacuoles. They measure 17.5 to 28 μ by 8.7-12.3 μ (average 24 × 11.1 μ). This isolate was considered as *P.cydoniae.* Goodling (1962) assigned stem canker of pigeonpea to *Physalospora cajani* only.

Khune and Kapoor (1981a) described *Phoma cajani* as *pycnidia* on leaves and stems, dark brown, globose, 45-130μ in diameter with conspicuous ostiole; *pycnidiospores* hyaline, round to ovate, one-celled, 2-6 × 1.5-2.5 μ and arise from dolliform conidiogenous cells lining the pycnidial cavity. On the basis of these characters, the fungus was identified as *Phoma* and matched with *Phyllosticta cajani* described from India. According to the present concept (Aa 1973), *Phyllosticta* is characterized in having much larger pycnidiospores than those of *Phoma,* being 1.5 to 2 times as long as wide and born on elongate to cylindric conidiogenous cells. They have a slimy envelop and an apical slimy appendage in most cases. On the other hand, *Pycnidiospores* in case of *Phoma* fall within the range of 2-10 × 1.5-4.5 μ and are born on dolliform conidiogenous cells lining the pycnidial cavity. Hence, transfer of this species from *Phyllosticta* to *Phoma* was proposed and named as *Phoma cajani* (Rangel) Comb. Nov.

Some of the isolates from pigeonpea seed were reported to be virulent while others non-virulent on Kaki cultivar of pigeonpea (Lopez 1969). The fungus grows well on PDA, corn meal agar, oat meal agar and pigeonpea pod agar media producing abundant pycnidia when plates were flooded with conidial suspension. Matured pycnidia appeared 44 h after inoculation. The discharge of pycnidiospores was greatly stimulated by chilling the cultures. The perfect stage, a heterothallic ascomycetes was observed on agar media and the ascospore cultures produced pycnidia in 4-5 days.

2.5.3 Disease Cycle and Epidemiology

The *Phoma* sp. has been found associated with 4% seeds of pigeonpea from stem canker affected crop and 1% from healthy crop in the same locality in Puerto Rico (Lopez 1969). Some of the isolates were extremely virulent producing lesions on stems within 48 h after inoculation although, all cankers healed 4 months after inoculation. Somani *et al.* (1981) and Agrawal and Nema (1988) could not find association of the pathogen with seeds of pigeonpea. It has been observed that the pathogen can survive in the diseased pigeonpea stubbles exposed to sun during the hot summer from harvest to the start of rains when new pigeonpea crop is sown in the field (Agrawal and Nema 1988). The symptoms of the disease on new crop in presence of the infected stubbles may appear 15 days after sowing on leaves as well as stems. The infection spreads, probably through splashing rains. The disease spreads very fast in the crop (Agrawal & Nema 1988).

2.5.4 Host Resistance

Singh *et al.* (1986) screened 153 genotypes of pigeonpea of which A 133, Al 136, ICPL 87, ICPL 148, ICPL 8304 and ICPL 4018 were found resistant while 20 lines were resistant to moderately resistant to Phoma leaf spot and stem canker. A 0-9 point scale was used for scoring as follows :

Grade	*Reaction*	*Diseased area (%) on stem/leaf*
0	Free	Nil
1	Resistant	0.1 to 5.0
3	Moderately resistant	5.1 to 10.0
5	Tolerant	10.1 to 25.0
7	Susceptible	25.1 to 50.0
9	Highly susceptible	Above 50 %

2.5.5 Control

The disease can be minimized by adopting certain general practices (Aponte and Aponte 1963). The important practices effective against the disease are as follows :

(i) Use healthy seed from healthy crop.
(ii) Destroy infected crop residues as soon as the harvesting of crop is completed.

(iii) Avoid damage/mechanical injury to plants during the agronomical operations specially interculture.
(iv) Rotate pigeonpea with other crops in areas with severe disease occurrence.

Efficacy of fungicides against the disease has been tested by Potdukhe *et al.* (1998). Out of six fungicides tested, carbendazim (0.1 and 0.05 %) was found best *in vitro* followed by Dithane M 45 (0.4 and 0.25 %) for inhibiting the growth of the pathogen. Seed treatment and two foliar application of Dithane M 45 and carbendazim at an interval of 15 days commencing from the first appearance of the disease was highly effective in significant reduction in disease incidence with increased yield and grain weight. Carbendazim was superior over Dithane M 45 in this respect.

2.6 Macrophomina Stem Canker

The first record of the pathogen of this disease seems to be from India (Sydow and Butler 1916) as *Macrophoma cajani* Syd. & Butler. It was reported to infect living stems of pigeonpea in India by Ashby (1927) who included it in the synonym of *Macrophomina phaseoli.* In Trinidad, Leach and Wright (1930) described a collar and stem canker disease of pigeonpea with which several fungi including *Macrophoma* sp. were found associated. He considered the pathogen as the stage of *Physalospora.* The disease was later reported from Jamaica (Leather 1967), Tanzania (Kannaiyan *et al.* 1981c), Nepal (Reddy *et al.* 1989c) and Malawi (Reddy *et al.* 1992d) where it is widespread. The land races of pigeonpea appeared to be tolerant to the disease but wilt resistant variety which performed well in Malawi was infected. The disease has also been reported from Australia, Myanmar, Sri Lanka, Vietnam and Zambia (Nene *et al.* 1996). In India, the disease occurs in the states of Bihar, Madhya Pradesh, Maharashtra, Orissa, Uttar Pradesh, Andhra Pradesh, Tamil Nadu, Gujarat and Rajasthan (Kannaiyan *et al.* 1981c). The disease has potential to cause heavy losses under favourable environmental conditions.

2.6.1 Symptoms

The symptoms of stem canker caused by *Macrophomina phaseolina* resemble with those caused by *Phoma cajani*. According to Reddy *et al.* (1989c), the symptoms may range from restricted spindle shaped lesions on the stem to extended lesions which may cause drying of whole of the plant. Agrawal and Gupta (1991) described the symptoms as greyish white elongated to elliptical lesions with dark brown margins showing small pin head size dark brown to black pycnidia. The small spots develop after 4-5 days of inoculation which later turn into characteristic lesions. The lesions sometimes coalesce, become sunken and black. The lesions may crack longitudinally after stoppage of rain resulting in exposure of internal woody portion of the stem. Some plants may break from the site of infection. In some cases, cracking of bark is followed by growth of callus forming knot.

2.6.2 Causal Organism

Macrophomina Phaseolina (Tassi) Goid.
Sclerotial stage : *Rhizoctonia bataticola* (Taub.) Britten Jones
Synonyms : *Macrophoma cajani* Syd. & Butler
Dothiorella cajani (Syd. & Butler) Petrak & Syd.
Macrophomina phaseoli (Maubl.) Ashby
Macrophoma phaseolina Tassi
Macrophoma cajanicola Pavgi & Singh

The fungus was recorded on pigeonpea by Sydow and Butler (1916) as *Macrophoma cajani* and simultaneously described as *D.cajani* (Petrak and Sydow 1925). These were later treated as synonyms to *M.phaseoli* by Ashby (1927) and finally the combination *M.phaseolina* was accepted. *Rhizoctonia bataticola* is the sclerotial stage of *M.phaseolina,* the pycnidial stage of the fungus.

The fungus associated with pigeonpea stem is described (Leach and Wright 1930) to have the *pycnidia* variable in size and structure with minute conidiophores on the whole of the inner surface, without papilla. The *conidia* are elongate, subellipsoidal to subrhomboid, obtuse, measuring 18.5 to 35 μ in length and average 24.5 × 7 μ, hyaline with non-vacuolated granular contents and mucilagenous envelop.

The *Macrophomina Phaseoli* isolate from pigeonpea stem produced culture with pycnidia on sterilized pigeonpea stems with *pycnospores* 16-27 by 5-11 μ (average 24 × 8 μ). On the maiz meal agar, pycnospores produced culture with pycnidia and sclerotia both (Haigh 1930). According to Agrawal and Gupta (1991), pigeonpea stem canker isolate had *pycnidia* globose, osteolate, thick walled, 105-197 μ in size. *Pycnidiospores* released in water were elliptical, single celled, hyaline, thin walled, 14.4 to 25.6 × 4.9 to 85 μ in size. On the PDA, typical culture of *R. bataticola* is produced.

The pathogen has a very wide host range, strain variability and environmental adoptability which make it an important plant pathogen.

2.6.3 Disease Cycle and Epidemiology

The pathogen has frequently been observed associated with seeds of pigeonpea and detected from seed coat, cotyledons and embryos (Bhaskara Reddy *et al.* 1992). The fungus also survives on the infected pigeonpea stems in the field for a long period in the form of mycelia and sclerotia. The population of sclerotia declines rapidly under high soil moisture and C : N ratio. The aerial strain of *R.bataticola* survives parasitically on a large number of hosts (Saksena 1980). The fungus is primarily pathogenic to young seedlings and immature tissues particularly those devitalized by abiotic stresses but in several cases the severity is found to increase in older plants causing root rots. The disease is favoured by a temperature around 30°C and high soil moisture.

2.6.4 Host Resistance

Screening of pigeonpea genotypes against Macrophomina stem canker indicated that resistance is available and can be utilized for developing suitable commercial varieties. The sources of resistance identified so far are compiled in Table 2.4.

Table 2.4 : Sources of resistance in pigeonpea against Macrophomina stem canker

Number of entries tested	*Entries resistant*	*Reference*
70	GP 125 D, ICP 8862, ICP 11289, ICP 8157	Anonymous (1982)
80	ICP Nos. 5701, 7855, 8798, 8863, 8864, 9120, 9126, 9134, 9142, 9144, 9147, 9156, 9159, 9168, 9174, 9175, 9177, 9213, 9758, 10269, 10958, 11290, 11299, GP 125D, K 70, MAUE 175, AWR 74/16, 79-7, P 76-56, 91-1, BDN 3, KSMR 8-3, C No. 74360	Anonymous (1983)
179	RGO 311, ICP 7035, PR 5106 and PR 5122	
254	MRG 66, ICP 29, 43, 102, 210, 268, 308 and ICPI 86005	Ramana *et al.* (1999)

For screening, a knife cut method has been developed at ICRISAT (Anonymous 1982) in which small amount of inoculum from PDA is taken and placed on the stem after split opening the bark with sharp blade or knife. The lesions develop 15 days after inoculation. Scoring is done on the basis of 9-point scale as follows :

> 1 = Resistant (No visible symptoms), 2-3 = Moderately resistant (1-5 cm long lesions), 4-5 = Tolerant (6-15 cm long lesions), 6-7 = Moderately susceptible (16-25 cm long lesions), 8-9 = Susceptible (above 25 cm long lesions and drying of branches).

2.6.5 Control

No specific control measure is recommended but selection of seed from disease-free crop, seed treatment with fungicide and sanitory practices after the crop harvest will minimize the disease.

2.7 Diplodia Stem Canker

The collar and stem canker of pigeonpea was first reported from Trinidad (Leach and Wright 1930) with which several fungi including *Diplodia* sp. were found associated. Later, the diseased plants were collected from Pusa, Bihar in India under natural condition showing death of some of the plants (Raychaudhury 1941, 1942). The disease may cause serious damage to pigeonpea crop (Purseglove 1968).

2.7.1 Symptoms

The fungus *Diplodia* sp. was reported to produce local cankers at the collar region of pigeonpea. The pathogen was thought to have induced carbonaceous appearance in the collar cankers caused by *Macrophoma*. The rapid enlargement of canker probably being due to the combined action of both the fungi (Leach and Wright 1930). However, Garcia (1960) observed the carbonaceous appearance of cankers in plants inoculated by *Phoma* sp. alone. The primary symptoms of the disease are thickening and distortion of the collar regions of the affected plants (Raychaudhury 1942). Elliptical lesions of various shapes and sizes with dark margins appear on thickened part of the stem. The affected parts are transformed into large deep seated cankers after 20-30 days, they spread and usually girdle the stem causing collapse of plants, although, partial recovery of plant may take place through callus formation. The cankerous part of the stem shows the twisted appearance due to unequal growth of the wood. The internal tissues of effected part show discolouration extending few cm above the lesion in advanced cases. The adventitious roots may be produced at the affected site. The mycelial growth may be observed in primary and secondary xylem vessels in the discoloured areas.

2.7.2 Causal Organism

Diplodia cajani Raychaudhury

The *Diplodia* sp. associated with pigeonpea had *spores* measuring 18.9-30.4 by 11.6-13 µ with average of 22.3 by 11.9 µ (Leach and Wright 1930). According to Raychaudhury (1942), *D.cajani* has the *mycelium* septate, hyaline but becoming olive-green to brown and finally black gradually; 2.6 to 8.6 µ in width (4.3 µ). The *pycnidia* are simple, globose, osteolate, immersed in the beginning but later emerging through the epidermis, glabrous and 301 to 464 µ (average 405 µ) in size. *Conidiophores* are short, needle shaped, pale to dark brown phialides on which 2 celled, ovoid to ellipsoid *conidia* are produced which measure 21.5-30.1 × 10.8-12.9 µ (average 25.1 × 12.7 µ). They are hyaline at first but turn dark brown later, attached to conidiophore from the side of narrower ends. The upper cell of the conidium germinate first by producing germ tube within 5 h while lower cell requires 15-20 h for this process. The fungus grows well on PDA at 20 - 35°C. Several strains of the fungus have been described from pigeonpea (Raychaudhury 1947).

2.7.3 Disease Cycle and Epidemiology

The pathogen is expected to survive on diseased stems of pigeonpea in soil. The plants injured during the field operations are prone to infection.

2.7.4 Control

The disease can be reduced by avoiding the injury to stems of plants during the cultural operations etc.

2.8 Crown Canker

A crown canker of pigeonpea was reported on pigeonpea variety Kaki from Puerto Rico (Kaiser *et al.* 1982). The incidence of the disease rarely exceeded 1 per cent and the disease has not been reported from any other country. The etiology of the disease and the host range of the pathogen responsible for the disease was studied by Kaiser *et al.* (1987).

2.8.1 Symptoms

The disease is characterized by the formation of reddish brown to dark brown cankers in the crown region of the plant or just below the soil surface level. The cankers may range in length from 0.5 to 10 mm and frequently girdle the stem causing the affected plants to wilt and/or lodge. The white mycelial strands of the fungus often extend above and below the cankers but no sclerotia or fruiting bodies are seen on affected part of the plant. On inoculation, more than one cankers often develop in the hypocotyl region. The symptoms of this disease resemble with those of collar rot/southern blight except that the sclerotia or any fruiting bodies are not formed on the affected part of the plant while mustard seed like sclerotia develop in case of collar rot. In general, collar rot merely affect the older plants while they are attacked by crown canker pathogen. However, fleshy bract like structures reminiscent of fruiting bodies were formed on inoculated hypocotyl beneath the soil surface. The fungus caused seed rot as well as post-emergence death.

2.8.2 Causal Organism

The causal fungus is a sterile white Basidiomycete which is morphologically similar to *S. rolfsii* but it did not form any sclerotia or fruiting bodies. However, it formed fleshy bract like structures reminiscent of fruiting bodies beneath the soil surface on hypocotyl of inoculated plants. These fleshy bodies were 3-9 mm broad × 10-20 mm wide × 2-5 mm thick with cream to tan colour. Hymenium was not seen on these structures and no basidia developed. The hyphal cells were binucleate with clamp connections.

2.8.3 Disease Cycle and Epidemiology

The fungus is soil borne and is able to remain viable even after 4 years at 23-25°C in the laboratory. In an inoculation test, the fungus was able to infect *Citrullus lanatus* var. *lanatus* 'Sugar baby', *Cucumis melo* 'Hales best', *Cucumis sativus* 'Ohio MR-17', *Cucurbita pepo* 'Early white bush', *Cajanus cajan* 'T 21', *Glycine max* 'Bragg', *Phaseolus vulgaris* 'Bountiful', *Vigna radiata* var. *radiata* 'Berkin', *Vigna unguiculata* subsp.

unguiculata 'California black eye', *Zea mays* 'Golden bantam' and *Lycopersicon lycopersicum* 'Rutgers' causing variable degree of mortality.

Pre-inoculation wounding of plant do not affect the number of diseased plants but it increased the length of the canker formed and the death of plants. The infection as well as mortality of plants due to this pathogen was favoured by a temperature of 30°C. No further work has been done on this disease.

2.9 Botryosphaeria Stem Canker

This is a minor disease first reported from Puerto Rico (Tucker 1927). He reported the fungus *Botryosphaeria xanthocephala* to be associated with the pigeonpea stem canker but did not demonstrate the pathogenicity of the fungus. The fungus has been found to cause the disease in pigeonpea in Fiji (Samuels and Singh 1986). They confirmed the genetic link between *B. xanthocephala* and *Macrophoma cajani* and thus proposed a new combination as *Fusicoccum cajani.* The fungus has been reported on twigs of pigeonpea in India (Butler and Bisby 1931) and also by the name *Physalospora xanthocephala* Syd. & Butler.

2.10 Phytophthora Stem Canker

Phytophthora stem canker of pigeonpea was first observed on Kaki variety in experimental crop and later in commercial crop in Puerto Rico (Kaiser and Melandez 1978). The disease is minor and not reported from any other country but it is capable of causing considerable losses under favourable weather conditions.

2.10.1 Symptoms

The disease is characterized by appearance of dark brown to black, necrotic and depressed lesions on the main stem, branches, twigs petioles etc. The lesions may be up to 6 cm long and may girdle the affected part which results in drying and death of the portion above the infection site. Sometimes the plant parts break at the infection site. The roots remain apparently healthy. The symptoms resemble with those of Phytophthora blight.

2.10.2 Causal Organism

Phytophthora parasitica Dastur

The fungus is treated as the synonym of *Phytophthora nicotianae* Breda de Hann. var. *parasitica* (Dastur) Waterhouse. It was isolated from pigeonpea, eggplant and tomatoes. All the isolates had papillate sporangia and formed chlamydospores on V 8 juice agar, typical of *P.parasitica.* Isolates from eggplant and tomatoes did not form oospores and grew best at 30°C. All the three isolates were pathogenic to pigeonpea although, those from pigeonpea were more virulent than others.

2.10.3 Disease Cycle and Epidemiology

The disease is favoured by wounds and a temperature of 25-30°C. The leaf scars are the favourable sites of infection in the field. The spread of the pathogen seems to be aided by rainfall as the inoculum is dispersed through water splash into the upper canopy of plants and its amount is affected by rains. The pathogen could be obtained from the rotting fruit of brinjal and tomatoes which were grown in rotation with pigeonpea. No work related to survival of the pathogen and the disease cycle has been reported.

2.10.4 Control

No control measures are recommended. No lesions of the disease were observed on some genotypes of the pigeonpea, namely 394-014, 396-356, 396-731, 396-295, 6AB-2 and 731 BD during the screening test (Rodriguez and Melandez 1985).

2.11 Stem Canker and Die Back

A stem canker and die-back disease of pigeonpea caused by *Colletotrichum capsici* was reported from Maharashtra, India (Somani *et al.* 1975) in September on variety Kaki and some other local varieties in the area. As early as 1923, similar disease of pigeonpea was reported from Kenya (McDonald 1924), the cause of which was mentioned to be *Vermicularia capsicae* which is considered as the synonym of *Collectotrichum capsici.*

2.11.1 Symptoms

Somani *et al.* (1975) described three types of symptoms of the disease as follows :

(i) *Stem canker* : Large number of brownish grey, oblong, slightly sunken and cankerous spots are formed on the main stem about

10 cm above the ground level. The cankers coalesce at advanced stage girdling the stem and exhibiting the grey colour in centre with dark brown margins (Fig 2.8). Minute black acervuli develop on these sunken centres. The affected part turns brittle and the plant breaks at the point of girdle. In some cases, amber coloured gum like exudation is also noticed. Branches of the plant may also be infected.

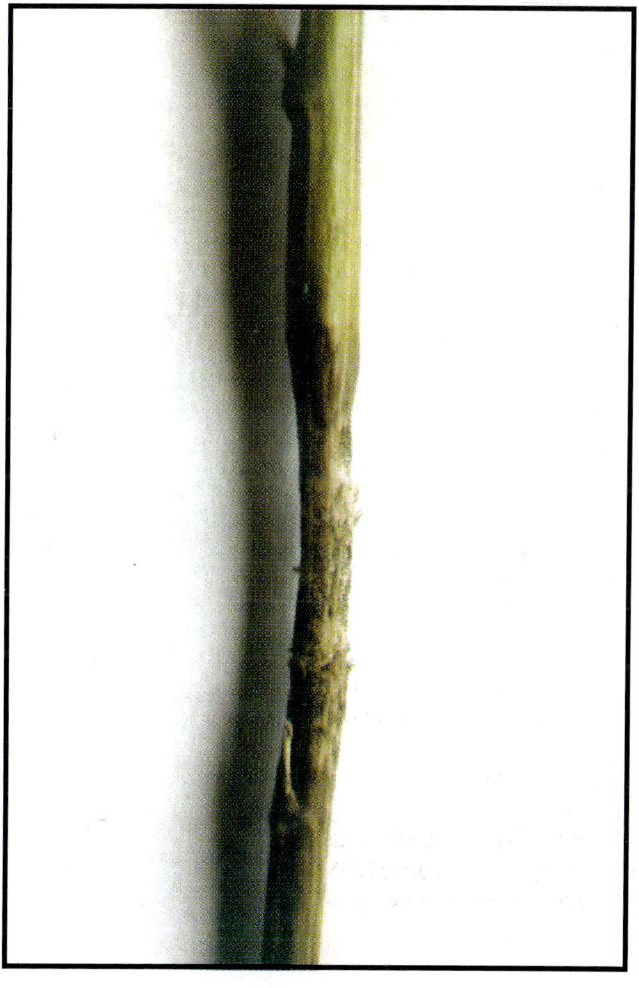

Fig. 2.8: Stem infection of pigeonpea by *Colletotrichum capsici*: Girdling of stem showing acervuli.

(ii) *Die-Back* : Drying and death of the branches from tip downwards is observed. The leaves shed and affected branches show distinct demarkation between healthy and diseased parts. Several minute, black acervuli with pinkish white, powdery mass of conidia are visible on dead twigs.

(iii) *Corky Splitting of the Stem* : The bark of the stem splits longitudinally and the splits are corky and localized. The splitted portion swells slightly at the centre and inner tissues are exposed. The symptoms of a bark disease similar to stem canker and die-back were described from Kenya as short longitudinal splits and stem pitting leading to die-back and coalesce of pigeonpea but cause of the disease was not identified (Nattrass 1958).

2.11.2 Causal Organism

Colletotrichum capsici (Syd.) Butler & Bisby

The fungus has very wide host range. The pigeonpea isolate of the fungus has been described by Somani *et al.* (1975) as *acervuli* setose, round, measuring up to 350 μ in diameter. The *setae* are brown in colour, dark at base and paler at tips with 1-5 septa and 264 × 5 m in size. *Conidia* sickel shaped to falcate, one-celled, hyaline, thin-walled and slender measuring 15-28 by 4-5 m in size.

This description does not agree with *colletotrichum cajani,* a conidial stage of *Glomerella cingulata* but agrees with *C.capsici*.

The fungus infects chillies producing typical die-back symptoms. Isolations from all the three types of symptoms on pigeonpea yielded *Colletotrichum* only.

2.11.3 Disease Cycle and Epidemiology

The pathogen is believed to survive on seed or diseased plant debris. The symptoms of the disease are produced within a week by inoculation of one and half month old plants with spray of spore suspension (Somani *et al.* 1975). No detailed work on epidemiology of the disease has so far been done.

2.11.4 Host Resistance

Godbole *et al.* (1977) developed a suitable technique for scoring the infection grades on pigeonpea and reported BDN 1, BDN 2 and C 11 to show moderate reaction while Prabhat and Kaki were highly susceptible to this disease.

2.11.5 Control

In the *in vitro* tests, Cuman, Benlate, Ziride and Captan were found highly effective for inhibiting the mycelial growth and spore germination of *C.capsici* from pigeonpea (Joshi and Wangikar 1977). Calixin was more effective against spore germination while Dithane Z 78, Macuprax, Bavistin and Dithane M 45 were more inhibitory to growth when used at lower concentrations.

Out of nine fungicides tested, Cuman, Calixin, Benlate, Ziride and Captan inhibited the spore germination completely at 10 ppm while others were effective at 200 ppm (Joshi and Wangikar 1978).

2.12 Stem Anthracnose

This is not a widespread disease and is reported from India only (Khan and Singh 1974). The disease was observed in the last week of September on some of the early maturing and medium duration varieties of pigeonpea and not on the late maturing ones.

2.12.1 Symptoms

The disease manifests in patches and the infection is confined to main axis and lateral branches of the plant (Khan and Singh 1974). The characteristic symptoms of the disease are blackening and drying of the cortical region of the stem and branches in the form of lesions which are distinctly marked from the healthy portion. The lesions on the stem spread from the lower portion and may extend up to upper most branches. On branches, the lesions are noticed at the point of their origin but later they traverse towards their tips. Outer surface of the stele is blackened which traverse towards the pith. Fungal growth or its fruiting bodies are not observed inside the cortical layer or on the outer surface of the stele but numerous acervuli may be seen on outer surface of the affected portion of stem and branches. In cases of severe infection, young branches and leaves show drying and drooping ultimately resulting in complete drying and defoliation.

2.12.2 Causal Organism

Colletotrichum truncatum (Schw.) Andrus and Moore

Colonies of *C. truncatum* on PDA growing at 25°C are dark brown to black with a felt of greyish mycelium through which tufted to irregular, often confluent black sclerotia are produced occasionally with scattered tufts of pale-grey to white mucelium. Conidial masses are honey coloured, sclerotia and setae abundant.

Khan and Singh (1974) described the pigeonpea isolate of *C.truncatum* as : *Acervuli* numerous, linear oval, black, scattered to gregarious, erumpent; *Setae* numerous, divergent, dark brown, filiform, variable in length, long and short intermixed, 95-360 × 3.6-9 μ in size; *Conidia* single celled, falcate to lanceolate, hyaline, 19-29.5 × 3.5-5.4 μ in size.

The fungus *C.truncatum* is not much different from *C.capsici* except that the former is restricted to Leguminosae while later has wide host range (Sutton 1980). Both these fungi differ from *C.dematium* on the basis of broader conidia of former (3.5-4μ) than later (2-2.5μ). Thus *C.capsici* as well as *C.truncatum* have been considered as synonyms of *C.dematium* (Kulshrestha *et al.* 1976). Singh and Shrivastava (1985) reported *C. dematium* to infect pigeonpea and suggested some characters for identification of *Colletotrichum* spp. infecting pulse crops. They suggested shape and size of conidia, presence and position of chlamydospores; shape, size and colour of appressoria and presence or absence of sclerotia to be the consistant characters.

2.12.3 Disease Cycle and Epidemiology

No work on this aspect has been done. The fungus is reported to be seed transmitted in several legumes. It may survive on infected stems/branches of pigeonpea in the field. The disease appears in patches and spreads under moist weather conditions. The spread of disease and its development is declined after the rains. Early and medium maturing varieties are affected more severely showing infection of stems and branches while in case of late maturing variety only main axis is affected.

2.12.4 Host Resistance

Hasan and Khan (1979b) screened 49 cultivars against *C.truncatum* and reported NPWR 15, Pant A9, Prabhat and 1234 to be immune while some were resistant.

2.12.5 Control

In the *in vitro* tests, the growth and sporulation of the pathogen were inhibited by Brassicol, Thiram, Coprantol, Dithane Z 78, Dithane M 45,

Agrosan GN, Captan and DDT. The Coprantol was best which did not allow growth even at 0.1% concentration (Hasan *et al.* 1975). The growth of the pathogen and spore germination was inhibited effectively by copper oxychloride, carboxin, benomyl, captan, mancozeb and thiram. All of these 6 fungicides had marked fungistatic effect on germ tubes and the colony characters.

In field, the above mentioned fungicides gave better control when used as prophylactic spray as compared to post-inoculation sprays (Hasan and Khan 1979a).

2.13 Collar Rot/Southern Blight

The first report of this disease seems to be from Puerto Rico by Cook (1939) who observed a serious stem disease of pigeonpea to be caused by *Sclerotium* sp. Later, a seedling blight was recorded in India and the causal fungus was identified as *Corticium rolfsii* (Malik 1945) and *Sclerotium rolfsii* (Patel *et al.* 1949). The disease has also been reported from Nicaraguan (Litzenberger and Stevenson 1957). However, the disease was studied in detail first in Trinidad under the name Southern blight (Phelps *et al.* 1974). The disease has so far been found occurring in Australia, India, Pakistan, Puerto Rico, Sri Lanka, Trinidad & Tobago, U.S.A., Venezuela and Zambia (Nene *et al.* 1996).

This disease has been mentioned to be of potential importance to the Caribbean region (Spence 1975). It may cause heavy losses under favourable weather conditions. Singh *et al.* (1987) observed 5-40% seedlings affected by this disease in Nagaland state of India while in some fields the incidence was as high as 70 per cent. Fortunately the disease is not serious in India but it cannot be considered as minor one in areas with climatic conditions like those of Nagaland. Introduction of new technology of the pigeonpea cultivation in post-rainy season created some new disease problems which otherwise were of minor importance.

2.13.1 Symptoms

The symptoms of the disease have been described in detail (Phelps *et al.* 1974, Ariyanayagam 1975). The young seedlings of 27-45 days age when attacked, show drooping of leaves which is more evident in lower leaves of older plants. The symptoms start as small, water soaked, grey lesion at the base of the stem close to the soil surface which later turns brown and girdles the stem causing rotting and wilting of seedling. The necrosis of the stem bark is evident (Singh *et al.* 1987). On the affected part, white feather like growth of the fungus is visible (Fig 2.9). Sometimes the mycelial growth may extend up on to the stem and spread on to the soil especially under wet weather conditions. Small round sclerotia of the fungus may be found associated with the mycelial growth which are white at first but gradually become brown like a seed of mustard and are the characteristic sign of the disease from the diagnosis point of view.

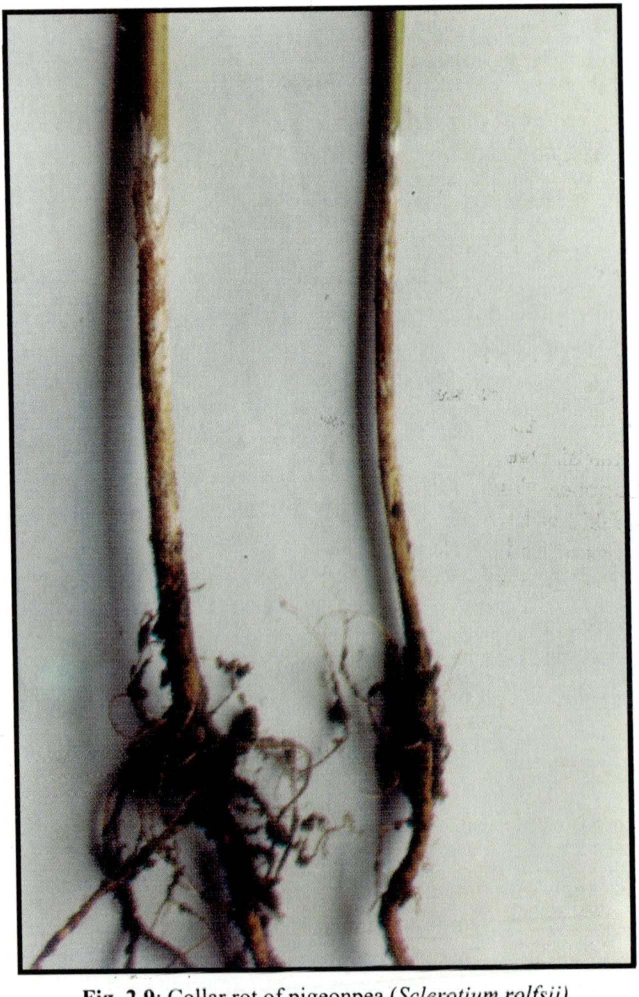

Fig. 2.9: Collar rot of pigeonpea (*Sclerotium rolfsii)*.

The leaves become yellow before collapse and root system is shredded (Iqbal *et al.* 1990). The affected plants can be uprooted easily but the lower part of their roots usually remain in soil. The patches of dead seedlings at the primary leaf stage can be seen over the field.

2.13.2 Causal Organism

Sclerotium rolfsii Sacc.
Teleomorph : *Athelia rolfsii* (Curzi) Tu & Kimbrough
(= *Corticium rolfsii* Curzi)

The fungus produces fan shaped, profuse, mycelial growth on PDA. The mycelium is hyaline, branched, septate, slender possessing clamp connections with a tendency to grow on the glass surface and to aggregate in to rhizomorph cords. The clamp connections may be absent in slender portion of the hyphae. The sclerotia are white in the beginning but later becoming brown, spherical and resembling seeds of mustard. They are easily detached from the mycelium and measure 0.5 to 0.8 mm in size.

The fungus has very wide host range belonging to different families. The perfect state of the fungus has not been observed commonly.

2.13.3 Disease Cycle and Epidemiology

The pathogen is mainly soil-borne in nature. The fungus actively colonizes the pieces of dead bamboo grass (*Paspalum fasciculatum*) from which it is able to attack the host plant (Phelps *et al.* 1974). The infection does not take place when the grass pieces are more than 2 cm away from the living host. The fungus grows only little in the soil without organic matter. The plants are more prone to attack of disease up to 27 days after germination. The plants show resistance between 27 and 45 days and become more or less immune after the age of 45 days. The disease is favoured by dense seeding and presence of undercomposed organic matter in the field (Anonymous 1982). High soil moisture and a temperature of about 30°C at sowing time pre-disposes seedlings to infection. In India, the disease is more of a problem in early sown (June) than in a later sown crop (Reddy *et al.* 1993c).

2.13.4 Host Resistance

All the determinate type of pigeonpea varieties have been found susceptible but some resistance appears to be in semi-determinate types

(Phelps *et al.* 1974). Tolerance against the collar rot has been reported in pigeonpea genotypes 10/246, 4/95, 5/119 (Ariyanayagam 1975), Azamgarh local, UPAS 120, Pant A2 and ICP 7239 (Gurha *et al.* 1983). In India, medium maturing entry ICPH 5 exhibited less than 10 % disease (Anonymous 1982, Kannaiyan *et al.* 1983a) although, it is considered that host resistance against *S.rolfsii* is very rare.

2.13.5 Control

Chemical : Captan as oil drench and thiram or Brassicol as seed dresser or soil drench are reported to control the disease to some extent (Anil Kumar *et al.* 1976). Other fungicides as effective seed dressers for the control of collar rot of pigeonpea are captafol and mancozeb (Zote *et al.* 1982); Bavistin and Benlate (Saraswathi and Pal 1986) while for soil drenching formaldehyde, Captan and PCNB were highly effective. Reddy *et al.* (1993c) recommended seed dressing with tolclophos methyl (Rhizolex), Captan or thiram @ 3 g/kg seed for control of collar rot of pigeonpea.

Cultural : Control of *S.rolfsii* field is often difficult, however, general sanitation and tillage methods that burry crop residues and weeds under the soil are effective. The cereal stubbles like that of *Sorghum* should not be left in the field. They should be collected and destroyed before sowing of pigeonpea (Reddy *et al.* 1993c).

Biological : *Trichoderma* as well as some species of bacteria have been found effective in checking the pathogen *S.rolfsii. Trichoderma harzianum* and *T.viride* are able to check the pathogen *in vitro* as well as *in vivo. T. harzianum* is reported to reduce the collar rot as well as seed rot of pigeonpea (Saraswathi and Pal 1986). The bacterial species *Pseudomonas aeruginosa* and *Bacillus subtilis* are able to inhibit the sclerotial germination, growth and the sclerotial production of *S. rolfsii* in soil (Brathwaite 1978). Inoculation of the fungus infested soil with both the bacteria prior to planting the pigeonpea increases the seedling emergence and reduces the disease. The inhibition by *P. aeruginosa* is reported to be due to production of an antibiotic pyocyanine.

2.14 Stem Rot/Sclerotinia Rot

Pigeonpea was recorded as new host of *Sclerotinia sclerotiorum* (Lib) de Bary by Waterson (1944) who reported infection of pods in Bermuda. The disease has also been reported from Australia, Malaysia and Zambia

(Nene *et al.* 1996). It is a minor disease and occurs in comparatively cooler areas. It is found to be the commonest disease at the experimental site in Australia (Akinola and Whiteman 1972).

The pigeonpea lines with yellow petals having light red veins and non-hard brown seeds were mostly susceptible to *Sclerotinia sclerotiorum*. On the other hand, all the accessions with completely red standard petals on the dorsal surface were unaffected. This correlation should be confirmed before selections and breeding for resistance to this disease is done (Akinola and Whiteman 1972).

No control measures are recommended. Burning of the infected crop residues, avoiding thick sowing and seed treatment with Captan or thiram @ 3 g/kg of seed helps in reducing the disease.

2.15 Dry Root Rot

The dry root rot of pigeonpea is reported to occur in India, Jamaica, Trinidad and Tobago, Australia, Malawi, Myanmar, Nepal, Sri Lanka, U.S.A. and Vietnam (Nene *et al.* 1996). The pathogen causing dry root rot is responsible for stem canker disease also which is described separately. The infection of living stem of pigeonpea by the root rot pathogen was first reported by Butler (1920) and the same could be isolated from the diseased roots of pigeonpea in Uttar Pradesh (Edward 1954). The disease has been described by the name wilt at Pantnagar, India (Rathi and Lal 1977). The disease is not serious for the normal rainy season crop of pigeonpea but it occurs severely in off-season irrigated crop in some parts of India (Reddy *et al.* 1990d). The production and productivity of pigeonpea can be increased in central and south India by taking an extra crop between November and April but it is seriously hit by this disease.

2.15.1 Symptoms

The seedling blight symptoms have been described by Ahmad (1974) which include discolouration and rotting of root and basal stem. The bark of the affected part rots and may exhibit splitting ultimately exposure of wood at many places at advanced stages of the disease. Large number of minute, black coloured sclerotia can be seen under the bark which look like the particles of charcoal. The affected roots of the aged plant become dry and brittle and the plant is killed prematurely specially when it faces the drought conditions. Seedlings are infected at early stages and collapse by rotting. The symptoms described by Rathi and Lal (1977) include wilting of the foliage followed by defoliation and death of infected plants. A number of discoloured areas having shades of brown to dark brown develop on main stem and branches. At later stage, numerous small brown to black sclerotia are observed on roots. Number and the size of pods on affected plants are reduced.

2.15.2 Causal Organism

Rhizoctonia bataticola (Taub.) Butler
Pycnidial stage : *Macrophomina phaseolina* (Maubl.) Ashby

R.bataticola, the sclerotial stage of the fungus has been found associated with the dry root rot or seedling blight symptoms. An isolate of the fungus from potato was able to infect the pigeonpea (Bhargava 1965). According to Rathi and Lal (1977), the pigeonpea isolate produced mouse coloured colonies with fluffy, abundant, light brown aerial hyphae without circular zonations. Numerous, black sclerotia are present. Mycelium hyaline, brown with age, septate, distance between two septa 13-15 μ; branches of the mycelium arising usually at right angles with a septum at some distance from point of origin, 3.5-5.8 μ wide. *Sclerotia* quite abundant, submerged, black, spherical to irregular, aggregated in groups or formed singly, texture loose, composed of pseudoparenchymatous cells, 65-100 μ in diameter; sporodochia and pycnidia not observed; *Chlamydospores* are observed in old culture. They are thick walled, smooth, round to irregular, dark brown, submerged, formed in chain of 3-6, occasionally singly, intercallary, 10-14.2 μ in size. The fungus is considered non-specific, although, the aggressiveness differs from isolate to isolate (Singh and Nene 1990). Some strains are reported to produce pycnidial stage, *M.phaseolina* while others may not.

2.15.3 Disease Cycle and Epidemiology

The fungus *M. Phaseolina (R. bataticola)* is basically soil borne but it has been found associated with seed coat, cotyledons and embryo of pigeonpea seed (Kannaiyan *et al.* 1980a, Bhaskara Reddy *et al.* 1992). It survives on infected plant debris in its sclerotial form in the soil. It is able to infect large number of weeds and other crop plants also.

The disease incidence has been found more on ratooned crop than on main crop; on extra short duration varieties than the medium and long duration ones; at pod filling stage of the crop than any other stage; in Vertisol than in Alfisol and in off-season irrigated crop in summer than rainy season crop. The disease is favoured at 30°C. The young seedlings or immatured tissues specially devitalized by adverse weather conditions are more prone to the attack of dry root rot pathogen.

2.15.4 Host Resistance

Out of 31 genotypes of pigeonpea evaluated, 12 were found tolerant to dry root rot (Kannaiyan and Haciwa 1990). In general, extra short duration genotypes are more susceptible than medium or long duration ones (Reddy *et al.* 1993b). They identified ICPL 86005, ICPL 86020, ICPL 87105, ICPH 149, ICPL 91028, ICPX 860200 and ICPX 870023 as resistant with less than 10 % disease incidence. The variety S 18 has been found to be resistant to dry root rot (Vidhyasekaran and Arjunan 1976).

2.15.5 Control

The seed treatment with Campogran M @ 1.5 g or Allisan 2.5 g or Busan 72 @ 0.3 g/kg seed is reported to protect the pigeonpea crop from *M.Phaseolina* effectively (Chaudhury and Ahmed 1977). Similarly mancozeb, captafol and carbendazim have also been found as good seed dressers for increasing the germination of pigeonpea (Bhaskara Reddy *et al.* 1992). The seedling infection by *M.Phaseolina* may be reduced greatly by seed treatment with benomy1, thiram, Benlate T and tolclofos methy1 (Rhizolex) as reported by Kannaiyan *et al.* (1980a).

2.16 Wet Root Rot

The wet root rot of pigeonpea was first reported as wilt caused by *Rhizoctonia* (*Corticium*) *solani* from Pusa, Bihar, India. The fungus was able to kill about 80% plants under inoculated (Mitra 1931) conditions. Simultaneously disease was reported from Sierra Leone where the fungus formed large sclerotia on pigeonpea (Deighton 1932). The disease occurs in Africa (Kaiser 1976) and Uganda also (Mukiibi 1976). It has been reported as wet root rot from Zambia (Kannaiyan and Haciwa 1990). The disease is minor one and not much work has been done on it.

2.17 Neocosmospora Root Rot

This disease has so far been reported from India only (Butler 1910). The pathogen infects the roots of pigeonpea and kills the plant , although, the disease is minor one (Mitra 1934). The disease has been studied under the name *Neocosmospora vasinfecta* disease at Madras, India (Sarojini 1954).

2.17.1 Symptoms

The symptoms are similar to those caused by *Fusarium udum*. The fungus infects seedlings at first leaf stage causing preliminary curling of leaf tips while older seedlings exhibit gradual yellowing of leaflets. The affected plants later wilt and collapse. The diseased portion of the hypocoty1 and root may show presence of numerous small perithecia of black colour.

2.17.2 Causal Organism

Neocosmospora vasinfecta Smith

The pathogen is the ascomycetous fungus. Sarojini (1954) obtained the conidial as well as chlamydospore isolates of the pathogen which were more virulent than its original isolate, its ascospore derivatives or *Fusarium udum*. The *perithecia* are gregarious, often closely crowded, bright red, smooth with prominent ostiole, flask shaped, 200-225 × 250-275 μ, *Asci* are nearly cylindrical, eight-spored and 85-90 × 12-15 μ in size. *Ascospores* uniceriate, globose, or sub-globose, at first hyaline but becoming brown with outer surface rough and wrinkled and 10 μ in diameter. *Paraphyses* are inconspicuous, simple and septate.

2.17.3 Control

The pathogen is mainly soil inhabiting facultative saprophyte and the disease is minor so no control measures are recommended.

2.18 Phytophthora Root Rot

It is the serious root rot of pigeonpea reported from Australia where it occurred in experimental fields after heavy rains or irrigation resulting in local water logging (Wearing and Birch 1988).

The affected plants exhibit wilting associated with chlorosis, loss of leaves and rotting of the tap as well as lateral roots. Dark brown lesions are observed extending from base up the stem. The affected plants are generally killed. It differs from the Phytophthora stem canker and Phytophthora blight diseases as roots do not rot in both of these cases as observed in case of root rot. On inoculation, the 5-day old seedlings of pigeonpea exhibited wilting, stem collapse and root rot within 3-5 days.

The disease is caused by *Phytophthora drechsleri* Tucker which was isolated from affected parts of the plant and the pathogenicity was tested. The disease is reported from U.S.A. also. No control measures are recommended.

2.19 Phellinus Root Rot

This is a minor disease reported from Papua New Guinea (Dennis 1994) on 18 months old pigeonpea growing in the area previously planted with Cocoa. The disease is reported to occur in Nigeria also (Bailey 1966).

The symptoms of the disease include reduced vigour of plants quickly followed by yellowing and wilting of leaves. The affected plants die within 3-4 weeks. The stem at ground level exhibit a brown-black fungal crust with coverage of root surface and a soil encrusted fungal sleeve. The disease has been observed in Cocoa and the symptoms on both resemble with each other.

The pathogen infects the tree stumps of Cocoa and then spreads by root to root contact. Hence, it is suggested to disinfect or remove the stumps before planting in infected area and also remove the infected roots for reducing the disease.

2.20 Rosellinia Root Rot

The roots of pigeonpea were found infected by *Rosellinia* sp. causing death of plants in West Indies (Nowell 1923). In the Antilles region of Caribbean, the root rot of pigeonpea was found to be caused by *Rosellinia bunodes* (Cook 1939).

2.21 Armillaria Root Rot

This disease has been reported from Nyasaland where it was found to kill the pigeonpea plants in a tea plantation infested by *Armillaria mellea* (Leach 1934). The disease has also been reported to occur in Africa (Kaiser 1976).

2.22 Collar Disease

A collar rot disease of pigeonpea has been reported from the island of Carriacon in the Granadines (Anonymous 1917). The infected plants were distributed unevenly in the field. The diseased plants showed lesion at the collar region and killed during the course of time. These lesions exhibited presence of pycnidia and perithecia in the bark of the affected area. It yielded the ascomycetous fungus consistantly. The *pycnospores* as well as *ascospores* were unicellular and hyaline. The identity of the fungus and its pathogenicity to pigeonpea was not confirmed. A similar disease has been reported from West Indies also (Nowell 1923). The fungus was not able to infect the plants when inoculated during the dry season.

2.23 Other Fungi Infecting Roots/Stems

The fungus *Corticium salmonicolor* was found associated with pigeonpea plants in Corledonia (Bugnicourt 1956). Similarly an unidentified fungal pathogen causing brown root rot of tobacco has been found pathogenic to pigeonpea (Johnson 1939).

Several other fungi have been found associated with the stem canker of pigeonpea. Leach and Wright (1930) observed numerous acervuli of *Myxosporium* sp. on dead twigs of pigeonpea. It has been reported that many fungi alone or in combination produce similar symptoms of stem canker in pigeonpea and also, the disease development and its severity is increased in cases of combined infections (Brathwaite 1981).

Stevenson (1917 and 1918) isolated several fungi from the dead wood and bark of pigeonpea plants in Puerto Rico some of which may be responsible for death and rotting of stems of mature plants. The isolated fungi were *Megalonectria pseudotrichia* (Schw.) Speg., *Creonectria grammicospora* (Ferd & Wing) Seaver (=*Nectria grammicospora* Ferd & Wing) and *Pleonectria megalospora* Speg (= *Thyronectria megalospora* (Speg.) Seavera & Chardon). However, he did not test the pathogenicity of these fungi. Other fungi isolated are *Dendrochium gigasporium* from drying pigeonpea stems in Uganda (Hansford 1943); *Alleschirina cajani* Syd. & Butler from bark of branches in India (Sydow and Butler 1911); *Nectria bolbophylli* P. Henn on stems in India (Butler and Bisby 1931).

The stem canker of pigeonpea has been reported to be caused by a complex of fungal pathogens and an unidentified bacterium (Kannaiyan and Haciwa 1990). The fungi involved are *Phoma sorghina* (Sacc.) Boerema *et al., Phomopsis cajani* Sydow & Sydow, *Cercospora canescens* Ellis & Martin, and *Colletotrichum crassipes* (Speg.) Arx. which is responsible to cause Colletotrichum stem canker disease of pigeonpea in Zambia (Nene *et al.* 1996). Infection of the stem of pigeonpea has also been reported by *Colletotrichum* sp. in Barbados (Dash 1917), *C. graminicola* in India (Nene *et al.* 1996). In Uganda, Hansford (1938) isolated various species of *Fusarium* belonging to *Hypomyces ipomoeae, Lisia* and *Gibberella* from pigeonpea plants showing die-back symptoms. This disease was different from wilt. The *Gibberella* spp. were found to be the primary parasite on pigeonpea.

REFERENCES

Aa, H.A. Vander 1973. Studies in Mycology. C.B.S., Netherlands (Baarn) 5 : 1-110.

Acland, J.D. 1971. East African crops. London, UK : Longman. pp 140-141.

Agnihothrudu, V. 1954. Soil conditions and wilt diseases in plants. Rhizosphere microflora in relation to fungal wilts. Ph.D. thesis. Madras University (cf. Sadasivan, T.S. and Subramanian, C.V. 1954. Recent advances in the study of soil-borne *Fusaria. Journal of the Indian Botanical Society* 33 : 162-176)

Agnihothrudu, V. 1955. Incidence of the fungistatic organisms in the rhizosphere of pigeonpea (*Cajanus cajan*) in relation to resistance and susceptibility to wilt caused by *Fusarium udum* Butler. *Naturwissenschaften* 42 : 1-2.

Agrawal, S.C. 1985. Studies on stem blight of pigeonpea caused by *Phytophthora drechsleri* Tucker f sp. *cajani (Mahendra Pal* et al.) Kannaiyan *et al.* Ph.D. thesis, JNKVV, Jabalpur, pp. 159.

Agrawal, S.C. 1987a. Fungicidal control of stem blight of pigeonpea caused by *Phytophthora drechsleri* f sp. *cajani. Indian Journal of Plant Protection* 15 : 35-37.

Agrawal, S.C. 1987b. Epidemiology of Phytophthora stem blight of pigeonpea. Pages 42-45 *in* Diseases of oilseed and pulse crops and their control: proceedings of symposium, 29-31 Jan. 1987, JNAU, Indore, India (S.C.Vyas and V.N. Shroff eds.).

Agrawal, S.C. 1989a. Effect of land slop on the severity of stem blight of pigeonpea caused by *Phytophthora drechsleri* f sp. *cajani. Indian Journal of Pulses Research* 2 : 179-180.

Agrawal, S.C. 1989b. Effect of stem inoculation of Phytophthora stem blight on phenol contents in pigeonpea. *Indian Journal of Pulses Research* 2 : 39-41.

Agrawal, S.C. 1990. Effect of Phytophthora stem blight on amino acids and protein contents of pigeonpea plants. *Indian Journal of Pulses Research* 3 : 171-174.

Agrawal, S.C. 1991. Effect of stem inoculation of pigeonpea plants by *Phytophthora drechsleri* f sp. *cajani* on their sugar content. *Indian Journal of Pulses Research* 4 : 225-226.

Agrawal, S.C., and Gupta, R.K. 1991, Stem canker of pigeonpea (*Cajanus cajan*) caused by *Macrophomina phaseolina. Indian Journal of Pulses Research* 4 : 124-125.

Agrawal, S.C., Gupta, R.K. and Prasad, K.V.V. 1991. Resistance in pigeonpea against Fusarium wilt. *Indian Journal of Pulses Research* 4 : 120-121.

Agrawal, S.C. and Khare, M.N. 1986. Variability in the sensitivity of some isolates of *Fusarium oxysporum* and *Sclerotium rolfsii* to some guazatine formulations. *Pestology* 10 (1) : 35-36.

Agrawal, S.C. and Khare, M.N. 1987a. Comparative epidemic growth of stem blight on four genotypes of pigeonpea. *Indian Journal of Mycology and Plant Pathology* 17 : 79-80.

Agrawal, S.C. and Khare, M.N. 1987b. Development of stem blight of pigeonpea in relation to environmental factor. *Indian Journal of Mycology and Plant Pathology* 17 : 305-309.

Agrawal, S.C. and Khare, M.N. 1988a. Survival of *Phytophthora drechsleri* f sp. *cajani* causing stem blight of pigeonpea. *Indian Phytopathology* 41 : 250-251.

Agrawal, S.C. and Khare, M.N. 1988b. Survey of stem blight *(Phytophthora drechsleri* f sp. *cajani*) of pigeonpea (*Cajanus cajan*) in Madhya Pradesh. *Agriculture Science Digest* 8 : 219-21.

Agrawal, S.C. and Nema, S. 1985. Occurrence of Phoma stem canker in pigeonpea in Madhya Pradesh, India. *International Pigeonpea Newsletter* 4 : 37-38.

Agrawal, S.C. and Nema, Sushma 1988, Survival of stem canker (*Phoma cajani*) in pigeonpea stubbles in the field. *Indian Journal of Pulses Research* 1 : 147-148.

Ahmed, T. 1974. Rhizoctonia seedling blight of pigeonpea and its control. M.Sc. thesis. Bidhan Chandra Krishi Vishwa Vidyalaya, Kalyani, West Bengal, India.

Akinola, J.O. and Whiteman, P.C. 1972. A numerical classification of *Cajanus cajan* (L.) Millsp. accessions based on morphological and agronomic attributes. *Australian Journal of Agricultural Research* 23 : 995-1005.

Amin, K.S., Baldev, B. and Williams, F.J. 1976. Differentiation of Phytophthora stem blight from Fusarium wilt of pigeonpea by field symptoms. *FAO Plant Protection Bulletin* 24 : 123-124.

Amin, K.S., Baldev, B. and Williams, F.J. 1978. *Phytophthora cajani* a new species causing stem blight of *Cajanus cajan. Mycologia* 70 : 171-176.

Amin, K.S., Reddy, M.V., Raju, T.N., Nene, Y.L., Singh, R.A., Pal, M., Rathi, Y.P.S., Agrawal, S.C. and Chauhan, V.B. 1993a. Multilocational evaluation of pigeonpea for resistance to Phytophthora blight. *Indian Journal of Plant Protection* 21(1): 26-27.

Amin, K.S., Reddy, M.V., Raju, T.N, Nene, Y.L., Singh, R.A., Zote, K.K., Bendre, N.J., Jha, D.K., Bidari, V.B., Naphade, S.D., Arjunan, G., Agrawal, S.C., Sinha, B.K., Mahendrapal, Grewal, J.S. and Anilkumar, T.B. 1993b. Multilocational evaluation of pigeonpea for broad-based resistance to Fusarium wilt in India. *Indian Journal of Plant Protection* 21 (1) : 28-30.

Anil Kumar, T.B., Hiremath, P.C. and Sulladmath, V.V. 1976. Fungicidal control of foot rot of pigeonpea. *Current Research* 5 : 98-99.

Anonymous. 1917. A collar disease of pigeonpea. *Agriculture News* (Barbados) 16 : 78.

Anonymous. 1931a. Review of Agricultural Operations in India, 1928-29. Pusa : Imperial Council of Agricultural Research, 251 pp.

Anonymous. 1931b. Work on *Cajanus cajan* at Pusa. Scientific Reports of the Imperial Institute of Agricultural Research, Pusa, 1929-30.

Anonymous. 1941. Agriculture and Animal Husbandry in India, 1938-39. Delhi : Imperial Council of Agricultural Research. 422 pp.

Anonymous. 1946. Scientific Reports of the Indian Agricultural Research Institute, 1945-46. 109 pp.

Anonymous. 1947a. Report on the Administration of the Department of Agriculture, United Provinces (India), 1944-45. 86 pp.

Anonymous. 1947b. Scientific Reports of the Indian Agricultural Research Institute, 1946-47. 131 pp.

Anonymous. 1948. Scientific Reports of the Indian Agricultural Research Institute, 1947-48.182 pp.

Anonymous. 1949. Report, Department of Agriculture, Uttar Pradesh, 1947-48.

Anonymous. 1950. Report, Department of Agriculture, Uttar Pradesh, 1948-49. 125 pp.

Anonymous. 1951. Scientific Reports of the Indian Agricultural Research Institute, 1948-49. pp 177-190.

Anonymous. 1952. Scientific Reports of the Indian Agricultural Research Institute, 1949-50, pp 81-88.

Anonymous. 1953. Scientific Reports of the Indian Agricultural Research Institute, 1950-51. pp 89-99.

Anonymous. 1954a. Scientific Report of the Indian Agricultural Research Institute, 1952-53. pp 78-89.

Anonymous. 1954b. Agricultural Research Report, Indian Council of Agricultural Research, 1951-52 pp. 11-53.

Anonymous. 1955. Scientific Reports of the Indian Agricultural Research Institute, 1953-54. pp 87-99.

Anonymous. 1956. Scientific Reports of the Indian Agricultural Research Institute, 1955-56. 142 pp.

Anonymous. 1964. Mycology and Plant Pathology Section. *Agricultural Research (India)* 4 : 209-222.

Anonymous. 1965. Improved crop varieties and their yields. *Indian Farming* 15 : 35-38.

Anonymous. 1976. Testing of Arhar (Pigeonpea) strains against wilt disease. *Pesticides* 10 :17.

Anonymous. 1982. Pulse Pathology (Pigeonpea), Report of work 1981- 82. Progress Report No. 23, ICRISAT, Patancheru, India, pp. 113.

Anonymous. 1983. Pulse Pathology (Pigeonpea) Report of work 1982-83. Progress Report No. 30, ICRISAT, Patancheru, India, pp. 187.

Anonymous. 1990. Identification of a multiple disease resistant pigeonpea line. *International Pigeonpea Newsletter* 12 : 4.

Anonymous. 1991. All India Coordinated Pulses Improvement Project. *International Pigeonpea Newsletter* 14 : 2-3.

Anonymous. 1992. AICPIP Kharif Pulses workshop 1992, Highlights. *International Pigeonpea Newsletter* 16 : 3-4.

Aponte Aponte, F. 1963. (Cultivation of pigeonpea in Puerto Rico). *Caribbean Agriculture* 1 : 191-197.

Ariyanayagam, R.P. 1975. Status of research on pigeonpea in Trinidad. Pages 131-140 *in* Proceedings of the International Workshop on Grain Legumes, 13-16 Jan. 1975. Patancheru, A.P., India : International Crops Research Institute for the Semi-Arid Tropics.

Armstrong, G.M. and Armstrong, J.K. 1950. Biological races of the Fusarrium causing wilt of cowpea and soybeans. *Phytopathology* 40 : 181-193.

Ashby, S.C. 1927, *Macrophomina phaseoli* (Maubl.) Comb. Nov : The Pycnidial stage of *Rhizoctonia bataticola* (Taub.) Butler. *Transaction of British Mycological Society* 12 : 141-147.

Asthana, Sudha, Singh, N.P., Gurha, S.N. and Asthana, A.N. 1998. *In vitro* selection of callus lines of pigeonpea against *Phytophthora drechsleri*. Page 68 *in* Proceedings National Symposium on Management of Biotic and Abiotic Stresses in Pulse Crops, 26-28 June 1998, Kanpur, U.P., India : Indian Institute of Pulses Research.

Babu, Suresh, Mthindi, G.B., Subramanyam, P., Soko. H.N. and Saka, V.W. 1992. Impact assessment of an ICRISAT wilt resistant pigeonpea cultivar in Malawi. *International Pigeonpea Newsletter* 16 : 75-78.

Bailey, A. G. 1966. Niger Federation Department of Agriculture Research Memoir 96 : 37.

Bajpai, G.C. and Tripathi, H.S. 1999. Phytophthora stem blight management and breeding for its resistance in pigeonpea: a review. *Agricultural Review* (*Karnal*) 20 : 63-67.

Baldev, B. and Amin, K.S. 1974. Studies on the existence of races in *Fusarium udum* causing wilt of *Cajanus cajan*. *SABRAO Journal* 6 : 201-205.

Bantilan, M.C.S. and Joshi, P.K. 1996. Returns to research and diffusion investments on wilt resistance in pigeonpea. *ICRISAT Impact Series No. 1*, 30 pp.

Bapat, Sangita and Shah, A.K. 2000. Biological control of fusarial wilt of pigeonpea by *Bacillus brevis*. *Canadian Journal of Microbiology* 46 129-132.

Bhargava, P.K. and Gupta, R.K. 1983. Reaction of pigeonpea varieties to phytophthora stem necrosis in field. *JNKVV Research Journal* 17 (3/4) : 301-303.

Bhargava, R.N. 1975. Two new varieties of Arhar for Bihar. *Indian Farming* 25 : 23.

Bhargava, S.N. 1965. Studies on the charcoal rot of potato, *Phytopathologische Zeitschrift* 53 : 35-44.

Bhargava, S.N., Shukla, D.N., Pandey, R.S. and Khati, D.V.S. 1981. New Seedling rot of pigeonpea and sesame (*Fusarium equiseti*). *Acta Botanica Indica* 9 : 131

Bhargava, S.N. and Singh, A.P. 1978. Survival studies on three species of *Fusarium* causing wilt of pigeonpea. Page 189 *in* Abstract of papers of the Third International Congress of Plant Pathology, 16-23 August 1978, Munich Federal, Republic of Germany. Berlin, Federal Republic of Germany: Paul Parey.

Bhaskaran, K. 1954. Crops and crop improvement in Hyderabad. *Agricultural College Journal*, Osmania University 1 : 60-63.

Bhaskara Reddy, M.V., Ghanekar, A.M. and Chakrabarty, S.K. 1992. Association of *Macrophomina phaseolina* (Tassi) Goid. and *Phomopsis* species with pigeonpea seed. *International Pigeonpea Newsletter* 15 : 21 - 23.

Bhatnagar, Himani 1996. Influence of environmental conditions on antagonistic activity of *Trichoderma* spp. against *Fusarium udum*. *Indian Journal of Mycology and Plant Pathology* 26 : 58 - 63.

Bhattacharya, P. 1998. Interaction of *Fusarium oxysporum* f sp. *udum* and *Rhizobium* on pigeonpea (*Cajanus cajan*). *Indian Agriculturist* 42 : 199-204.

Bidari, V. B. 1995. Incidence and distribution of pigeonpea wilt in Karnataka. *Indian Journal of Pulses Research* 8 : 166-168.

Bidari, V.B., Dayanand, M. and Mannur, D.M. 1991. Management of Pigeonpea wilt through intercropping. *Indian Journal of Pulses Research* 4 : 185-187.

Bidari, V.B., Dayanand, M., Patil, J.R. and Mannur, D.M. 1994. Identification and development of pigeonpea genotypes against Fusarium wilt in Karnataka. *Indian Phytopathology* 47 : 332.

Bidari, V.B., Dayanand, M., Patil J.R. and Anahosur, K.H. 1995. Reaction of extra early maturing pigeonpea genotypes against wilt in Karnataka, India. *International Chickpea and Pigeonpea Newsletter* 2 : 70-71.

Bidari, V.B., Dayanand, M., Conda, C.R., Patil. J.R. and Rao, T.M. 1996a. Field evaluation of short, medium and long duration pigeonpeas against wilt in Karanataka, India. *International Chickpea and Pigeonpea Newsletter* 3 : 88.

Bidari, V.B., Dayanand, M. and Vishwa Dhar. 1996b. Stable Fusarium wilt resistance in pigeonpea. *Indian Journal of Pulses Research* 9 : 213-214.

Bidari, V.B. and Gundappagol, R.C. 1997. *Trichoderma viride* in the integrated management of pigeonpea wilt under dryland cultivations. *Advances in Agricultural Research in India* 7 : 65-69.

Bisht, V.S., Kannaiyan, J. and Nene, Y.L. 1988. Methods of metalaxyl application to control Phytophthora blight of pigeonpea. *International Pigeonpea Newsletter* 8 : 9-10.

Bisht, V.S., Krishna, K.R. and Nene, Y.L. 1985. Interaction between vesicular-arbuscular mycorrhiza and *Phytophthora drechsleri* f. sp. *cajani. International Pigeonpea Newsletter* 4 : 63-64.

Bisht, V.S. and Nene, Y.L. 1986. Phytophthora blight of pigeonpea survival spread of pathogen. *Indian Phytopathology* 39 : 145

Bisht, V.S. and Nene, Y.L. 1988. A selective medium for *Phytophthora drechsleri* f sp. *cajani* causing pigeonpea blight. *International Pigeonpea Newsletter* 8 : 12-13.

Bisht, V.S. And Nene, Y.L. 1990. Studies on survival and dispersal of Pigeonpea *Phytophthora. Indian Phytopathology* 43 : 375 - 381.

Biswas, K.K. and Das, N.D. 1999. Biological control of pigeonpea wilt caused by *Fusarium udum* with *Trichoderma* spp. *Annals of Plant Protection Sciences* 7 : 46-50.

Booth, C. 1971. The genus *Fusarium,* Kew, Surrey, UK : Commonwealth Mycological Institute, p. 114.

Bose, R.D. 1938. The rotation of tobacco for the control of wilt disease in pigeonpeas (*Cajanus cajan* (L.) Millsp.). *Agriculture and Livestock in India* 8 : 653-668.

Brathwaite, C.W.D. 1978. Inhibition of *Sclerotium rolfsii* by *pseudomonas aeruginosa* and *Bacillus subtilis* and its significance in the biological control of Southern blight of pigeonpea (*Cajanus cajan* (L.) Millsp.). Page 197 *in* Abstracts of papers of the Third International Congress of Plant Pathology, 16-23 August 1978, Munich, Federal Republic of Germany, Berlin, Federal Republic of Germany : Paul Parey.

Brathwaite, C.W.D. 1981. Diseases of pigeonpea in the Caribbean region. Pages 129-136 *in* Proceedings of the International Workshop on Pigeonpeas, 15-19 December 1980, ICRISAT Centre, volume 1. Patancheru, India : International Crops Research Institute for semi-Arid Tropics.

Bugnicourt, F. 1956. (Parasitic fungi of cultivated plants in New Caledonia). Noumida, France : Institut Francais d'Oceanie. 23 pp.

Butler, E.J. 1906. The wilt disease of pigeonpea and pepper. *Agricultural Journal of India* 1 : 25-36.

Butler, E.J. 1908. Selection of pigeonpea for wilt disease. *Agricultural Journal of India* 3 : 182-183.

Butler, E.J. 1910. The wilt disease of pigeonpea and the parasitism of *Neocosmospora vasinfecta* Smith. *Memoirs of the Department of Agriculture in India, Botanical Series* 2 : 1-64.

Butler, E.J. 1918. Fungi and Diseases in Plants. Thacker Spink & Co. Calcutta, 547 pp.

Butler, E.J. 1920. Report of the Imperial Mycologist. *In* Reports of the Agricultural Research Institute and College, Pusa 1919-1920, pp 58-67.

Butler, E.J. 1926.The wilt disease of cotton and sesamum in India. *Agricultural Journal of India* 21 : 268-273.

Butler, E.J. and Bisby, G.R. 1931. The Fungi of India. Imperial Council of Agricultural Research India, Science Monograph i, XVIII. pp 237.

Chadha, K.C. and Raychaudhuri, S.P. 1965. Interaction between sterility virus and *Fusarium udum* Butler in pigeonpea. *Indian Journal of Agricultural Sciences* 36 : 133-139.

Chakrabarti, S. and Nandi, P. 1969. Effect of griseofulvin on *Fusarium udum* Butler and its host pigeonpea (*Cajanus cajan* (L.) Millsp.). *Proceedings of the Indian Science Congress* 56 : 288.

Chakraborti, A. 1987. Some factors affecting production and germination of chlamydospores of *Fusarium oxysporum* f sp. *udum,* causal organism of wilt of pigeonpea, M.Sc. Ag. thesis, Bidhan Chandra Krishi Vishwa Vidyalaya, 1-50 pp.

Chakraborti, A. and Gupta, P.K.S. 1991. Germination of chlamydospores of *Fusarium udum*, the causal organism of pigeonpea wilt. *Journal of Mycopathological Research* 29 (2) : 165-170.

Chakraborty, A. and Gupta, P.K.S. 1995a. Factors affecting cross protection of *Fusarium* wilt of pigeonpea by soil borne non-pathogenic fungi. *Phytoparasitica* 23 (4) : 323-334.

Chakraborty, A. and Gupta, P.K.S. 1995b. Factors affecting chlamydospore formation by *Fusarium udum,* the causal organism of wilt of pigeonpea. *Journal of Mycopathological Research*. 33 : 71-75.

Chakraborty, A.S., Saha, A.K. and Gupta, P.K.S. 1992. Germination of chlamydospores of *Fusarium udum* adjacent to roots of pigeonpea. *Soil Biology and Biochemistry* 24 : 927-928.

Chari, S.K.V.K., Kannaiyan, J., Nene, Y.L. and Nunn, E.W. 1984. Technique to detect infection by *Fusarium* in pigeonpea before symptom appearance. *Tropical Agriculture* (Trinidad) 61:257-260.

Chattopadhyay, S.B. and Sengupta, P.K. 1967. Studies on wilt diseases of pulses. I. Variation and Taxonomy of *Fusarium* species associated with wilt disease of pulses. *Indian Journal of Mycological Research* 5 : 45-53.

Chaube, H.S., Singh, U.S. and Sinha, P.K. 1984 : Translocation and persistence of metalaxyl in pigeonpea. *Indian Journal of Agricultural Sciences* 59 : 777-779.

Chaube, H.S., Singh, V.S., Rajdan, V.K. and Kumar, S. 1987a. Studies on uptake, translocation, distribution and persistence of 14 C - metalaxyl in pigeonpea. *Indian Phytopathology* 40 : 507-513.

Chaube, H.S., Rajdan, V.K. and Singh, U.S. 1987b. Effect of metalaxyl on growth, sporulation and sporangial germination of *Phytophthora drechsleri* f sp. *cajani*. *International Pigeonpea Newsletter* 6 : 59-61.

Chaudhary, R.G. and Kumar, Kumud. 2000. Role of width of xylem and root vascular bundles of pigeonpea resistance to wilt. *Annals of Plant Protection Sciences* 8 : 102-104.

Chaudhary, R.G., Kumar, Kumud and Naimuddin. 2000. Association of dates of sowing, flowering and wilt incidence in pigeonpea. *Indian Journal of Agricultural Sciences* 70 : 452-454.

Chaudhary, R.G., Naimuddin, Singh, K.K. and Ali, M. 1998. Effect of mungbean on the population of *Fusarium udum* Butler in pigeonpea under intercropping system. page 58 *in* Abstracts of National Symposium on Management of Biotic and Abiotic

Stresses in Pulse Crops, 26-28 June 1998, Indian Institute of Pulses Research, Kanpur, India.

Chaudhary, S. and Ahmed, T. 1977. Fungicides for the control of Rhizoctonia seedling blight of pigeonpea. *Pesticides* 11:23-25.

Chaudhary, S.K. and Prasad, M. 1974. Variations in sugar contents of healthy and *Fusarium oxysporum* f sp. *udum* infected plants of *Cajanus cajan*. *Phytopathologische Zeitschrift* 80 : 303-305.

Chaudhary, S.K. and Prasad, M. 1975. Effects of micronutrients and intermittent sunlight on growth and sporulation of *Fusarium oxysporum* f *udum*. *Phytopathologische Zeitschrift* 82 : 287-290.

Chauhan, V.B. and Shaha, Subrata, 1999. Influence of environmental factors on Phytophthora blight of pigeonpea. *Indian Journal of Pulses Research* 12 : 206-210.

Chauhan, V.B. and Singh, U.P. 1987. A naturally occurring resistant forma specialis of *Phytophthora drechsleri* f sp. *cajani* to metalaxy1. *Phytopathologische Zeitschrift* 120 : 93.

Chauhan, V.B. and Singh, U.P. 1991a, Effect of weed infestation on the severity of Phytophthora blight of pigeonpea. *Plant Disease* 75 : 1230-1232.

Chauhan, V.B. and Singh, U.P. 1991b. Control of Phytophthora blight of pigeonpea (*Cajanus cajan* (L.) Millsp.) by metalaxy1. *New Agriculturist* 2 (2) : 109-112.

Chauhan, V.B. and Singh, U.P. 1991c. Effect of pH and light on the germination of zoospores of *Phytophthora drechsleri* f sp. *cajani*. *Indian Phytopathology* 44 : 193 - 196.

Chauhan, Y.S. 1991. Possible influence of competition from weeds and increased plant population on wilt incidence in pigeonpea. *International Pigeonpea Newsletter* 14 : 26-27.

Chaurasia, S. and Rathi, Y.P.S. 1993. Management of Phytophthora stem blight of pigeonpea. *Indian Phytopathology* 44 & 45 (Suppliment) : LXV-LXVI(Abstracts).

Chaurasia, S., Rathi, Y.P.S., Srivastava, A., Sand, N.K. and Gupta, K.C. 1993. The role of phenolic acids in Phytophthora blight resistance. *International Pigeonpea Newsletter* 17 : 29-31.

Chavan, P.N., Gahukar, K.B. and Raut, B.T. 1995. Reaction of pigeonpea cultivars/lines to Fusarium wilt in wilt sick plot. *PKV Research Journal* 19 : 200-201.

Cook, M.T. 1939. (Diseases of economic plants in the Antilles). Monograph Series B.No. 4. Rio Piedras, Puerto Rico : University of Puerto Rico. 530 pp.

Das, N.D. and Gupta, S.K. 1992. Evaluation of some pigeonpea lines for resistance to wilt and sterility mosaic. *International Pigeonpea Newsletter* 15 : 23-24.

Das, S.K. and Sengupta, P.K. 1998. Variability in *Fusarium udum*, the causal organism of wilt of pigeonpea. *Journal of Mycopthological Research*, 36 : 7-11.

Dasgupta, A., Chakraborty, A. and Gupta, P.K.S. 1992s. Effect of crop sequence on the population of *Fusarium udum* Butler in soil. *Journal of Mycological Research* 30(1) : 37-42.

Dasgupta, A. and Sengupta, P.K. 1988. Reaction of pigeonpea (*Cajanus cajan*) lines to wilt pathogen *Fusarium udum*. *Indian Journal of Agricultural Science* 58 : 546-548.

Dasgupta, A. and Sengupta, P.K. 1989. Effect of different soil amendments on wilt of pigeonpea (*Cajanus cajan* (L.) Hath.) caused by *Fusarium udum* Butler. Beitrag. Trop. Landwirtsch. Vet. med. 27 : 341-345.

Dasgupta, A. and Sengupta, P.K. 1993. Some factors affecting growth of *Fusarium udum* in soil. *Journal of Mycopathological Research* 31(2): 93-97.

Dash, J.S. 1917. Crop diseases. Report of the Department of Agriculture, Barbados, 1915-16. pp. 37-38.

Dastur, J.F. 1946. Report of the Imperial Mycologist. Scientific Reports of the Indian Agricultural Research Institute, 1944-45. pp. 66-72.

Daya Ram. 1994. Field evaluation of fungicides and natural products to control Phytophthora blight of pigeonpea. *Indian Phytopathology* 47 : 318 (abstract).

Deighton, F.C. 1932. Mycological work. Report, Agricultural Department, Sierra Leone, 1931. pp. 20-25.

Dennis, J.J.C. 1994. First report of pigeonpea root rot caused by *Phellinus noxius* in Papua New Guinea. *Plant Disease* 78: 316.

Deodikar, G.B. and Thakar, C.V. 1956. Cyto-taxonomic evidence for the affinity between *Cajanus indicus* Spreng, and certain erect species of *Atylosia* W. and A. *Proceedings of the Indian Academy of Sciences, Section* B 43 : 37-45.

Desai, B.G., Vora, M.S. and Patel, J.C. 1981. A note on survey of pigeonpea diseases in Gujrat State. *Pulse Crop Newsletter* 1(3) : 54.

Deshpande, R.B., Jeswani, L.M. and Joshi, A.B. 1963. Breeding of wilt resistant varieties of pigeonpea. *Indian Journal of Genetics and Plant Breeding* 23 : 58-63.

Dey, P.K. 1947. Plant Pathology. Report, Department of Agriculture, Uttar Pradesh, 1944-45. pp 38-40.

Dey, P.K. 1948, Plant Pathology. Report, Department of Agriculture, Uttar Pradesh, 1946-47. pp. 39-42.

Dwivedi, R.K., Upadhyay, K.D. and Dwivedi, K. 1992. Interaction of root knot nematode, *Meloidogyne incognita* and fungus *Fusarium oxysporum* f sp. *udum* on pigeonpea. *Indian Journal of Nematology* 22 : 96-100.

Dwivedi, S., Faris, D.G. and Jain, K.C. 1989. Gamma ray induced Fusarium wilt resistance in pigeonpea (*Cajanus cajan* (L.) millsp.). pages 781-784 *in* Proceedings of 6th International Congress of SABARAO, Tsukuba, Japan.

Edward, J.C. 1954. *Macrophomina* and *Botryodiplodia*, two distinct genera of *Sphaeropsidaceae*. *Allahabad Farmer* 28 : 5.

Edward, J.C. and Singh, K.P. 1979. Interaction between *Heterodera cajani* and *Fusarium udum* on pigeonpea. *Allahabad Farmer* 50 : 23.

Gangawane, L.V. 1995. Management of fungicide resistance in soilborne pathogens. *Indian Journal of Mycology and Plant Pathology* 25 : 49-50 (Abstract).

Gangawane, L.V., Waghmare, Suman and Kareppa, B.M. 1988. Studies on benomyl resistance in *Phytophthora drechsleri* f. sp. *cajani*. *Indian Phytopathology* 41 : 299 (Abstract).

Gangawane, L.V., Waghmare, Suman and Kareppa, B.M. 1989. Breakdown of benomyl resistance in *Phytophthora drechsleri* f sp. *cajani* by alternate and joint action of fungicides. *Indian Phytopathology* 42 : 353-354 (Abstract).

Garcia, L.A.A. 1960. Phoma canker of pigeonpea in Puerto Rico. *Journal of Agriculture of the University of Puerto Rico* 44 : 28-30.

Gaur, Vinod Kumar, and Sharma, L.C. 1988. Screening of Pigeonpea for resistance to Fusarium wilt. *Indian Journal of Mycology and Plant Pathology* 18 : 206.

Gaur, Vinod Kumar and Sharma, L.C. 1989. Prevalence of Fusarium wilt of pigeonpea in Rajasthan. *Indian Phytopathology* 42 : 468.

Gaur, V.K. and Sharma, L.C. 1990. Estimation of ascorbate from root exudates of pigeonpea. *Indian Journal of Mycology and Plant Pathology* 20 : 89 (Abst.).

Ghosh, M.K. and Sinha, A.K. 1981. Laboratory evaluation of some systemic fungicides against Fusarium wilt of pigeonpea. *Pesticides* 15 : 24-27.

Godbole, G.M., Dake, G.N. and Mayee, C.D. 1977. Quantitative estimation of pigeonpea stem canker intensity. *Research Bulletin of the Marathwada Agricultural University* 1 : 135-136.

Goodling, H.J. 1962. The agronomic aspects of pigeonpeas. *Field crop Abstracts* 15 : 1-5.

Goudar, S.B. and Kulkarni, Srikant. 1998. Effect of organic amendments on *Fusarium udum Butler. Karnataka Journal of Agricultural Sciences* 11 : 690-692.

Goudar, S.B. and Kulkarni, Srikant. 1999. Compatibility effect of antagonists and seed dressers against *Fusarium udum*—the causal agent of pigeonpea wilt. *Karnataka Journal of Agricultural Sciences* 12 : 197-199.

Goyal, S.N., Patel, B.S. and Nigama, J.R. 1991. Response of pigeonpea to fusarium wilt and insect pests. *International Pigeonpea Newsletter* 14 : 17-19.

Gupta, A.K., Singh, I.S., Reddy, M.V. and Bajpai, G.C, 1996. Nature of resistance to Phytophthora blight in Pigeonpea-breeding implications. *International Chickpea and Pigeonpea Newsletter* No. 3 : 69-71.

Gupta, M.C. 1987. Influence of fungicides on growth and sporulation of wilt causing species of *Fusarium. Indian Journal of Mycology and Plant Pathology*. 17 : 103-104 (Abst.).

Gupta, M.C. 1993. Effect of fungicides on population of two wilt causing species of *Fusarium* in soil. *Indian Phytopathology* 44 & 45 (Suppl.) : LXVIII -LXIX (Abst.).

Gupta, Om, Kotasthane, S.R. and Khare, M.N. 1988. Strain variation in *Fusarium udum* in Madhya Pradesh, India. *International Pigeonpea Newsletter* 7 : 22-25.

Gupta, S.L. 1961. The effect of mixed cropping of arhar (*Cajanus indicus* Spreng.) with Jowar (*Sorghum vulgare* pers.) on incidence of arhar wilt. *Agriculture and Animal Husbandry in Uttar Pradesh* 3 (10-12) : 31-35.

Gurha, S.N., Singh, R.N. and Kinra, K.L. 1983. Reaction of post rainy season pigeonpea to collar rot. *International Pigeonpea Newsletter* 2 : 52.

Haider, M.G., Singh, R.K., Prasad, H., Nath, R.P. and Sharma, R.N. 1978. Effect of some common fungicides on the incidence of pigeonpea wilt. *Indian Phytopathology* 31 : 511-512.

Haigh, J.C. 1930. *Macrophomina phaseoli* (Maubl.) Ashby and *Rhizoctonia bataticola* (Taub.) Butler. *Annals of the Royal Botanical Gardens of Peradenia* 11 : 213-249.

Hansford, C.G. 1938. Annual Report of the Plant Pathologist 1936. Report of the Department of Agriculture, Uganda, 1936-37. Part 2, pp. 43-49.

Hansford, C.G. 1943. Contributions towards the fungus flora of Uganda. 5. Fungi imperfecti. *Proceedings of the Linnean Society of London,* 1942-43. pp. 34-67.

Haque, F. (Md.), Jha, D.K. and Mukharjee, A.K. 1984. Evalution of ICRISAT germplasm for wilt incidence in the plateau region of Chota Nagpur in India. *International Pigeonpea Newsletter* No. 3 : 36-37.

Hasan, A. 1984. Synergism between *Heterodera cajani* and *Fusarium udum* attacking *Cajanus cajan. Nematologia Mediterranea* 12: 159-162.

Hasan, A. and Khan, A.M. 1979a. On the fungicidal control of anthracnose disease of arhar. *Indian Journal of Mycology and Plant Pathology* 9 : 156-159.

Hasan, A. and Khan, A.M. 1979b. Varietal screening for anthracnose disease of arhar. *Acta Botanica Indica* 7 : 126-128.

Hasan, A., Khan, M.W., Rashid, A. and Abrar, M.K. 1975. Relative efficacy of certain fungicides against *Colletotrichum* spp. *Indian Journal of Mycology and Plant Pathology* 5 : 41.

Haware, M.P. 1993. Fusarium disease of crops in India. *Indian Phytopathology* 46 : 101-109.

Haware, M.P. and Kannaiyan, J. 1992. Seed transmission of *Fusarium udum* in pigeonpea and its control by seed treatment fungicides. *Seed Science and Technology* 20 : 597-601.

Haware, M.P. and Nene, Y.L. 1982. Symptomless carriers of the chickpea wilt *Fusaruim*. *Plant Disease* 66 : 250-251.

Haware, M.P. and Nene, Y.L. 1994. A rapid method for pigeonpea wilt resistance screening. *Indian Phytopathology* 47 : 400-402.

ICRISAT. 1986. Pigeonpea. Disease and Mycorrhizas. Annual Report 1984-85, pp. 182-189.

ICRISAT. 1987. Pulse Pathology (Pigeonpea), Report of Work 1986-87, Progress Report No. 50, pp. 1-78.

Ingham, J.L. 1976. Induced isoflavonoids from fungus infected stems of pigeonpea (*Cajanus cajan*). *Zeitschrift fur Naturforschung* C 31 : 504-508.

Iqbal, S.M., Hussain, S. and Khan, H.R. 1990. Collar rot of pigeonpea in Pakistan. *International Pigeonpea Newsletter* 11:47.

Jain, K.C., Kannaiyan, J. and Faris, D.G. 1983. ICRISAT breeding lines show promise for Fusarium wilt resistance. *International Pigeonpea Newsletter* 2 : 43.

Jain, K.C. and Reddy, M.V. 1995. Inheritance of resistance to Fusarium wilt in pigeonpea (*Cajanus cajan* (L.) Millsp.). *Indian Journal of Genetics and Plant Breeding* 55 : 434-437.

Jain, K.C. and Sharma, S.B. 1996. Loss of Fusarium wilt resistance in a pigeonpea line ICPL 270 in reniform nematode infested soil at ICRISAT Asia centre. *International Chickpea and Pigeonpea Newsletter* 3 : 90.

Jehle, R. A. and Wood, J.I. 1926. Diseases of field and vegetable crops in the United States in 1925. *Plant Disease Reporter* 45 (Suppl.) : 152.

Jeswani, M.D. and Gemawat, P.D. 1981. Seed borne nature of wilt of arhar. Pages 162 *in* Abstracts of papers of the Third International Symposium of Plant Pathology, 14-18 December 1981, New Delhi, India : Indian Phytopathological Society.

Jeswani, M.D., Prasad, N. and Gemawat, P.D. 1975. Morphological variability in *Fusarium lateritium* f *cajani*. *Indian Journal of Mycology and Plant Pathology* 5 : 4.

Johnson, J. 1939. Studies on the nature of brown root rot of tobacco and other plants. *Journal of Agricultural Research* 58 : 843-63.

Joshi, A.B. 1957. Genetics of resistance to diseases and pests. *Indian Journal of Genetics and Plant Breeding* 17 : 305-317.

Joshi, C.G. and Wangikar, P.D. 1977. Efficacy of fungicides against stem canker and die-back disease of *Cajanus cajan* caused by *Colletotrichum capsici*. *Indian Phytopathology* 30 : 148.

Joshi, C.G. and Wangikar, P.D. 1978. Efficacy of fungicides against *Colletotrichum capsici*. *Indian Phytopathology* 31 : 222-223.

Kaiser, S.A.K.M. and Sengupta, P.K. 1969. Cross protection against wilt disease caused by *Fusarium oxysporum* f sp. *udum* in pigeonpea. *Indian Journal of Mycological Research* 7 : 38-39.

Kaiser, S.A. K.M. and Sengupta, P.K. 1975. Infection and Pathological histology of pigeonpea (*Cajanus cajan* (L.) Millsp.) plants inoculates with pathogenic and non-pathogenic formae speciales of *Fusarium oxysporum*. *Zeitschrift fur Pflanzenkrankheiten und Pflanzenschutz* 82 : 485-492.

Kaiser, S.A.K.M. and Sengupta, P.K. 1976. Serological and electorphoratic studies of three formae speciales of *Fusarium oxysporum*. *Transaction of the British Mycological Society* 67 : 33-37.

Kaiser, S.A.K.M. and Sengupta, P.K. 1977. Inhibition of wilt symptoms by *Fusarium oxysporum* f sp. *udum* in pigeonpea (*Cajanus cajan*) induced by other formae speciales of *Fusarium oxysporum*. *Phytopathologia Mediterranea* 16 : 1-4.

Kaiser, S.A.K.M. and Sengupta, P.K. 1979. Role of pectolytic enzymes in pathogenesis by different formae speciales of *Fusarium oxysporum* on pigeonpea. *Indian Phytopathology* 32 : 311-313.

Kaiser, W.J. 1976. Important diseases and pest of bean (*Phaseolus vulgaris*), Lima bean (*Phaseolus lunatus*) and pigeonpea (*Cajanus cajan*) in Africa. *African Journal of Plant Protection* 1: 97-102.

Kaiser, W.J. and Melendez, P.L. 1978. A Phytophthora stem canker disease of pigeonpea in Puerto Rico. *Plant Disease Reporter* 62 : 240-242.

Kaiser, W.J., Melendez, P.L. and Zapate, M. 1982. Crown Canker disease of pigeonpea caused by a sterile Basidiomycete in Puerto Rico (Abstr.). *Phytopathology* 72 : 994.

Kaiser, W.J., Melendez, P.L., Hannan, R.M. and Rapate, M. 1987. Crown canker of pigeonpea caused by a sterile white Basidiomycete in Puerto Rico. *Plant Disease* 71 : 1006-1009.

Kalyansundaram, R. 1952. Ascorbic acid and *Fusarium* wilted plants. *Proceedings of the Indian Academy of Sciences, Section* B 36 : 102-104.

Kamble, S.V. and Gangawane, L.V. 1994. Effect of passage on the development of benomyl resistance in *Fusarium udum in vitro. Indian Phytopathology* 47 : 354 (Abstract).

Kannaiyan, J., Erwin, D.C., Ribeiro, O.K. and Nene, Y.L. 1979. *Phytophthora drechsleri* f sp. *cajani,* the causal organism of blight of pigeonpea in India. *Phytophthora Newsletter* 7 : 32-33.

Kannaiyan, J. and Haciwa, H.C. 1990. Diseases of Pigeonpea in Zambia. *International Pigeonpea Newsletter* 12 : 22-23.

Kannaiyan, J., Jain, K.C., Raju, T.N. and Nene, Y.L. 1983a. Sclerotium blight of pigeonpea. *International Pigeonpea Newsletter* No. 2 : 51-52.

Kannaiyan, J., Jain, K.C., Raju, T.N. and Nene, Y.L. 1983b. Wilt resistance sources in vegetable pigeonpea. *International Pigeonpea Newsletter* 2 : 42-43.

Kannaiyan, J. and Nene, Y.L. 1978. Screening of pigeonpea for resistance to Phytophthora blight. Page 302 *in* Abstracts of papers of the Third International Congress of Plant Pathology, 16-23 August 1978, Munich, Federal Republic of Germany. Berlin, Federal Republic of Germany : Paul Parey.

Kannaiyan, J. and Nene, Y.L. 1979. Association of different *Fusarium* species with wilt disease of pigeonpea. *Tropical Grain Legume Bulletin* 15 : 26-27.

Kannaiyan, J. and Nene, Y.L. 1981a. Field and Greenhouse techniques to screen pigeonpea for resistance to wilt. Pages 277-280 *in* Proceedings of the International Workshop on Pigeonpeas, 15-19 December 1980, ICRISAT Centre, India. Volume 2. Patancheru A.P. 502324, India : International Crop Research Institute for the Semi-Arid Tropics.

Kannaiyan, J. and Nene, Y.L. 1981b. Greenhouse and field techniques to screen pigeonpea for resistance to Phytophthora blight. Pages 281-284 *in* Proceedings of the International Workshop on Pigeonpeas, 15-19 Dec. 1980, ICRISAT Centre. Volume 2. Patancheru, A.P. 502324, India : International Crops Research Institute for the Semi-Arid Tropics.

Kannaiyan, J. and Nene, Y.L. 1981c. Influence of wilt at different growth stages on yield loss in pigeonpea. *Tropical Pest Management* 27 : 141.

Kannaiyan, J. and Nene, Y.L. 1984. Efficacy of metalaxyl for control of Phytophthora blight of pigeonpea. *Indian Phytopathology* 37 : 506-510.

Kannaiyan, J. and Nene, Y.L. 1985a. *Atylosia scarabaeoides* an alternate host to *Phytophthora drechsleri* f sp. *cajani. International Pigeonpea Newsletter* 4 : 35-36.

Kannaiyan, J. and Nene, Y.L. 1985b. Effect of sowing dates on wilt incidence in pigeonpea. *International Pigeonpea Newsletter* No. 4 : 33-35.

Kannaiyan, J., Nene, Y.L. and Bisht, V.S. 1984a. Ridomil application methods for the control of pigeonpea Phytophthora blight. *Indian Phytopathology* 37 : 384 (Abstract).

Kannaiyan, J., Nene, Y.L. and Raju, T.N. 1985. Host specificity of pigeonpea wilt pathogen, *Fusarium udum. Indian Phytopathology* 38 : 553-554.

Kannaiyan, J., Nene, Y.L., Raju, T.N. and Sheila, V.K. 1981a. Screening for resistance to Phytophthora blight of pigeonpea. *Plant Disease* 65 : 61-62.

Kannaiyan, J., Nene, Y.L. and Reddy, M.V., 1981b. Survival of pigeonpea wilt *Fusarium* in Vertisols and Alfisols. Pages 291-295 *in* Proceedings of the International Workshop on Pigeonpeas. 15-19 December 1980, ICRISAT Centre, India. Volume 2. Patancheru A.P. 502324, India : International Crops Research Institute for the Semi-Arid Tropics.

Kannaiyan, J., Nene, Y.L., Reddy, M.V. and Raju, T.N. 1981c. International Survey of pigeonpea diseases. Pulse Pathology Progress Report No. 12. Patancheru, A.P. 502324, India : International Crops Research Institute for the Semi-Arid Tropics, 82 p.

Kannaiyan, J., Nene, Y.L. Reddy, M.V., Ryan, J.G. and Raju, T.N. 1984b. Prevalence of pigeonpea diseases and associated crop losses in Asia, Africa and the Americas. *Tropical Pest Management* 30 : 62-71.

Kannaiyan, J., Nene, Y.L. and Sheila, V.K. 1980a. Control of mycoflora associated with pigeonpea seeds. *Indian Journal of Plant Protection.* 8 : 93-98.

Kannaiyan, J., Nene, Y.L. and Sheila, V.K. 1980b. Longevity of *Phytophthora drechsleri* f sp. *cajani in vitro. Phytophthora Newsletter* 8 : 7.

Kannaiyan, J., Raju, T. N. and Nene, Y.L. 1983. Survival of Pigeonpea Phytophthora blight fungus in infected stubbles. *International Pigeonpea Newsletter* 2 : 49-50.

Kannaiyan, J., Ribeiro, O.K., Erwin, D.C. and Nene, Y.L. 1980c. Phytophthora blight of pigeonpea in India. *Mycologia* 72 : 169-181

Kannaiyan, J. and Sharma, H.C. 1992. New record of Fusarium wilt and Web blight in Zambia. *International Pigeonpea Newsletter* 15 : 18.

Kannaiyan, J., Sheila, V.K. and Nene, Y.L. 1994. A technique for *Phytophthora drechsleri* f sp. *cajani* sporangia and zoospores production. *International Chickpea and Pigeonpea Newsletter* No. 1 : 36-37.

Kant, L., Bajpai, G.C. and Singh, D.P. 1998. Screening for resistance to Phytophthora stem blight in pigeonpea. Page 37 *In* Abstracts of papers on National Symposium on Management of Biotic and Abiotic Stresses in Pulse Crops, 26-28 June 1998, Indian Institute of Pulses Research, Kanpur, India.

Khan, M.W. and Singh, R.K. 1974. Anthracnose of arhar incited by *Colletotrichum truncatum. Indian Phytopathology* 27 : 622-624.

Khan, T.N. and Ashley, J.M. 1975. Factors affecting Plant stand in pigeonpea. *Experimental Agriculture* 11 : 315-322.

Khare, N. and Lakpale, N. 1997. Sources of resistance in pigeonpea for Phytophthora stem blight in Chhatisgarh region of India. *Journal of Soils and Crops* 7 : 99-100.

Khune, N.N. 1990. Transmission studies of *Fusarium udum* Butler in pigeonpea. *PKV Research Journal* 14 (2) : 213-214.

Khune, N.N. and Kapoor, J.N. 1981a. A new disease of pigeonpea. *Indian Phytopathology* 34 : 258-260.

Khune, N.N. and Kapoor, J.N 1981b. Phoma canker : a new disease of pigeonpea. *PKV Research Journal* 5 : 101-102.

Konda, C.R., Parameswarappa, R. and Rao, T.S. 1986. Pigeonpea ICP 8863 - A boon to Fusarium wilt endemic areas of Karnataka. *International Pigeonpea Newsletter* 5 : 36-37.

Kotasthane, S.R. and Gupta, Om 1981. Trend in wilting in pigeonpea varieties of variable maturity. Pages 161-162 *in* Abstracts of papers of the Third International Symposium of Plant Pathology, 14-18 December 1981, New Delhi, India. New Delhi, India : Indian Phytopathological Society.

Kotasthane, S.R. and Gupta, Om. 1983. Studies on root exudates of susceptible and resistant cultivars of pigeonpea. *Indian Phytopathology* 36 : 195 (Abstract).

Kotasthane, S.R. and Gupta, Om 1984. Studies on biochemical aspects of resistance in pigeonpea against Fusarium wilt. *Indian Phytopathology* 37 : 396 (Abstract).

Kotasthane, S.R., Gupta, Om and Khare, M.N. 1987. Influence of fungicidal seed treatment and soil amendment on the development of *Fusarium udum* propagules in soil and pigeonpea wilt. *Indian Phytopathology* 40 : 197-200.

Kotasthane, S.R., Gupta, Om and Lal, M.S. 1981. Wilt resistance sources in pigeonpea (*Cajanus cajan* (L.) Millsp.). *Pulse Crop Newsletter* 1 (4) : 52-53.

Kotasthane, S.R., Gupta, Om, Tiwari, D.P. and Khare, M.N. 1983. Studies on root exudates of susceptible and resistant cultivars of pigeonpea. *JNKVV Research Journal* 17(1/2): 141-144.

Kotwal, I., Vyas, S.C. and Jain, A.C. 1981. Translocation and persistence of acylon in pigeonpea. *Indian Phytopathology* 34 : 492-493.

Kulshrestha, D.D., Mathur, S.B. and Paul, Neergaard. 1976. Identification of seed borne species of *Collectotrichum. Friesia* 11 : 116-125.

Kumar , J., Dutta, M. and Prasad, Rajendra. 1991. Pigeonpea diseases at different altitudes in Garhwal hills, India. *International Pigeonpea Newsletter* 14 : 16-17.

Kumar, Kumud, Chaudhary, R.G. and Prajapati, R.K. 1998a. Transmission of *Fusarium udum* Butler from seed to seedlings. Page 116 *in* Abstract of papers of National Symposium on Management of Biotic and Abiotic Stresses in Pulse Crops, 26-28 June 1998, IIPR, Kanpur, India. Kanpur: Indian Society of Pulses Research and Development.

Kumar, Kumud, Chaudhary, R.G. and Prajapati, R.K. 1998b. Variations in seed borne infection of *Fusarium udum* Butler in pigeonpea seed. Page 116 *in* Abstracts of papers of National Symposium on Management of Biotic and Abiotic Stresses in Pulse Crops, 26-28 June 1998, IIPR, Kanpur, India. Kanpur, India : Indian Society of Pulses Research and Development.

Kumar, L.S.S., Thombre, M.B. and D'Cruz, R. 1958. Cytological studies of an intergeneric hybrid of *Cajanus cajan* (L.) Millsp. and *Atylosia lineata* W. & A., *Proceedings of the Indian Academy of Sciences, Section* B 47 : 252-262.

Kumar, Vinod and Sharma, L.C. 1994. Biochemical changes in root exudates of pigeonpea in relation to Fusarium wilt resistance. *Indian Journal of Mycology and Plant Pathology* 24 : 74-75.

Leach, R. 1934. Report of the Mycologist for 1933. Annual Report of the Department of Agriculture, Nyasaland, pp. 54-55.

Leach, R. and Wright, J. 1930. Collar and stem canker of pigeonpea (*Cajanus cajan*) caused by a species of *Physalospora. Memoirs of the Imperial College of Tropical Agriculture, Trinidad, Mycological Series no.* 1, 12 p.

Leather, R.I. 1967. A catalogue of some plant diseases and fungi in Jamaica. *Bulletin*, Ministry of Agriculture, Jamaica, New Series No. 61.

Litzenberger, S.C. and Stevenson, J.A. 1957. A preliminary list of Nicaraguan Plant diseases. *Plant Disease Reporter* 243 (Suppl.) : 4-19.

Lopez Rosa, J.H. 1969. *Phoma* sp. the causal agent of pigeonpea canker. *Phytopathology* 59 : 1348.

Magdum, J.A. and Nair, L.N. 1988. Biochemical changes during wilt *of Cajanus cajan* (L.) Millsp. *Indian Journal of Mycology and Plant Pathology* 18 : 85.

Mahalinga, D.M., Suryanarayana, V., Gundappagol, R.C. and Jayalaxmi, S.K. 1998. Status of Pigeonpea diseases in northern Karnataka. Page 113 *in* Abstracts of papers of National Symposium on Management of Biotic and Abiotic stresses in Pulse Crops, 26-28 June 1998, IIPR, Kanpur, India. Kanpur, India: Indian Society of Pulses Research and Development.

Mahmood, M. 1964. Factors governing the production of antibiotic bulbiformin and its use in the control of pigeonpea wilt. *Science and Culture* 30 : 352.

Maitra, A. and Sinha, A.K. 1973. Partial inhibition of Fusarium wilt symptoms in pigeonpea by non-pathogenic formae of *Fusarium oxysporum*. *Current Science* 42 : 654-656.

Malik, R.P. 1945. Collar rot of pigeonpea caused by *Pythium aphanidermatum* (Edson) Fitz. *Indian Journal of Agricultural Sciences* 15 : 92-93.

Marley, P.S. and Hillocks, R.J. 1993. The role of phytoalexins in resistance to fusarium wilt in pigeonpea (*Cajanus cajan*). *Plant Pathology* 42 : 212-218.

Marley, P.S. and Hillocks, R.J. 1994. Effect of root knot nematode on cajanol accumulation in the vascular tissues of pigeonpea after stem inoculation with *Fusarium udum*. *Plant Pathology* 43 (1) : 172-176.

Marley, P.S. and Hillocks, R.J. 1996. Effect of root knot nematodes (*Meloidogyne* spp.) on Fusarium wilt in pigeonpea (*Cajanus cajan*). *Field Crops Research*. 46 : 15 - 20.

Mathur, R.S. 1954. Disease of pulse crops in Uttar Pradesh. *Agriculture and Animal Husbandary in India* 5 : 24-28.

Mbwaga, A.M. 1995. Fusarium wilt screening in Tanzania. Pages 101-103 *in* Improvement of pigeonpea in Eastern and Southern Africa, Annual Research Planning Meeting 1994, Nairobi, Kenya, 21-23 Sep. 1994 (Eds. S.N. Silim, S.B. King and S. Tuwafe). Patancheru, India. International Crops Research Institute for the Semi-Arid Tropics.

McDonald, J. 1924. Annual Report of the Mycologist for the year 1923. Annual Report, Department of Agriculture, Kenya, 1923, pp. 81-85.

McRae, W. 1923. Report of the Imperial Mycologist. Scientific Reports, Agriculture Research Institute, Pusa, 1922-23, 53-60 pp.

McRae, W. 1924. Report of the Imperial Mycologist. Scientific Reports of the Agricultural Research Institute, Pusa, 1923-24. pp 41-51.

McRae, W. 1926. Report of the Imperial Mycologist. Scientific Reports of the Agricultural Research Institute, Pusa, 1925-26. pp. 54-69.

McRae, W. 1928a. Report of the Imperial Mycologist. Scientific Reports of the Agricultural Research Institute, Pusa, 1926-27. pp. 45-55.

McRae, W. 1928b. Report of the Imperial Mycologist. Scientific Reports of the Agricultural Research Institute, Pusa, 1927-28. pp. 56-70.

McRae, W. 1930. Report of the Imperial Mycologist. Scientific Reports of the Agricultural Research Institute, Pusa, 1928-29. pp. 51-66.

McRae, W. 1931. Note on wilt in arhar in permanent plots in Pusa. Proceedings of the Board of Agriculture of India, 1929. pp. 236-241.

McRae, W. 1932. Report of the Imperial Mycologist. Scientific Reports of the Agricultural Research Institute, Pusa, 1930-31. pp. 73-86.

McRae, W. and Shaw, F.J.F. 1926. Report on Experiments with *Cajanus indicus* (arhar) for resistance to *Fusarium vasinfectum* (Wilt disease). Scientific Reports of the Agricultural Research Institute, Pusa, 1925-26. pp. 208-212.

McRae, W. and Shaw, F.J.F., 1933. Influence of manures on the wilt disease of *Cajanus indicus* Spreng, and isolation of types resistant to the disease. Part II. The isolation of resistant types. Scientific Monograph, Imperial Council of Agricultural Research Pusa, 7 : 37-68.

Mehrotra, R.S. 1992. Status of *Phytophthora* research in India. *Indian Phytopathology* 45 : 1-18.

Mishra, A.N. and Shukla, P. 1986a. Relation between the age of pigeonpea plant and its susceptibility to phytophthora blight. *Indian Journal of Mycology and Plant Pathology* 16 : 292.

Mishra, A.N. and Shukla, P. 1986b. Screening of pigeonpea germplasm against phytophthora blight. *Farm Science Journal* 1 : 84-85.

Mishra, A.N. and Shukla, P. 1987. Prevalence of Phytophthora blight of pigeonpea in Uttar Pradesh. *Indian Phytopathology* 40-56-58.

Mishra, A.N. and Shukla, P. 1989. Evaluation of fungicides against *Phytophthora drechsleri* f sp. *cajani*. *Farms Science Journal* 4 : 21-27.

Mitra, M. 1925. Report of the Imperial Mycologist. Scientific Reports of the Agricultural Research Institute, Pusa 1924-25. pp. 45-57.

Mitra, M. 1931. Report of the Imperial Mycologist. Scientific Reports of the Agricultural Research Institute, Pusa, 1929-30, pp. 58-71.

Mitra, M. 1934. Wilt disease of *Crotalaria juncea* (Sunnhemp). *Indian Journal of Agricultural Sciences* 4 : 701 - 714.

Mohanty, U.N. 1946. The wilt disease of pigeonpea with special reference to the distribution of causal organism in the host tissues. *Indian Journal of Agricultural Sciences* 16 : 379-390.

Mukherjee, D., De, T.K. and Parui, N.R. 1971. A note on the screening of arhar against wilt disease. *Indian Phytopathology* 24 : 598-601.

Mukhopadhyay, D. and Sengupta, P.K., 1991. Factors affecting competitive saprophytic activity of *Fusarium udum*, the causal organism of wilt of pigeonpea. *Indian Phytopathology* 43 : 73-79.

Mukiibi, J. 1976. Possible relationship between intercropping and plant disease problems in Uganda. Paper presented at the Symposium on Intercropping for Semi-arid Areas, University of Darres-Salam, 10-12 May 1976, Morogoro, Tanzania.

Mundkur, B.B. 1935. Influence of temperature and maturity on the incidence of sunnhemp and pigeonpea wilt at Pusa. *Indian Journal of Agricultural Sciences* 5 : 606-618.

Mundkur, B.B. 1938. Phytopathology-Mycology : Pigeonpea, *Annual Review of Biochemical and Allied Research in India* 9 : 112.

Mundkur, B.B., 1946. Report of the Imperial Mycologist. Scientific Reports of the Indian Agricultural Research Institute, 1944, pp. 57-63.

Murthy, G.S. 1975. Studies on the nature of resistance in *Cajanus cajan* (L.) Millsp. against wilt caused by *Fusarium udum* Butler. *Mysore Journal of Agricultural Sciences* 9 : 716-717.

Murthy, G.S. and Bagyaraj, D.J. 1978. Free amino nitrogen and amino acids in *Cajanus cajan* in relation to Fusarium wilt resistance. *Indian Phytopathology* 31 : 482-485.

Murthy, G.S. and Bagyaraj, D.J. 1980. Flavanol and alkaloid content of pigeonpea cultivars resistant and susceptible to *Fusarium udum*. *Indian Phytopathology* 33 : 633-634.

Murthy, G.S. and Bagyaraj, D.J. 1983. Nature of resistance in *Cajanus cajan* in relation to fusarial wilt. *Mysore Journal of Agricultural Sciences* 17 : 144-146.

Nafde, S.D., Mevada, K.D. and Patel, T.C. 1998. Effect of cultural practices to control wilt of pigeonpea. Pages 222 in Abstract of papers of National Symposium on Management of Biotic and Abiotic Stresses in Pulse Crops, 26-28 June 1998, IIPR, Kanpur, India. India: Indian Society of Pulses Research and Development.

Naik, M.K. and Reddy, M.V. 1992. Pathometry of Fusarium wilt of Pigeonpea. Pages 35-40 *in* Proceedings Annual Meeting of the IPS, 29-30 November, 1991, Directorate of Rice Research, Rajendranagar, Hyderabad, India. Indian Phytopathological Society.

Naik, M.K. and Reddy, M.V. 1993a. Pathometry of Fusarium wilt of pigeonpea. *Indian Phytopathology* 44 & 45 (Suppl.) : CXLI.

Naik, M.K., and Reddy, M.V. 1993b. Relationship between Fusarium wilt incidence and yield loss in pigeonpea. *International Pigeonpea Newsletter* 17 : 25-26.

Naik, M.K., Reddy, M.V. and Smith, D.H. 1992. Inoculum density and disease relationship in Fusarium wilt in pigeonpea. *International Pigeonpea Newsletter* 15 : 25-26.

Naik, M.K., Reddy, M.V. and Rego, T.J. 1994. Influence of production system on Fusarium wilt of pigeonpea. *Indian Phytopathology* 47 : 325 (Abstract).

Naik, M.K., Reddy, M.V. and McDonald, D. 1995. Ecology of Fusarium wilt of pigeonpea. *Indian Journal of Mycology and Plant Pathology* 25 : 50 (Abstract).

Naik, M.K., Reddy, M.V., Raju, T.N. and McDonald, D. 1997. Wilt incidence in sole and sorghum intercropped pigeonpea at different inoculum densities of *Fusarium udum*. *Indian Phytopathology* 50 : 337-341.

Natrajan, M., Kannaiyan, J., Willey, R.W. and Nene, Y.L. 1985. Studies on the effect of cropping system on Fusarium wilt of pigeonpea. *Field Crops Research* 10 : 333-346.

Nattrass, R.M. 1958. Report of the senior Plant Pathologist. Report Department of Agriculture, Kenya, 1956, Pt. 2. pp 9-14.

Nema, A.G. 1992. Studies on pectinolytic and cellulolytic enzymes produced by *Fusarium udum* causing wilt of pigeonpea. *Indian Journal of Forestry* 15 : 353-355.

Nene, Y.L. and Kannaiyan, J. 1982. Screening pigeonpea for resistance to Fusarium wilt. *Plant Disease* 66 : 306-307.

Nene, Y.L., Kannaiyan, J., Haware, M.P. and Reddy, M.V. 1980. Review of the work done at ICRISAT on soil borne disease of pigeonpea and chickpea. Pages 3-47 *in* Proceedings of the Consultants' Group Discussion on the Resistance to soil-borne Diseases of Legumes, 8-11 January 1979, ICRISAT, Hyderabad, India. Patancheru, A.P. 502324, India : International Crops Research Institute for the Semi-Arid Tropics.

Nene, Y.L., Kannaiyan, J. and Reddy, M.V. 1981a. Pigeonpea diseases : resistance-screening techniques. *Information Bulletin No. 9.* Patancheru, A.P., India : International Crops Research Institute for the Semi-Arid Tropics. 14 pp.

Nene, Y.L., Kannaiyan, J. and Reddy, M.V. 1981b. Resistance to major pigeonpea disease. Pages 121-128 *in* Proceedings of International Workshop on Pigeonpea, Vol. 1, 15-19 December 1980, ICRISAT Centre, Patancheru, India. India : International Crops Research Institute for Semi-Arid Tropics.

Nene, Y.L., Kannaiyan, J., Reddy, M.V., Zote, K.K., Mahmood, M., Hiremath, R.V., Shukla, P., Kotasthane, S.R., Sengupta, K., Jha, D.K., Haque, M.F., Grewal, J.S. and Pal, M. 1989. Multilocational testing of pigeonpea for broad based resistance to Fusarium wilt in India. *Indian Phytopathology* 42 : 449-453.

Nene, Y.L., Sarkar, Nandita, Bisht, V.S. and Sheila, V.K. 1992. Variability in growth characteristics of *Phytophthora drechsleri* f sp. *cajani* isolate. *International Pigeonpea Newsletter* 15 : 18-20.

Nene, Y.L., Sheila, V.K., Sarkar, Nandita and Reddy, M.V. 1991. Pathogenic variability among the isolates of *Phytophthora drechsleri* f sp. *cajani*. *International Pigeonpea Newsletter* No. 14 : 23-24.

Nene, Y.L., Sheila, V.K. and Sharma, S.B. 1996. A world list of chickpea and pigeonpea pathogens (Fifth edition). Patancheru, A.P., India. International Crops Research Institute in Semi Arid Tropics. pp. 27.

Nowell, W. 1923. Diseases of crop plants in the Lessey Antilles. London, UK : West Indian Comm. 383 pp.

Okirar, M.A. and Kimani P.M. 1997. Pathogenic variation of *Fusarium udum* of pigeonpea. *Indian Journal of Genetics and Plant Breeding* 57 : 186-192.

Okirar, M.A. 1999. Evaluation of pigeonpea germplasm for resistance to Fusarium wilt. *Indian Journal of Agricultural Sciences.* 69 : 600-601.

Padule, D.N., Newase, A.G. and Patil, B.P. 1982. Survey for incidence of Fusarium other diseases of pigeonpea in central parts of western Maharashtra. *Journal of Maharashtra Agricultural Universities* 7 (2) : 159-161.

Padwick, G.C. 1939. Report of the Imperial Mycologist. Scientific Reports of the Imperial Agricultural Research Institute, Pusa, 1937-38. pp. 105-112.

Padwick, G.W. 1940. The genus *Fusarium*. 5. *Fusarium udum* Butler. *F. vasinfectum* Atk. and *F.lateritium* var. *uncinatum* Wr. *Indian Journal of Agricultural Sciences* 10 : 863-878.

Padwick, G.W., Mitra, M. and Mehta, P.R. 1940. The genus *Fusarium*. IV. Infection and cross infection tests with isolates from cotton (*Gossypium* spp.), pigeonpea (*Cajanus cajan*) and sunnhemp (*Crotalaria juncea*). *Indian Journal of Agricultural Sciences*. 10 : 707-715.

Pal, B.P. 1934. Recent progress in Plant Breeding at Pusa-arhar. *Agriculture and Livestock in India* 4 : 511-512.

Pal, B.P., Shukla, A. and Rathi, Y.P.S. 1989a. Reaction of pigeonpea lines to sterility mosaic and phytophthora stem blight. *International Pigeonpea Newsletter* 10 : 25-26.

Pal, D., Kumar, Prashant, Sengupta, P.K. and Gupta, S. 1996. A comparative assessment of efficacy of conidia and chlamydospores of *Fusarium udum* in inducing wilt of pigeonpea. *Journal of Mycological Research* 34 : 87-92.

Pal, M. and Grewal, J.S. 1975a. Utilization of different nitrogen sources by *Phytophthora drechsleri* var *cajani*. *Indian Phytopathology* 28 : 499-501.

Pal, M. and Grewal, J.S. 1975b. Resistance of pigeonpea to phytophthora blight. 1. Total phenolic contents. *Indian Phytopathology* 28 : 559-560.

Pal, M. and Grewal, J.S. 1975c. Physiological studies on *Phytophthora drechsleri* var. *cajani*. *Indian Phytopathology* 28 : 479-482.

Pal, M. and Grewal, J.S. 1976a. Effect of NPK fertilizers on the Phytophthora blight of pigeonpea. *Indian Journal of Agricultural Sciences* 46 : 32-35.

Pal, M. and Grewal, J.S. 1976b. Resistance of pigeonpea to phytophthora blight. II. Total reducing and non-reducing sugars. *Indian Phytopathology* 29 : 429-431.

Pal, M. and Grewal, J.S. 1978. Growth of *Phytophthora drechsleri* var. *cajani* on different vitamins. *Indian Phytopathology* 31 : 356-538.

Pal, M. and Grewal, J.S. 1983. Chemical control of Phytophthora blight of Pigeonpea.*Indian Phytopathology* 36 : 380-381.

Pal, M. and Grewal, J.S. 1984. Zoosporangia formation of *Phytophthora drechsleri* var. *cajani* the causal organism of Phytophthora blight of pigeonpea. *Indian Phytopatholgy* 37 : 69-74.

Pal, M., Singh, Birendra and Bakshi, S.K. 1987. Evaluation of important varieties/lines of pigeonpea against Phytophthora blight and wilt. *Indian Phytopathology* 40 : 285.

Pal, M., Singh H., and Singh, Birendra, 1989b. Screening of pigeonpea genotypes for resistance to Phytophthora blight. *Indian Phytopathology* 42 : 296.

Pandey, B.K., Chaube, H.S. and Tripathi, H.S. 1987. Phytophthora blight of pigeonpea - a serious threat to pigeonpea cultivation in Tarai area of Nainital. *Indian Journal of Mycology and Plant Pathology* 17 : 110-11.

Pandey, D.K., Chandra, H. and Tripathi, N.N. 1982. Volatile fungitoxic activity of some higher plants with special reference to that of *Collistemone lanceolatus* DC. *Phytopathologische Zeitschrift* 105 : 175-182.

Pandey, D.K. Chandra, N., Tripathi, N.N. and Dixit, S.N. 1983. Toxicity of the essential oil of *Ageratum houstonianum* against *Fusarium lateritium* f sp. *cajani*. *Beitrage zur Biologie der Pflanzen* 58 : 115-122.

Pandey, K.K., Mishra, G.S. and Grover, S.K. 1976. Some studies on chemoserilants. I. Thiourea as fungus growth inhibitor. *Science and Culture* 42 : 476-477.

Pandey, K.K. and Upadhyay, J.P. 1999. Comparative study of chemical, biological and integrated approach for management of Fusarium wilt of pigeonpea. *Journal of Mycology and Plant Pathology* 29 : 214-216.

Pandey, R.N., Pawar, S.E. and Bhatia, C.R. 1995a. Effect of culture filtrate of *Fusarium udum* and fusaric acid on wilt susceptible and resistant pigeonpea cultivars. *Indian Phytopathology* 48 (4) : 444-448.

Pandey, R.N., Pawar, S.E. and Bhatia, C.R. 1995b. Improved laboratory screening technique for Fusarium wilt resistance in pigeonpea. *Indian Journal of Pulses Research* 8 : 45-49.

Pandey, R.N., Pawar, S.E. and Bhatia, C.R. 1996a. Inheritance of wilt resistance in pigeonpea. *Indian Journal of Genetics and Plant Breeding* 56 : 305-308.

Pandey, R.N. Pawar, S.E., Wanjari, K.B., Raut, B.T. and Bhatia, C.R. 1996b. Breeding pigeonpea for resistance to *Fusarium* wilt. *Indian Journal of Pulses Research*. 9 : 6-10.

Pandey, R.N., Pawar, S.E. and Bhatia, C.R. 1997. Interaction between *Fusarium udum* and wilt susceptible and resistant pigeonpea genotypes: Fungal growth and histopathology. *Indian Phytopathology* 50 : 53-58.

Parameswarappa, R., Rao, T.S. and Konda, C.R. 1987. ICPL 270 : a high yielding, wilt resistant variety of pigeonpea. *International Pigeonpea Newsletter* 6 : 20.

Parameswarappa, R., Rao, T.S., Konda, C.R., Rao. T.M., Raghumurthy, M., Emimath, V.S. and Sangappa, H.K. 1986. Maruthi—a wilt resistant red gram variety. *Current Research*, UAS Bangalore 15 (7/8) : 69-70.

Parveen, Kahkashan, Habib, Akhtar and Shukla, Prabhat Kumar. 1998. Effect of *Meloidogyne incognita* and *Fusarium udum* on disease development and growth of pigeonpea. Page 115 *in* the Abstract of papers of National Symposium on Management of Biotic and Abiotic Stresses in Pulse Crops, 26-28 June 1998, IIPR, Kanpur, India. India : Indian Society of Pulses Research and Development.

Patel, J.A., Nafde, S.D., Patel, D.B., Zaberi, P.P. and Pathak, A.R. 1988. Field screening of pigeonpea lines for resistance to wilt at Vadodara, Gujarat, India. *International Pigeonpea Newsletter* 27 : 27-28.

Patel, J.C., Vora, M.S. and Desai, B.G. 1981. Screening of pigeonpea lines for resistance to *Fusarium* wilt (*Fusarium udum* Butler) under natural conditions. *Pulse Crop Newsletter* 1 (4) : 51.

Patel, M.K. and Kamat, M.N. 1950. Control of plant disease through disease resistance in Bombay. *Poona Agricultural College Magazine* 40 : 6-11.

Patel, M.K., Kamat, M.N. and Bhide, V.P. 1949. Fungi of Bombay, Supplement I. *Indian Phytopathology* 2 : 149.

Patel, M.K. and Kulkarni, Y.S. 1949. Nitrogen utilization by *Xanthomonas malvacearum* (SM) Dowson. *Indian Phytopathology* 2 : 62-64.

Pathak, G.N. 1970. Redgram. Pages 14-53 *in* Pulse crops of India. ICAR, New Delhi, India.

Patil, B.G. and Sable, J.E. 1973. A note on the screening of tur against wilt disease. *Punjabrao Krishi Vidyapeeth Research Journal* 2 : 73-76.

Patil, P.Y. and Patil, B.P. 1993. Studies on wilt disease of pigeonpea with reference to physiologic races. *Indian Phytopathology* 44 & 45 (Suppl.) : XXI.

Pawar, K.B., Bendre, N.J. and Deshmukh, R.B. 1992. Screening of pigeonpea lines against *Fusarium* wilt. *International Pigeonpea Newsletter* 16 : 17.

Pawar, K.B., Bhor, S.B., Bendre, N.J. and Deshmukh, R.B. 1993. Evaluation of pigeonpea lines for wilt resistance. *Indian Journal of Pulses Research* 6 : 112 - 114.

Pawar, N.B. and Banchod, S.B. 1994. Screening of pigeonpea genotypes against *Fusarium* wilt. *Indian Phytopathology*. 47 : 348.

Pawar, N.B. and Mayee, C.D. 1983a. Combining ability analysis of resistance in pigeonpea (*Cajanus cajan* (L.) Millsp.) to wilt caused by *Fusarium udum* Butler. *Indian Phytopathology* 36 : 185.

Pawar, N.B. and Mayee, C.D. 1983b. Virulence differences in *Fusarium udum* isolates from Maharashtra State. *International Pigeonpea Newsletter* 2 : 41-42.

Pawar, N.B. and Mayee, C.D. 1986. Reaction of pigeonpea genotypes and their crosses to *Fusarium* wilt. *Indian Phytopathology* 39 : 70-74.

Petrak, F. and Sydow, H. 1925. Krtisch Systematische Originluntersuchungen uber Pyrenomyzeten, Sphaeropsideen, und Melanconieen. *Annals, Mycol* 23 : 209-294.

Phelps, R.H., Oudit, I.L. and Page, C. 1974. Sclerotium blight, *Sclerotium rolfsii*, a new disease of pigeonpea, *Cajanus cajan*. Proceeding of the Caribbean Crop Protection Symposium on Horticultural Crops. pp. 63-70.

Plymen, F.J. 1933. Report of the Department of Agriculture, Central Provinces, Nagpur, 1932-33, pp. 40.

Podile, A.R. and Dube, H.C. 1987. Antagonism of *Bacillus subtilis* to *Phytophthora drechsleri* f sp. *cajani*. *Indian Phytopathology* 40 : 503-506.

Potdukhe, S.R., Raut, B.T. and Sonwane, G.J. 1998. Effect of seed treatment and foliar application of fungicides on stem canker of pigeonpea. Pages 85-86 *in* Abstract of papers of National Symposium on Management of Biotic and Abiotic Stresses in Pulse Crops, 26-28 June 1998, IIPR, Kanpur, India. India : Indian Society of Pulses Research and Development.

Prasad, G.S., Podile, A.R. and Dube, H.C. 1988. Regulation of xylanase synthesis and activity in *Fusarium oxysporum* f sp. *udum*. *Indian Phytopathology* 41 : 443 - 449.

Prasad, Laxman and Khan, R.U. 1998. Influence of different levels of inoculum of *Fusarium udum* on mortality and final plant stand of pigeonpea. Page 117 *in* Abstract of papers of National Symposium on Management of Biotic and Abiotic Stresses in Pulse Crops, 26-28 June 1998, IIPR, Kanpur, India. India: Indian Society of Pulses Research and Development.

Prasad, M. and Chaudhary, S.K. 1965. Studies on the effects of carbon and nitrogen on macro-conidial, micro-conidial and chlamydospore production in *Fusarium udum* Butler. Proceedings of the National Academy of Sciences of India, Section B 35 : 171 - 181.

Prasad, M. and Chaudhary, S.K. 1966. Studies on the effect of different phosphorus concentrations on the production of chlamydospores, micro-conidia and macro-conidia in the culture of *Fusarium udum* Butler. *Proceedings of the National Academy of Sciences, India, Section* B 36 : 43-48.

Prasad, M. and Chaudhary, S.K. 1967. Effect of sulphur on sporulation of *Fusarium udum* Butler. *Journal of the Indian Botanical Society 46* : 45-51.

Prasad, M. and Chaudhary, S.K. 1973. Variations in amino acids and sugars and their effect on growth and sporulation in *Fusaruim oxysporum* f. *udum*. Phytopathologische Zeitschrift 78 : 147-151.

Prasad, M. and Chaudhary, S.K. 1974a. Amino acids and fusaric acid production in tissues of *Cajanus cajan* infected with *Fusarium oxysporum* f. *udum* pathogenic fungi. *Phytopathologische Zeitschrift* 81 : 339-345.

Prasad, M. and Chaudhary, S.K. 1974b. *In vitro* production of fusaric acid and its impact on growth and sporulation in *Fusarium oxysporum* f. *udum*. *Phytopathologische Zeitschrift* 80 : 279-282.

Prasad, M. and Chaudhary, S.K. 1975. Influence of vitamins on growth and sporulation of *Fusarium oxysporum* f *udum*. *Phytopathologische Zeitschrift* 82 : 56-62.

Prasad, M. and Chaudhary, S.K. 1976. Influence of IAA and GA on mycelial output and sporulation of varied spore forms of *Fusarium oxysporum* f *udum*. *Indian Phytopathology* 29 : 193-194.

Prasad, M. and Chaudhary, S.K. 1977a. Effect of different concentrations of D1-isoleucine, D1-valine and D1-alanine on growth and sporulation in *Fusarium oxysporum* f *udum* (Butl.) Sn. et H. *Zentralblatt fur Bakterialogie, Parasitenkunde, Infections Krankheiten und Hygiene* 132 : 735-739.

Prasad, M. and Chaudhary, S.K. 1977b. Relations of pH levels and varied nutrients media to growth and sporulation of *Fusarium oxysporum* f *udum* (Butler) Sn. et H. *Research Journal of Ranchi University* 13 : 214-222.

Prasad, M. and Chaudhary, S.K. 1978. Effect of C.C.C.2-(Chloroethyl), trimethyl Ammonium chloride on growth and sporulation in *Fusarium oxysporum* f *udum* (Butler) Sn. et H. *Zent Bacteriol Parasiten Infect. Hygiene* 133 : 86.

Prasad, N. 1978. Status of fusarial wilts. *Indian Journal of Mycology and Plant Pathology* 8 : 5-18.

Preston, N.W. 1977. Cajanone : an antifungal isoflavanone from *Cajanus cajan*. *Phytochemistry* 16 : 144-145.

Purkayastha, R.P. and Chattopadhyay, M. 1975. Antibiotic sensitivity of normal and amino-deficient mutants of *Fusarium udum* in relation to control of wilt disease of *Cajanus cajan* (L.) Millsp. *Indian Journal of Experimental Biology* 13 : 58-60.

Purkayashtha, R.P. and Das, A. 1973. Amino acids associated with pathogenicity of UV-induced mutants of *Fusarium udum* inciting wilt of pigeonpea. *Proceedings of the Indian Science Congress* 60 : 357 (Abstract).

Purseglove, J.W. 1968. Tropical crops, Dicotyledons 1. London, UK: Longmans, p. 240.

Raguchander, T. and Arjunan, G. 1996. Performance of pigeonpea genotypes against wilt. *Current Research* UAS 25 (1) : 21.

Rai, Bharat and Upadhyay, R.S. 1979a. *Micromonospora globosa* Krassilnikov : destructive parasite of *Fusarium udum* Butler. *Microbios Letters* 8 : 123-128.

Rai, Bharat and Upadhyay, R.S. 1979b. Discovery of prefect state of *Fusarium udum* Butler. Proceedings of the Annual Conference of the Society of Advance Botany 5 : 25.

Rai Bharat and Upadhyay, R.S. 1982. *Gibberella indica* perfect state of *Fusarium udum*, *Mycologia* 74 (2) : 343 - 346.

Rai, Bharat and Upadhyay, R.S. 1983. Competitive saprophytic colonization of pigeonpea substrate by *Fusarium udum* in relation to environmental factors, chemical treatments and microbial antagonism. *Soil Biol. Biochemistry* 15 : 187.

Rai, Bharat, Upahdyay, R.S. and Gupta, R.C. 1978. Resting body formation by *Fusarium udum* inside sporangiophores of *Rhizopus nigricans* during hyphal parasitism. *Microbios Letters* 6 : 125-27.

Rai, P.K. 1994. Effect of some plant growth regulators on *Phytophthora drechsleri* f sp. *cajani*. *Crop Research (Hisar)* - 8 : 155-158.

Rai, P.K. and Singh, K.P. 1995. Efficacy of certain oil cake amendments on *Heterodera cajani, Fusarium udum* and associates wilt of pigeonpea. *International Journal of Tropical Plant Diseases* 13 (2) : 213-219.

Rai, P.K. and Singh, K.P. 1996. Pathogenicity and histopathology of *Heterodera cajani* and two isolates of *Fusarium udum* on pigeonpea. *National Academy of Science Letters* 19 : 4-7.

Raina, Rajni and Singh, U.P. 1996. Inheritance of wilt resistance in pigeonpea. *Indian Journal of Pulses Research* 9 : 187-188.

Rajdan, V.K. 1985. Studies on phytophthora blight of pigeonpea with special reference to survival and control. M.Sc. thesis G.B.P. U. A. Technology, Pantnagar, 111 pp.

Rajendra, M.M. 1993. Pathogenic variation in wilt of pigeonpea in summer and kharif seasons. *Indian Phytopathology* 44 & 45 (Suppl.) : XXI (Abstract).

Rajendra, M.M. and Patil, P.L., 1992a. Interaction studies on *Fusarium udum* causing wilt of pigeonpea. *Journal of Maharashtra Agricultural Universities* 17 : 350-351.

Rajendra, M.M. and Patil, P.L. 1992b. Morphological, cultural and physiological variation in *Fusarium udum* Butler. *Journal of Maharashtra Agricultural Universities* 17 : 465-467.

Rajendra, M.M. and Patil, P.L. 1993a. Reaction of some pigeonpea cultivars to Fusarium wilt. *Journal of Maharashtra Agricultural Universities* 18 : 116-117.

Rajendra, M.M. and Patil, P.L. 1993b. A Study of Fusarium wilt pathogen of pigeonpea. *Journal of Maharshtra Agricultural Universities* 18 : 123-124.

Rajkule, P.N., Goyal, S.N. and Vala, D.G. 1989. Screening of pigeonpea varieties against *Fusarium* wilt. *International Pigeonpea Newsletter* 9 : 24.

·Raju, T.N. and Reddy, M.V. 1993. Integrated management of phytophthora blight of pigeonpea. *Indian Phytopathology* 44 & 45 (Suppl.) : VIII.

Ramana, M.V., Rao, C.R. and Reddy, M.V. 1999. Sources of resistance to macrophomina stem canker in red gram. *Agricultural Science Digest (Karnal)* 19 : 15-17.

Rangel, E. 1915. Fungus parasites of pigeonpea (*Cajanus indicus* Spreng.). *Boletim de Agricultura Sao Paulo* 16 : 145-156.

Rathi, Y.P.S. and Lal, S. 1977. Wilt disease of pigeonpea caused by *Macrophomina phaseoli. Acta Botanica Indica* 5 : 83-84.

Raut, N.K. and Bhombe, B.B. 1971. A review of the work of selection of tur varieties resistant to Fusarium wilt at College of Agriculture, Parbhani (MS.). *Magazine, College of Agriculture Parbhani* 12 : 37-42.

Ravishankar, 1936. Isolation of wilt resistant tur. *Nagpur Agricultural College Magazine* 10 : 162-167.

Raychaudhuri, S.P. 1941. Studies on the canker disease of pigeonpea (*Cajanus cajan* (L.) Millsp.) caused by *Diplodia cajani* Nov. sp. Thesis, Indian Agricultural Research Institute, New Delhi, India.

Raychaudhuri, S.P. 1942. A disease of pigeonpea (*Cajanus cajan* (L.) Millsp.) caused by *Diplodia cajani* Spec. Nov. *Indian Journal of Agricultural Sciences* 12 : 837-847.

Raychaudhuri, S.P. 1947. Further studies on *Diplodia cajani* Raychaudhuri. *Journal of the Indian Botanical Society* 26 : 221-225.

Raychaudhuri, S.P. 1968. Diseases of pulse pose a challenge to Plant Pathologists, breeders. *Indian Farming* 17 : 39-43.

Reddy, M.V. and Jain, K.C., 1992. Recent advances in breeding for disease resistance in pigeonpea. Pages 77-83 *in* New Frontiers in Pulses Research and Development : Proceedings of National Symposium, 10-12 November, 1989 at DPR, Kanpur, India.

Reddy, M.V., Narayana Rao, J. and Krishna, R.K. 1989a. Influence of vesicular and arbuscular mycorrhyzae on Fusarium wilt of pigeonpea. *International Pigeonpea Newsletter* 9 : 23.

Reddy, M.V., Nene, Y.L., Kannaiyan, J., Raju, T.N., Saka, V.W., Daudi, A.T., Songa, W.P. and Omanga, P. 1990a. Pigeonpea lines resistant to wilt in Kenya and Malawi. *International Pigeonpea Newsletter* 12 : 25-26.

Reddy, M.V., Nene, Y.L., Raju, T.N., Sheila, V.K., Kannaiyan, J. and Beniwal, S.P.S. 1989b. Evaluation of pigeonpea lines for resistance to wilt, sterility mosaic and phytophthora blight. *International Pigeonpea Newsletter* 10 : 22-24.

Reddy, M.V., Nene, Y.L., Raju, T.N., Sheila, V.K., Sarkar, Nandita, Remanandan, P. and Amin, K.S. 1991. Pigeonpea lines field resistant to phytophthora blight. *International Pigeonpea Newsletter* 13 : 20-22.

Reddy, M.V. and Raju, T.N. 1993. Investigations on pathogenic variability in the pigeonpea wilt pathogen, *Fusarium udum*. *Indian phytopathology* 44 & 45 (Suppl.) : CXI.

Reddy, M.V., Raju, T.N. 1996. Infection and colonization of pigeonpea genotypes with different degrees of susceptibility to wilt by *Fusarium udum*. *Indian Phytopathology* 49 : 384-386.

Reddy, M.V., Raju, T.N. and Chauhan, Y.S. 1994. More pigeonpea biomass more Fusarium wilt susceptibility - a hypothesis. *International Chickpea and Pigeonpea Newsletter* 1 : 35-36.

Reddy, M.V., Raju, T.N. and Naik, M.K. 1993a. Infection and colonization of *Fusarium udum* in pigeonpea. *Indian Phytopathology* 46 : 268 (Abst.).

Reddy, M.V., Raju, T.N., Naik, M.K., Chauhan, Y.S., Ariyanayagam, R.P. and Singh, N.B. 1993b. Field resistance in extra short duration pigeonpea lines to dry root rot. *International Pigeonpea Newsletter* 17 : 32-33.

Reddy, M.V., Raju, T.N. and Nene, Y.L. 1988. Low wilt incidence in short duration pigeonpeas. *International Pigeonpea Newsletter* 7 : 26.

Reddy, M.V., Raju, T.N. and Nene, Y.L. 1990b. Disease debris field inoculation technique for phytophthora blight of pigeonpea. *International Pigeonpea Newsletter* 12 : 23 - 25.

Reddy, M.V., Raju, T.N. and Saxena, K.B. 1992a. Effectiveness of hill plots in screening pigeonpea for resistance to Fusarium wilt. *Indian Journal of Pulses Research* 5 : 45-48.

Reddy, M.V., Raju, T.N., Sharma, S.B., Nene, Y.L. and McDonald, D. 1993c. Handbook of pigeonpea diseases. Patancheru, India : *ICRISAT Information Bulletin* No. 42. pp 61.

Reddy, M.V., Raju, T.N. and Sheila, V.K. 1996. Phytophthora blight resistance in wild pigeonpea. *International Chickpea and Pigeonpea Newsletter* 3 : 52-53.

Reddy, M.V., Raju, T.N., Sheila, V.K., Sarkar, Nandita, Nene, Y.L., Remanandan, P. and Amin, K.S. 1990c. Identification of pigeonpea lines field tolerant to phytophthora blight. *Indian Phytopathology* 43 : 243.

Reddy, M.V. Sarkar, Nandita, Nene, Y.L. and Raju, T.N. 1992b. Predisposing factors for phytophthora blight of pigeonpea. *Indian Phytopathology* 45 : 268-270.

Reddy, M.V., Sharma, S.B., Jaysekara, S.J.B.A. and Faris, D.G. 1992c. Assessment of diseases on short duration pigeonpea in Sri Lanka. *International Pigeonpea Newsletter* 15 : 15- 17.

Reddy, M.V., Saxena, K.B., Singh, O., Karna, R.S.L., Sahu, R., Bharti, M.P. and Sah, R.P. 1989c. Macrophomina stem canker of pigeonpea in Nepal. *International Pigeonpea Newsletter* 9 : 22-23.

Reddy, M.V., Sharma, S.B. and Nene, Y.L. 1990d. Pigeonpea disease management. Pages 303-348 *in* Pigeonpea (Eds. Y.L. Nene, Susan D. Hall and V.K. Sheila). CAB, International, U.K., ICRISAT, Patancheru, India.

Reddy, M.V. and Sheila, V.K. 1994. Phytophthora blight of pigeonpea: Present status and future priorities. *International Journal of Pest Management* 40 : 98-102.

Reddy, M.V., Subramanayam, P., Likoswe, A.A., Saka, V.W. and Msuku, W.A.B. 1992d. Survey of pigeonpea diseases in Malawi. *International Pigeonpea Newsletter* 15 : 24-25.

Reddy, M.V., Subramanyam, P., Likoswe, A.A., Saka, V.W., Msuku, W.A.B. 1993d. Pigeonpea diseases in Malawi. *FAO Plant Protection Bulletin* 41 : 101-106.

Reddy, N.P.E. and Chaudhary, K.C.B. 1985. Variation in *Fusarium udum*. *Indian Phytopathology* 38 : 172-173.

Reddy, N.P.E. and Chaudhary, K.C.B. 1990. Effect of culture filtrate of *Fusarium udum* on the seeds of pigeonpea. *Madras Agricultural Journal* 77 : 109-111.

Rodriguez, R. and Melendez, P.L. 1985. Identification of *in vitro* resistance to pigeonpea (*Cajanus cajan* (L.) Millsp.) to phytophthora stem canker. *The Journal of Agricultural University, Puerto Rico* 69 : 11-17.

Sadasivan, T.S. and Subramanian, C.V. 1954. Recent advances in the study of soil borne *Fusaria. Journal of the Indian Botanical Society* 33 : 162- 176.

Saka, V.W., Msuku, W.A.B., Subramanyam, P., Tuwafe, S. and Banda, A.C. 1995. Pathogenic variability in *Fusarium udum*, the incitant of wilt of pigeonpea. Pages 64-68, *in* Improvement of pigeonpea in eastern and southern Africa: Annual Research Planning Meeting 1994, Nairobi, Kenya, 21-23 Sept. 1994 (Eds. S.N.Silim, S.B. King and S. Tuwafe). Patancheru, India, International Crops Research Institute for the Semi-Arid Tropics.

Saksena, H.K. 1980. Epidemiology of diseases caused by *Rhizoctonia* spp. Pages 59-64 *in* Proceedings of the Consultants Group Discussion on the Resistance to Soil-borne Diseases of Legumes, 8-11 Jan. 1979, ICRISAT, Hyderabad, India.

Salam, M.A. and Khan, M.W. 1986. Reaction of some cultivars of pigeonpea against *Fusarium udum* and *Meloidogyne javanica*. *International Nematological Network Newsletter* 3 : 16-17.

Samajpati, J. 1973. Interaction of near ultraviolet radiation and hydrogen-ion concentration on growth and sporulation of *Fusarium udum* Butler. *Science and Culture* 39 : 127-129.

Samuels, G.J. and Singh, B. 1986. *Botryosphaeria xanthocephala,* cause of stem canker in pigeonpea. *Transaction of British Mycological Society* 86 : 295-299.

Saraswathi, T. and Pal, M. 1986. Chemical and biological management of collar rot of pigeonpea caused by *Sclerotium rolfsii. Indian Phytopathology* 39 : 146.

Sarkar, Nandita 1988, Taxonomic and epidemiological studies on phytophthora blight of pigeonpea. Pulse Pathology (Pigeonpea) Progress Report 52, Patancheru, A.P., India, Legume Programme, ICRISAT, 43 pp.

Sarkar, Nandita, Nene, Y.L., Reddy, M.V. and Sheila, V.K. 1992. Influence of Plant age on susceptibility of pigeonpea to Phytophthora blight. *Indian Phytopathology* 45; 426-429.

Sarkar, Nandita, Sheila, V.K. and Nene, Y.L. 1991. Host range of pigeonpea *Phytophthora. International Pigeonpea Newsletter* 14 : 24-25.

Sarojini, T.S. 1950. Soil conditions and root diseases I. Micronutrients - elements and disease development of *Fusarium udum* on red gram. *Journal of the Madras University,* Section B 19 : 1-32.

Sarojini, T.S. 1951. Soil conditions and root diseases. II. *Fusarium udum* disease of red gram (*Cajanus cajan* (L.) Millsp.). *Proceedings of the Indian Academy of Sciences*, Section B 33 : 49-68.

Sarojini, T.S. 1954. Soil conditions and root diseases. XI. *Neocosmospora vasinfecta* Smith disease of *Cajanus cajan*. *Journal of the Madras University*, Section B 24 : 137- 142.

Sarojini, T.S. and Yogeswari, L. 1947. Aeration affecting growth and sporulation of some Fusaria in liquid cultures. *Proceedings of the Indian Academy of Science*, Section B 26 : 69-76.

Satyanarayana, G. and Kalyanasundaram, R. 1952. Soil conditions and root disease. V. Symptomatology of wilted cotton and red gram. *Proceedings of the Indian Academy of Sciences*, Section B 36 : 54-58.

Saxena, K.B., Reddy, M.V., Bhagwat, V.R. and Sharma, S.B. 1996. Preliminary studies on the incidence of major diseases and insects in *Cajanus platycarpus* germplasm at ICRISAT Asia Centre.

Saxena, Moly, Saxena, D.R. and Kataria, V.P. 1998. Response of pigeonpea genotypes to biotic stresses. Page 38-39. *in* Abstracts of papers of National Symposium on Management of Biotic and Abiotic stresses in Pulse Crops, 26-28 June 1998, IIPR, Kanpur, India. Indian Society of Pulses Research and Development.

Sen Gupta, P.K. 1974. Plant Pathogenic species of the genus *Fusarium* in India. *Nova Hedwigia* 25 : 699-717.

Sethuraman, K. and Vidyasekaran, P. 1994. Effective control of pigeonpea wilt by *Pseudomonas fluorescens. Indian Phytopathology* 47 : 289.

Sharma, D., Kannaiyan, J. and Reddy, L.J. 1982. Inheritance of resistance to blight in pigeonpea. *Plant Disease* 66 : 22-25.

Sharma, H.C. 1963. Growth and sporulation of *Fusarium udum* in relation to C/N ratio and nitrogen sources. *Physiologia Plantarum* 16 : 276-280.

Sharma, H.C. 1988. Selection and development of wilt resistant pigeonpea lines for Tawa command area in central India. *International Pigeonpea Newsletter* 7 : 9-10.

Sharma, H.C., Dixit, J.P. and Saran, R.N. 1987. Effect of inter-crops and irrigation levels on the incidence of pigeonpea wilt caused by *Fusarium udum* Butler. *Indian Journal of Agricultural Sciences* 57 : 650-652.

Sharma, N.D., Joshi, L.K. and Vyas, S.C. 1977. A new stem inoculation technique for testing Fusarium wilt of pigeonpea. *Indian Phytopathology* 30 : 406-407.

Sharma, R.P.R. 1980. Red gram breaks the rule. *Seed and Farms* 6 : 29-30.

Sharma, S.B. and Nene, Y.L. 1989. Interrelationship between *Heterodera cajani* and *Fusarium udum* in pigeonpea. *Nematologia* 19 : 21-28.

Sharma, S.B. and Nene, Y.L. 1990. Effect of *Fusarium udum* alone and in combination with *Rotylenchulus reniforms* or *Meloidogyne* spp. on wilt incidence, growth of pigeonpea and multiplication of nematodes. *International Journal of Tropical Plant Disease* 8 : 95-101.

Sharma, Y.R. and Singh, Harjinder. 1996. Survival of *Phytophthora drechsleri* f sp. *cajani* in the infected stubbles of pigeonpea. *Indian Journal of Pulses Research* 9 : 217-218.

Shaw, F.J.F. 1936. Studies in Indian pulses : The inheritance of morphological characters and wilt resistance in arhar (*Cajanus indicus* Spreng.). *Indian Journal of Agricultural Sciences*. 6 : 139-187.

Shaw, F.J.F. and Kashi Ram 1934. Improved varieties of crops produced at Pusa. *Agriculture and Livestock in India*, 4 : 465-480.

Sheila, V.K. and Nene, Y.L. 1987. Effect of phytoalexin formulation against *Phytophthora drechsleri* f sp. *cajani. International Pigeonpea Newsletter* 6 : 61-62.

Sheila, V.K., Nene, Y.L. and Kannaiyan, J. 1983. A simple culture medium for *Phytophthora drechsleri* f sp. *cajani. Indian Phytopathology* 36 : 152-154.

Sheldrake, A.R., Narayanan, A. and Kannaiyan, J. 1978. Some effects of the physiological state of pigeonpea on the incidence of the wilt disease. *Tropical Grain Legume Bulletin* 11. 1224-25.

Shinde, V.K. and Zote, K.K. 1993. Management of wilt and sterility mosaic through resistance breeding in pigeonpea (*Cajanus cajan*). *Indian Journal of Pulses Research* 6 : 60-63.

Shirshikar, S.P. and Ashtaputre, J.U. 1993. Effect of different crop rotations on the incidence of Fusarium wilt in pigeonpea. *Indian Phytopathology* 44 & 45 (Suppl.) . XXI.

Shrishikar, S.P., Ashtaputre, J.U., Shinde, V.K. and Deshmukh, R.B. 1990. Screening of pigeonpea entries against wilt and sterility mosaic disease. *Indian Phytopathology* 43 : 307.

Shit, S.K. and Sen Gupta, P.K. 1978. Possible existence of physiological races of *Fusarium oxysporum* f sp. *udum*, the incitant of the wilt of pigeonpea. *Indian Journal of Agricultural Sciences* 48 : 629-632.

Shit, S.K. and Sen Gupta, P.K. 1980. Pathogenic and enzymic variation in *Fusarium oxysporum* f sp.*udum*. *Indian Journal of Microbiology* 20 : 46-48.

Shukla, D.S. 1975. Incidence of Fusarium wilt of pigeonpea in relation to soil composition. *Indian Phytopathology* 28 : 395-396.

Siddiqui, Z.A. and Mahmood, I. 1996a, Biological control of *Heterodera cajani* and *Fusarium udum* on pigeonpea by *Glomus mosseae, Trichoderma harzianum* and *Verticillium chlamydosporium*. *Israel Journal of Plant Sciences* 44 : 49-56.

Siddiqui, Z.A. and Mahmood, I. 1996b. Effect of *Heterodera cajani, Meloidogyne incognita* and *Fusarium udum* on the wilt disease complex of pigeonpea. *Indian Journal of Nematology* 26 : 102-104.

Sideris, C.P. 1929. Pythiaceous root parasites of various agricultural plants. *Phytopathology* 19 : 1140.

Sideris, C.P. 1932. Taxonomic studies in the family Pythiaceae. II. *Pythium*. *Mycologia* 24 : 14-61.

Singh, A.P. and Bhargava, S.N. 1981. Survival studies on three species of *Fusarium* causing wilt of pigeonpea. *Phytopathologische Zeitschrift* 100 : 300 - 311.

Singh Birendra, Chaturvedi, S.N. and Singh, R.H. 1999. Effect of metalaxyl on phytophthora blight, seed germination and seedling vigour of pigeonpea. *Seed Research* 27 : 213-216.

Singh, Birendra, Chaturvedi, S.N. and Singh, R.H. 1999a. Influence of herbicides on the antifungal activity of some fungicides against phytophthora blight of pigeonpea. *Indian Phytopathology* 52 : 59-62.

Singh, B.V., Pandya, B.P. and Rathi, Y.P.S. 1985. Field screening of pigeonpea lines for resistance to phytophthora blight at Pantnagar, India. *International Pigeonpea Newsletter* 4 : 34 - 35.

Singh, D.V. and Mishra, A.N. 1976. Search of wilt resistant varieties of red gram in Uttar Pradesh. *Indian Journal of Mycology and Plant Pathology* 6 : 89.

Singh, G., Kapoor, Shashi, Verma, M.M. and Bhan, L.K. 1986. Field resistance of pigeonpea varieties to Phoma stem canker and leaf spot caused by *Phoma cajani*. *International Pigeonpea Newsletter* 5 : 34-36.

Singh, G.P. and Hussain, A. 1962. Production of pectic and cellulolytic enzymes by arhar wilt fungus. *Current Science* 31 : 110-112.

Singh, G.P. and Hussain, A. 1964. Presence of fusaric acid in wilt affected pigeonpea plants *Current Science* 33 : 287.

Singh, G.P. and Hussain, A. 1968. Role of enzymes in pathogenesis by *Fusarium lateritium* f *cajani*. *Indian Phytopathology* 21 : 361-73.

Singh, G.P. and Hussain, A. 1970. Role of toxic metabolites of *Fusarium lateritium* f *cajani* (Padw.) Gord. in the development of pigeonpea wilt. *Proceedings of the National Academy of Sciences of India,* Section B 40 : 9-15.

Singh, Harjinder and Sharma, Y.R. 1996. Efficacy of fungicides for the control of phytophthora blight of pigeonpea. *Plant Disease Research* 11 : 59-62.

Singh, H.B., Upadhyay, D.N. and Saha, L.R. 1987. Collar rot of pigeonpea in Nagaland, India. *International Pigeonpea Newsletter* No. 6 : 52-53.

Singh, I.P. and Vishwadhar. 1997. Allelic relationship among genes for resistance to Fusarium wilt of pigeonpea. *Indian Journal of Pulses Research* 10 : 74-77.

Singh, K.P. 1980. The association of *Gibberella udum* with the wilted arhar plants recorded again. *Indian Phytopathology* 33 : 161.

Singh, K.P. and Edward, J.C. 1978. *Gibberella* associated with wilted plants of arhar with its asexual *Fusarium* stage. *Allahabad Farmer* 49 : 91-94.

Singh, K.P. and Singh, R.S. 1987. Development of suppressiveness in two wilt sick soils. *Indian Journal of Mycology and Plant Pathology,* 17: 104 (Abstract).

Singh, Leena, and Shrivastava, S.N. 1985. Studies on the morphology and taxonomy of *Colletotrichum* spp. parasitizing pulse crops in northern India. *Indian Phytopathology* 38 : 616-617.

Singh, N. and Singh, R.S. 1970. Development of wilt causing species of *Fusarium* in fungicide treated soils. *Indian Phytopathology* 23 : 545-552.

Singh, N. and Singh, R.S. 1980a. Inhibition of *Fusarium oxysporum* fsp. *udum* by soil bacteria. *Indian Phytopathology* 33 : 356-357.

Singh, N. and Singh, R.S., 1980b. Lysis of *Fusarium oxysporum* f sp. *udum* caused by soil amendments with organic matter. *Indian Journal of Mycology and Plant Pathology* 10 : 146.

Singh, N. and Singh, R.S. 1981. Lysis of mycelium of *Fusarium oxysporum* f sp. *udum* in soil amended with organic matter. *Plant and Soil* 59 : 9.

Singh, N. and Singh, R.S. 1982a. Population dyanamics of *Fusarium udum* in saw dust amended soil. *Acta Botanica Indica* 10 (2) : 267-272.

Singh, N. and Singh, R.S. 1982b. Effect of oil cake amended soil atmosphere on pigeonpea wilt pathogen. *Indian Phytopathology* 35 : 300-305.

Singh, N. and Singh, R.S. 1983a. Development of *Fusarium udum* (Pigeonpea wilt pathogen) in oil cake amended soil. *Indian Botanical Reporter* 2 : 116.

Singh, N. and Singh, R.S. 1983b. Abundance of *Fusarium udum* in rice husk amended soil. *Indian Phytopathology* 36 : 307-311.

Singh, N. and Singh, R.S. 1983c. Chlamydospore formations in *Fusarium udum* by soil bacteria. *Indian Phytopathology* 36 : 164-167.

Singh, N. and Singh, R.S. 1983d. Inhibition of *Fusarium udum* (pigeonpea wilt pathogen) by ether distillate of margosa cake amended soil. *Indian Journal of Mycology and Plant Pathology* 13 : 329-330.

Singh, N.B., Reddy, M.V., Nageswara Rao, A., Raju, T.N., Singh Laxman and Gupta, S.C. 1996a. Newly developed extra short duration and short duration lines with combined resistance to wilt and sterility mosaic. *International Chickpea and Pigeonpea Newsletter* 3 : 87.

Singh, P., Vasudeva, R.S. and Bajaj, B.S. 1965. Seed bacterization and biological activity of bulbiformin. *Annals of Applied Biology* 55 : 89-97.

Singh, R., Jariwala, S. and Rai, B. 1996b. Effect of soil solarization on wilt disease of pigeonpea (*Cajanus cajan* (L.) Millsp). *Phytopathologia Polonica* 12 ; 139-146.

Singh, R.H. and Pal Mahendra 1990. Occurrence of pathological strains of *Fusarium udum* causing wilt of pigeonpea. *Indian Phytopathology* 43 : 255 (Abstract).

Singh, R.H. and Singh, U.P. 1994. Studies on the nutrition of *Phytophthora drechsleri* f sp. *cajani* causing pigeonpea blight. *Indian Phytopathology* 47 : 296 (Abst.).

Singh, R.S. 1974. Effect of host and non-host crops seeds on vegetative growth and sporulation of *Fusarium udum* in soil. *Indian Phytopathology* 27 : 553-557.

Singh R.S. and Singh, N. 1970. Effect of oil-cake amendment of soil on population of some wilt causing species of *Fusarium*. *Phytopathologische Zeitschrift* 26 : 160-167.

Singh, S.K. and Nene, Y.L. 1990. Cross inoculation studies on *Rhizoctonia bataticola* isolates from different crops. *Indian Phytopathology* 43 : 446-448.

Singh, U.P. and Chauhan, V.B. 1985a. Relationships between field levels and light and darkness on the development of phytophthora blight of pigeonpea (*Cajanus cajan* (L.) Millsp.). *Phytopathologische Zeitschrift* 114 : 160-167.

Singh, U.P. and Chauhan, V.B. 1985b. A suitable criterion for identifying resistance in pigeonpea against *Phytophthora drechsleri* f sp. *cajani*. *Agricultural Research and Rural Development* 8 : 46.

Singh, U.P. and Chauhan, V.B. 1988a. Oospore formation in *Phytophthora drechsleri* f sp. *cajani*. *Phytopathologische Zeitschrift* 123 : 89.

Singh, U.P. and Chauhan, V.B. 1988b. Effect of temperature on germination of zoospores of *Phytophthora drechsleri* f sp. *cajani*. *Indian Phytopathology* 41 : 80-85.

Singh, U.P. and Chauhan, V.B. 1992. Phytophthora blight of pigeonpea. Pages 375-387 in Plant Diseases of International Importance (Eds. U.S. Singh, A.N. Mukhopadhyay, J.Kumar and H.S. Chaube) Englewood Cliffs, New Jersy, USA : Prantice Hall Inc.

Singh, U.P., Chauhan, V.B., Wanger, K.G. and Anil Kumar. 1992. Effect of ajoene, a compound derived from garlic (*Allium sativum*) on *Phytophthora drechsleri* f sp. *cajani*. *Mycologia* 84 : 105-108.

Singh, U.P., Prithiviraj, B., Khiste, S., Kumar, Vinod, Srivastava, J.S. and Manickam, M. 1999b. Effect of *Cyperus rotundus* rhizome extract on *Fusarium udum*. *Indian Phytopathology* 52 : 18-23.

Sinha, A.K. 1974. The use of benomyl fungicide against *Fusarium oxysporum* f sp. *udum* wilt of pigeonpea. *Zeitschrift fur Pflanzenkrankheiten and Pflanzenschutz* 81 : 571-574.

Sinha, A.K. 1975. Control of Fusarium wilt of pigeonpea with Bavistin a systemic fungicide. *Current Science* 44 : 700-701.

Sinha, P.K. 1983. Studies on phytophthora blight of pigeonpeas. M.Sc thesis, GBPU of Agriculture and Technology, Pantnagar, 110 pp.

Small, W. 1922. On the occurrence of a species of *Fusarium* in Uganda. *Kew Bulletin* 9 : 269-291.

Snyder, W.C. and Hansen, H.N. 1940. The species concept in *Fusarium*. *American Journal of Botany* 27 : 64-67.

Somani, R.B., Khune, N.N. and Wangikar, P.D. 1981. Phoma stem canker a new menace to arhar crop in Vidarbha. Pages 88-89 *in* Abstract of papers of the Third International Symposium of Plant Pathology, 14-18 Dec. 1981. New Delhi, India. New Delhi, India: Indian Phytopathological Society.

Somani, R.B., Wangikar, P.D. and Shukla, V.N. 1975. A new stem canker and die-back disease of pigeonpea. *Indian Phytopathology* 28 : 436-437.

Somasekhara, Y.M., Anilkumar, T.B. and Siddaramaiah, A.L. 1996. Biocontrol of pigeonpea (*Cajanus cajan* (L.) Millsp.) wilt *Fusarium udum* Butler. *Mysore Journal of Agricultural Sciences* 30 (2) : 159-162.

Songa, W.A., Omanga, P. and Reddy, M.V. 1991. Survey of pigeonpea wilt and other diseases in Machakos and Kitui district of Kenya. *International Pigeonpea Newsletter* 14 : 25-26.

Spence, J.A. 1975. The importance of disease in relation to grain legume research programme in the eastern Caribbean. Pages 151-155 *in* Tropical diseases of legumes (Eds. J. Bird,

K. Marmorosch). New York, USA, Academic Press.

Stevenson, J.A. 1917. Disease of vegetables and garden crops. *Journal of the Department of Agriculture, Puerto Rico* 1 : 93 - 117.

Stevenson, J.A. 1918. A check list of Puerto Rican Fungi and host index. *Journal of the Department of Agriculture, Puerto Rico* 2 : 125-264.

Subramanian, C.V. 1955a. Studies on south Indian *Fusaria.* IV. The "Wild Type" in *Fusarium udum* Butler. *Journal of the Indian Botanical Society* 34 : 29-36.

Subramanian, C.V. 1955b. The ecological and taxonomic problems in *Fusarium. Proceedings of the Indian Academy of Sciences*, Section B 41 : 102-109.

Subramanian, S. 1961. Nutritional Studies on *Fusarium udum* Butler. *Proceedings of the Indian Academy of Sciences*, Section B 54 : 295 - 305.

Subramanian, S. 1963a. Fusarium wilt of pigeonpea. II. Changes in the host metabolism. *Proceedings of the Indian Academy of Sciences*, Section B 57 : 178-194.

Subramanian, S. 1963b. Fusarium wilt of pigeonpea. III. Manganese nutrition and diseases resistance. *Proceedings of the Indian Academy of Sciences*. Section B 57: 259 - 274.

Subramanian, S., 1963c. Fusarium wilt of pigeonpea. I. Symptomatology and infection studies. *Proceedings of the Indian Academy of Sciences,* Section B 57 : 134 - 138.

Subramanyam, P., Reddy, M.V., Likoswe, A.A., Saka, V.W. and Msuku, 1992. Diseases of pigeonpea in Malawi. *International Pigeonpea Newsletter* 16 : 75.

Sumitha, R. and Gaikwad, S.J. 1995a. Checking Fusarium wilt of pigeonpea by biological means. *Journal of Soils and Crops* 5 : 163-65.

Sumitha, R. and Gaikwad, S.J. 1995b. Efficacy of some fungicides against *Fusarium udum* in pigeonpea. *Journal of Soils and Crops* 5 (2) : 137-140.

Sutton, B.C. 1980. The Coelomycetes. CMI, Kew Surrey, London, UK.

Sydow, H. and Butler, E.J. 1911. Fungi Indiae orientalis, Part III. *Annals of Mycology* 9 : 372-421.

Sydow, H. and Butler, E.J. 1916. Fungi Indiae orientalis, Part V. *Annals of Mycology* 14 : 177-220.

Tucker, C.M. 1927. Report of the Plant Pathologist. Report of the Puerto Rico Agricultural Experiment Station 1925, pp. 24-40.

Upadhyay, R.S. 1987. Tolerance to higher temperature by *Aspergillus nidulans* and its possible implication on biological control of wilt disease of pigeonpea. *Plant and Soil* 97 : 273.

Upadhyay, R.S. and Rai, B. 1978. *Micromonospora globosa* Krass : A destructive parasite of *Fusarium udum* Butler. *Microbios Letters* 8 : 123.

Upadhyay, R.S. and Rai, B. 1981a. Fungistatic activity of different Indian soils against *Fusarium udum* Butler. Plant & Soil 63 : 407.

Upadhyay, R.S. and Rai, B. 1981b. Effect of cultural practices and soil treatments on incidence of wilt disease of pigeonpea. *Plant & Soils* 62 : 309-312.

Upadhyay, R.S. and Rai, B. 1982a. Ecology of *Fusarium udum* causing wilt disease of pigeonpea, population dynamics in the root region. *Transaction of British Mycological Society* 78 : 209.

Upadhyay, R.S. and Rai, B. 1982b. A possible mode of dispersion of *Fusarium udum* Butler in soil by termites. *Science and Culture* 48 : 207-208.

Upadhyay, R.S. and Rai, B. 1983a. A new disease cycle of wilt of pigoenpea. *Current Scinece*, 52 : 978-981.

Upadhyay, R.S. and Rai, B. 1983b. Competitive saprophytic ability of *Fusarium udum* in relation to some micro fungi of root region of pigeonpea. *Indian phytopathology* 36 : 539-544.

Upadhyay, R.S. and Rai, B. 1985. Antagonistic behaviour of root region of microfungi of pigeonpea against *Fusarium udum*. Page 131 *in* Ecology and Management of Soil-borne Plant Pathogens (Eds. C.A. Parker, A.D. Rovira, K.J. Moore, P.T.W. Wong and J.F. Kollmorgen). The American Phytopathological Society (St. Paul, Minnesota), USA, 131 pp.

Upadhyay, R.S. and Rai, B. 1982b. Studies on antagonism between *Fusarium udum* Butler and root region microflora of pigeonpea. *Plant and Soil* 101 : 79.

Upadhyay, R.S. and Rai, B. 1989. Wilt disease of pigeonpea and its causal organism *Fusarium oxysporum* f *udum* in perspective of Phytopathology (Eds. V.P. Agnihotri, U.S. Singh, H.S. Chaube, N. Singh and T.S. Trivedi), New Delhi : Today & Tomorrows Printers and Publishers.

Upadhyay, R.S. and Rai, B. 1992. Wilt of pigeonpea. Pages 388-414 *in* Plant diseases of International importance, Vol. I. Diseases of cereals and pulses (Eds. U.S. Singh, A.N. Mukhopadhyay, J. Kumar and H.S. Chaube). Englewood Cliff, New Jersey, USA: Prentice Hall Inc. USA.

Upadhyay, R.S., Rai, B. and Gupta, R.C. 1979a. Formation of reproductive bodies by *Fusarium udum* with in *Cunninghamella echinulata* during parasitism. *Microbios Letters* 11 : 69-75.

Upadhyay, R.S., Rai, B. and Gupta, R.C. 1979b. Hyphal parasitism and reproductive bodys formation by *Fusarium udum* with in *Cunninghamella èchinulata* during parasitism, *Microbios Letters* 11 : 69.

Upadhyay, R.S., Rai, B. and Gupta, R.C. 1981a. *Fusarium udum* parasitic on *Aspergillus luchuensis* and *Syncephalastrum racemosum*. *Plant & Soil* 63 : 407-413.

Upadhyay, R.S., Rai, B. and Gupta, R.C. 1981b. *Fusarium udum* as mycoparasite of *Mortierella subtilissima*. *Plant & Soil* 60 : 49-51.

Upadhyay, R.S., Rai, B. and Gupta, R.C. 1983. A possible mode of survival of *Fusarium udum* Butler as mycoparasite. *Acta Mycologia* 19 : 115.

Upadhyay, Shiv Kumar, Bajpai, G.C., Saad, N.K. and Tripathi, H.S. 1998. Inhibitory effect of some plant extracts against Phytophthora stem blight of pigeonpea. Page 83 *in* Abstract of papers of National Symposium on Management of Biotic and Abiotic Stresses in Pulse Crops, 26-28 June 1998, IIPR, Kanpur, India. India : Indian Society of Pulses Research and Development.

Uppal, B.N. and Kulkarni, N.T. 1935. Fusarium wilt in Sunnhemp. *Current Science* 5 : 314-315.

Vaheeduddin, S. 1956. Selection of tur (*Cajanus cajan*) resistance varieties against *Fusarium udum* Butler. *Agricultural College Journal, Osmania University* 3 : 12-13.

Vaheeduddin, S. 1958. Evolving wilt resistant strains in red gram. *Andhra Agricultural Journal* 5 : 163-164.

Vaheeduddin, S. and Nanjundiah, S.M. 1956. Evolving wilt resistant strains in tur (*Cajanus cajan* L.). *Proceedings of the Indian Science Congress* 43 (4) : 20.

Vasudeva, R.S. 1949. Soil borne plant diseases and their control. *Current Science* 18 : 114-115.

Vasudeva, R.S. 1958a. Report of the Division of Mycology and Plant Pathology. Scientific Reports of the Indian Agricultural Research Institute, 1956-57. pp. 86-100.

Vasudeva, R.S. 1958b. Report of the Division of Mycology and Plant Pathology. Scientific Reports of the Indian Agricultural Research Institute, 1955-56. pp. 85-104.

Vasudeva, R.S. and Govindaswamy, C.V. 1953. Studies on the effect of associated oil microflora of *Fusarium udum* Butler, the fungus causing wilt of pigeonpea (*Cajanus cajan* (L) Millap.) with special reference to its pathogenicity. *Annals of Applied Biology* 40 : 573-583.

Vasudeva, R.S., Jain, A.C. and Nema, K.G. 1952. Investigations of the inhibitory action of *Bacillus subtilis* on *Fusarium udum* the fungus causing wilt of pigeonpea. *Annals of Applied Biology* 39 : 229-238.

Vasudeva, R.S. and Roy, T.C. 1950. The effect of associated soil microflora on *Fusarium udum* Butler, the fungus causing wilt of pigeonpea (*Cajanus cajan* (L.) Millsp.). *Annals of Applied Biology* 37 : 169-178.

Vasudeva, R.S., Singh, G.P. and Iyengar, M.R.S. 1962. Biological activity of bulbiformin in soil. *Annals of Applied Biology* 50 : 113-119.

Vasudeva, R.S., Singh, P., Sengupta, P.K. and Mahmood, M. 1963. Further studies on the biological activity of bulbiformin. *Annals of Applied Biology* 51 : 415-423.

Vasudeva, R.S., Subbaiah, T.V., Sastry, M.L.N., Rangaswamy, G. and Iyenger, M.R.S. 1958. "Bulbiformin" an antibiotic produced by *Bacillus subtilis. Annals of Applied Biology* 46 : 336-345.

Venkataram, C.S. 1955. Soil *Fusaria* and their pathogenicity. *Proceedings of the Indian Academy of Sciences,* Section B 42 : 129-144.

Verma, Alpana and Singh, R.B. 1998. Effect of soil amendment of *Clorodendron aculeatum* and *Clorodendron fragrans* on disease incidence of pigeonpia wilt. *National Academy Sciences Letters* 21(1/2) : 9-13.

Verma, Alpana and Singh, R.B. 1997. Inhibitory properties of *Clarodendrum fragrans* against *Fusarium oxysporum* f. sp. *udum. Annals of Plant Protection Sciences* 5(2) : 190-193.

Verma, G. 1955. Mixed cropping with arhar. *Agriculture and Animal Husbandry in Uttar Pradesh* 6 : 70-80.

Vidyasekaran, P. and Arjunan, G. 1976. A new redgram pigeonpea variety resistant to root rot (*Macrophomina phaseolina*). *Madras Agricultural Journal* 63 : 175-176.

Vidyasekaran, P., Sethuraman, K., Rajappan, K. and Vasumathi, K. 1997. Powder formulations of *Pseudomonas fluorescens* to control pigeonpea wilt. *Biological Control* 8(3) : 166-171.

Vyas, S.C., Vadhera, I., Singh, R. and Khare, M.N. 1983. Ambimobility movement and persistence of metalaxyl in pigeonpea and its effect on Modulation. *Indian Journal of Mycology and Plant Pathology* 13 : 265-271.

Wallace, G.B. 1932. Tanganyika territory fungus list, Recent records. 10. Mycological Circulars, Department of Agriculture, Tanganyika 23 : 1-5.

Waterston, J.M. 1944. Plant Pathology, Report, Department of Agriculture, Bermuda, 1943. pp. 7-8.

Wearing, A.H. and Birch, C.J. 1988. Root rot of pigeonpea. International Pigeonpea Newsletter 8 : 13.

Williams, F.J., Amin, K.S. and Baldev, B. 1975. Phytophthora stem blight of *Cajanus cajan. Phytopathology* 65 : 1029-1030.

Williams, F.J., Grewal, J.S. and Amin, K.S. 1968. Serious and new diseases of pulse crops. *Plant Disease Reporter* 52 : 300-304.

Wiehe, P.O. 1939. Division of Plant Pathology. Report, Department of Agriculture, Mauritious, 1938. pp. 34-39.

Wollenweber, H.W. 1931. "*Fusarium*-Monographic. Fungi Parasitici et Saprophytici". Z. *Parasitenkol.* 3 : 269.

Wollenweber, H.W. 1938. (*Fusaria* of pigeonpea, *Cajanus cajan*). *Arbeitan aus der Biologischen Reichsanstalt fur Land-u-Forstwirtschaft* 22 : 339-347.

Wollenweber, H.W. and Reinking, O.A. 1935. Die Fusarien, ihre Beschreibung, Schadewirkung and Bekanpfung, Berlin, 355 pp.

Yogeswari, L. 1948. The element nutrition of fungi. I. The effect of boron, zinc and manganese on *Fusarium* species. *Proceedings of the Indian Academy of Sciences*, Section B 28 : 177-201.

Zaberi, P.P., Shah, R.M., Pathak, A.R., Patel, J.A., Kher, H.R., Patel, R.S. and Tikka, S.B.S. 1986. BDN 2, a wilt tolerant superior cultivar for Gujarat. *International Pigeonpea Newsletter* No. 5 : 38-39.

Zote, K.K., Dandnaik, B.P., Deshmukh, R.V. and Shaikh, M.H. 1990. Management of wilt of pigeonpea through resistance breeding. *Indian Phytopathology* 43 : 307.

Zote, K.K., Dandnaik, B.P., Khalikar, P.V. 1983a. Reaction of Maharashtra Pigeonpea cultivars to wilt and sterility mosaic. *International Pigeonpea Newsletter* 2 : 44-45.

Zote, K.K., Dandnaik, B.P. and Khalikar, P.V. 1986. Sources of resistance of some pigeonpea lines to wilt disease. *Indian Journal of Mycology and Plant Pathology* 16 : 144-145.

Zote, K.K., Dandnaik, B.P. and Khalikar, P.V. 1987a. Reaction of pigeonpea varieties/ lines to Fusarium wilt disease. *Journal of Maharashtra Agricultural Universities* 12 : 102-103.

Zote, K.K., Dandnaik, B.P., Khalikar, P.V. and Olekar, S.S. 1983b. Reaction of some pigeonpea lines to wilt. *International Pigeonpea Newsletter* 2 : 42.

Zote, K.K., Dandanaik, B.P., Shinde, V.K. and Raut, K.G. 1987b. Screening against wilt. and sterility mosaic of pigeonpea at Badnapur. *Indian Phytopathology* 40 : 285.

Zote, K.K., Khalikar, P.V. and Dandnaik, B.P. 1982. Evaluation of seed dressers against collar rot of pigeonpea. *Madras Agricultural Journal* 70 : 275-276.

Zote, K.K., Mayee, C.D. and Shaikh, M.H. 1993a. Survival of *Fusarium udum* a causal organism of pigeonpea wilt disease. *Indian Phytopathology* 44 & 45 (Suppl.) : XXI-XXII.

Zote, K.K., Pawar, B.R. and Shaikh, M.H. 1993b. Pathogenic variability in *Fusarium udum*: A casual organism of pigeonpea wilt. *Indian Phytopathology* 44 & 45 (Suppl.) : CXV.

Zote, K.K., Pawar, N.B., Dandnaik, B.P. and Shrirame, M.D. 1995. Crop improvement through resistance breeding in pigeonpea. *Indian Journal of Mycology and Plant Pathology* 25 : 100.

3

Fungal Diseases of the Foliage

Large number of fungal pathogens occur on the foliage of pigeonpea resulting in blight, leaf spots, mildews, rust, anthranose etc. However, only few of them cause diseases of some economic importance while others are minor and very much restricted in their occurrence geographically. Many of the pathogens have been reported for once only. The diseases having the potential to damage the pigeonpea crop are Alternaria blight, powdery mildew, rust, Cercospora leaf spot but they are not widespread. These diseases require specific environmental conditions for their development as epiphytotic. Secondly, pigeonpea crop is planted at wider spaces which probably do not allow very thick canopy of crop so as to develop suitable micro environment for development of foliar fungal diseases. However, looking to fast changing crop cultivation technology with newer varieties, the foliar fungal diseases, should not be ignored. This chapter deals with the diseases of foliage of pigeonpea as available in the literature.

3.1 Alternaria Blight/Leaf Spot

The Alternaria leaf spot of pigeonpea caused by *Alternaria tenuissima* was described by Kannaiyan and Nene (1977) who claimed it as the first record on pigeonpea, although, infection of pigeonpea by this fungus has already been noticed earlier by Hasija (1964) at Raipur (M.P.) followed by Pavgi and Singh (1971) at Varanasi (U.P.). The disease has been reported to occur in Puerto Rico, U.S.A. and Zambia (Nene *et al.* 1996). A similar leaf spot disease of pigeonpea caused by *Alternaria alternata* was reported to occur on the experimental crop of pigeonpea at Dholi, Bihar by Mehta and Sinha (1982). It also occurs in Australia (Nene *et al.* 1996). Alternaria blight/leaf spot has been reported from Kenya, Malawi and Sri Lanka also but the species of the fungus has not been identified. In India, the disease has been reported to occur in the states of Andhra Pradesh, Bihar, Gujarat and Rajasthan also (Kannaiyan *et al.* 1981). It is considered to be a potential problem of pigeonpea crop in the state of Gujarat (Desai *et al.* 1981) and higher elevations of Garhwal hills (Kumar *et al.* 1991). Alternaria blight has been considered to be the most serious disease of the post-rainy season pigeonpea in north-eastern India and epiphytotic of the disease has been reported from parts of the Bihar state (Mahmood *et al.* 1983). In Rajasthan, the disease occurred severely on July sown crop (Gurjar 1988). The disease has great potential to cause widespread losses to pigeonpea crop specially under changing varietal and environmental patterns in India. Severe infections in a susceptible cultivar like Bahar and Basant can destroy the crop completely (Venkateswarlu *et al.* 1981).

3.1.1 Symptoms

The Symptoms produced by *A. tenuissima* have been described by Kannaiyan and Nene (1977). Initially, small, light brown to dark brown necrotic spots appear on leaves which gradually increase in size to characteristic lesions with dark and light brown concentric rings having a wavy outline and a purple margin. As the infection progresses, the lesions enlarge, become darker in colour and coalesce. The disease is confined mostly to older leaves in adult plants but may infect new leaves of young plants particularly in the post-rainy season crop. According to Gurjar (1988), the initial symptoms on leaves include numerous dark spots extending rapidly to form large concentric rings after which they dry, curl and defoliate rapidly. The lesions are formed on stems, branches also which later cause splitting of the bark in the infected portions. The severe infections may cause complete defolation and destruction of the crop. Spots are formed on pods also infecting seeds.

The infections caused by *A. alternata* are characterized by brownish black spots with prominent black dots appearing on leaves (Mehta and Sinha 1982). The diseased plants are completely blighted due to coalescing of several spots in tender leaves and shoots. The disease starts as pin head size yellow halos 0.5 to 1 mm in diameter which gradually enlarge, turn reddish brown with black dots and measuring 2-13 mm with various shapes. The black dots on spots are mostly arranged in ring form.

3.1.2 Causal Organism

1. *Alternaria tenuissima* (Kunze ex Pers) Wiltshire
2. *Alternaria alternata* (Fr.) Keissler

The pathogen *A. tenuissima* from pigeonpea has been studied and described in detail by Pavgi and Singh (1971) and Kannaiyan and Nene (1977) as follows:

The *mycelium* is cottony, smoke grey and tufty on malt agar medium. *Conidiophores* fasciculate, simple or branched, straight or flexuous, septate, dark coloured, geniculate with 1-6 lateral spore scars, 30-60 µm × 4-5µm in size. *Conidia* smooth, obclavate, solitary or in short chains, muriform with several septa, slightly or not constricted at the septa, 33-103 × 13-30 µm is size. The fungus is commonly recorded on a very wide host range, usually as a secondary invader rather than a primary parasite. The optimum temperature for its growth on V 8 juice agar was 25-30°C (Anonymous 1983). It sporulates well on PDA at 25°C under 8 h near UV for 20 days (Anonymous 1986).

The *mycelium* of *A. alternata* from pigeonpea is olivaceous brown, turning dark brown with the age (Mehta and Sinha 1982). The cross walls are prominent. *Conidiophores* reddish brown, straight, branched, 28.4 to 170.4 µ in length and 3.54 to 7.1 µ in width having 2-12 cross septa. *Conidia* muriform, dark brown with ill-defined beak and produced in chains. They are 28.4 to 113.6 µ × 7.1 to 21.3 µ with 2-8 cross septa and 1-4 logitudinal septa.

3.1.3 Host Parasite Interaction

Pigeonpea isolate of *A. tenuissima* is reported to produce tenuzonic acid (TA) and host specific toxin (S) in culture (Nutsugah *et al.* 1993a). The TA was found toxic to pigeonpea leaves at 200-500 µg/ml and to other plants at 100-1000µg/ml or above. The host specific toxin extracted from the spore germinating fluid (SGF) of *A. tenuissima* induced necrosis on susceptible pigeonpea leaves at 5 µg/ml while resistant lines or non-host tolerated 20000 times higher concentration of the toxin (Nutsugah *et al.* 1994). A concentration of 10 µg/ml of toxin induced susceptibility in pigeonpea to non-pathogenic isolate of *A. alternata.* The toxin was released within 3 h of incubation and the concentration reached 6 times to that required for necrosis. The toxin did not induce necrosis if treated leaves were exposed to fluorescent light but necrosis was caused if leaves were shifted to dark (Nutsugah *et al.* 1993b). The toxin caused disappearance of mitochondrial matrics and disruption of cristae within 5 h of treatment and 100 % mitochondria were affected within 39 h in case of susceptible variety of pigeonpea (Nutsugah *et al.* 1993c). However, it did not affect other organelles of the host cells.

3.1.4 Disease Cycle and Epidemiology

The fungus *A. tenuissima* has been reported to be associated with pigeonpea seed internally as well as externally and exhibited negative correlation with the emergence of seed (Ellis *et al.* 1978). Similarly *A. alternata* has been found associated with pigeonpea seed (Kumar and Verma 1979) and the extent of infection differed in different varieties. The infected seeds exhibit discolouration and shrivelling (Kumar and Patnaik 1985).

It has been reported that the spores of *A. tenuissima* remain viable on leaves throughout summer when the temperature rises up to 45°C on surface of the soil (Singh and Fazili 1988). The pathogen attacked chickpea variety JG 62 severely and produced mild symptoms on *Vigna aconitifolia* and *Vicia faba* which may serve as the collateral hosts for survival of the pathogen (Kannaiyan and Nene 1986).

The disease development has been correlated with the meteorological parameters in Bihar (Sinha and Mahmood 1993). The disease appeared in 2nd week of November when temperature and RH were 24.04°C and 72.5% respectively without rains. The infection started at the average temperature between 15.33 to 32.67°C and RH 94%. The highest disease intensity was in February when mean temperature, RH and precipitation were 17.14°C, 81.39% and 1.67 mm respectively. The disease increased and spread from December to February when mean temperature, RH and precipitation were 9.22°C, 83.12 % and 2.86 mm respectively.

Singh *et al.* (1986) studied the progress of the disease in relation to growth of the foliage in pigeonpea taking into account the leaf fall due to disease in susceptible variety Bahar and concluded that the disease intensity increases despite the host growth indicating the epidemic of the disease.

Tremendous increase in the disease has been observed in areas where post-rainy season pigeonpea introduced or increased (Narula 1983). In September sown pigeonpea the disease appeared in December becoming severe by middle of January. Under such circumstances, medium and late maturing varieties like Bahar suffer more while early varieties like ICPL 86, ICPL 87 and ICPL 81 escape the losses. Such varieties reach towards maturity when the period favourable for disease development starts.

3.1.5 Host Resistance

Sources of Resistance : Kannaiyan and Nene (1977) searched 51 promising pigeonpea lines against *A. tenuissima* under field conditions and reported 25 lines to be free from the disease while cultivars like NPWR 15, Sharda and BDN 1 were susceptible. Large number of sources of resistance against Alternaria blight have been identified in India which are compiled in Table 3.1.

Table 3.1: Source of resistance against Alternaria blight of pigeonpea

Number of entries tested	*Entries found resistant*	*Reference*
—	MA 128-1, MA 128-2, DA 2, and 20-105 were free	Venkateswarlu *et al.* (1981)
39	ICPL 6 and 146 were resistant; Hy 8 and PDA 7 were MR	Reddy *et al.* (1984)
15	DA 2, 20(105), MA 128-2	Singh *et al.* (1986)
84	RNA 56, RNA 4 were least susceptible	Gurjar (1988), Pathak and Gurjar (1989)
—	62 lines/cultivars and 8 wild species including *Cajanus albicans, C. cajanifolia, C. lineata, C.platycarpa, C. scarabaeoides, C. sericea, C. viscidus,* and *C. volubilis* were resistant	Kannaiyan and Nene (1986)
84	128-2, DA 2, 4726, 4726 selfed, 129 A 4, 125 B, 125 C 2, 127, 133 B, 127 TTGP, 128-1, *Atylosia cajanifolia, A. scarabaeoides, A. sericea*	Singh *et al.* (1984)

Screening Technique: In most cases screening of pigeonpea against *A. tenuissima* has been done under natural infection. However, Kannaiyan and Nene (1986) used a pot culture technique using isolation plant propagator in a greenhouse. Twenty seeds of each test entry are sown in 15 cm diameter pot containing a mixture of autoclaved sand and vermiculite in a ratio of 3 : 1. The culture of *A. tenuissima* is multiplied on PDB at 28-30°C for 15 days. The mycelium and spores of the fungus are filtered and macerated intermittently in waring blender, diluted with tap water to have

3.25×10^4 conidia/ml. This suspension is sprayed on 2 weeks old seedlings which are covered by clear plastic to maintain nearly 100% RH. The observations are recorded 10 days after inoculation and percentage of blighted seedlings is calculated. Looking to the heterogenity due to crop being cross pollinated, the test lines can be classified as follows:

* Resistant (0-20 % plants infected)
* Moderately resistant (21-50% plants infected)
* Susceptible (51-100 % plants infected)

Singh *et al.* (1984) adopted 0-5 scale for scoring of plants where 0 = No disease (Highly Resistant), 1 = 0.1 - 5 % leaf area affected (Resistant), 2 = 5.1-10 % leaf area affected (Moderately Resistant), 3 = 10.1-25 % leaf area affected (Moderately Susceptible), 4 = 25.1-50 % leaf area affected (Susceptible) and 5 = more than 50 % leaf area affected (Highly Susceptible). Similarly, Reddy and Jain (1992) recommended a 9-point scale on the basis of extent of defoliation as the main criterion as follows:

Rating	*Reaction category*	*Defoliation %*
1	Highly Resistant (HR)	0
2	HR to Resistant	1 - 5
3	Resistant	6 - 10
4	Moderately Resistant (MR)	11 - 20
5	Tolerant	21 - 30
6	Moderately Susceptible	31 - 50
7	Susceptible (S)	51 - 70
8	S - Highly Susceptible	71 - 100
9	Highly Susceptible	Plant killed

Inheritance of Resistance: According to Singh *et al.* (1986) the resistance or susceptibility to *A.tenuissima* is not controlled by the genes responsible for plant height or days to flowering. In a stand of three crosses of pigeonpea, the resistance to *A. tenuissima* was found to be governed by a recessive gene abr 1 (Sharma *et al.* 1987). Singh *et al.* (1988) also concluded resistance to *A. tenuissima* to be monogenic and recessive in nature which is designated as al 1 al 1. In the same way Ojha *et al.* (1993) reported it to be monogenic and recessive in nature.

3.1.6 Control

Not much work has been done on control aspect of this disease. Suitable resistant varieties like ICPL 366, DA 2, and DA 11 may be used.

The seed infection of *A. tenuissima* is reported to reduce greatly by seed treatment with Bavistinl T @ 250 g/100kg while pelleting seed @ 500 g/100 kg eliminated seed borne inoculum completely (Pal 1984). According to Kumar and Patnaik (1985), *A. alternata* could be recovered from the seed coat only and the seed treatment with Bavistin or Difolatan reduced the seed infection greatly improving its germination. Of 10 fungicides tested, 7 improved the germination significantly and increased root and shoot length and dry weight of seedlings (Kumar and Patnaik 1986). Solanke *et al.* (1990) reported carbendazim + thiram to be the best for seed treatment.

Lal *et al.* (1998) tested 8 leaf extracts and 2 pure chemicals of plant origin against *A. tenuissima* and found *Achyranthes* to be the best followed by *Azadirachta.* Their foliar spray gave 40.1 and 37.97% protection of plants respectively. Spray of p-Hydroxybenzoic acid checked the disease in field increasing yield.

Out of 4 homeodrugs, Symphyticum reduced growth of *A. tenuissima in vitro*. In field, the disease was reduced maximum by Symphyticum followed by China @ 1 ml/l (Lal *et al.* 1999).

Since the inoculum of the pathogen has been reported to survive on the infected leaves in the field, their destruction will help in reducing the inoculum build up in the crop.

3.2 Cercospora Leaf Spots

Cercospora leaf spot is an important foliar disease of pigeonpea occurring in most of the pigeonpea growing areas of the world. The disease was first reported from Brazil (Rangel 1915). Out of several species of Cercospora occurring on pigeonpea, *Cercospora cajani* (= *Vellosiella cajani*) is very widespread and has been found occurring in Puerto Rico (Stevenson 1917), U.S.A. (Jehle and Wood 1926), Dominican Republic (Ciferri 1927, Ciferri *et al.* 1927), Tanzania (Wallace 1930), Venezuella (Muller and Chupp 1945), Guatemala (Muller 1950), Rhodesia and Nyasaland (Bates 1957), Kenya (Nattras 1958), Mauritius (Telix 1960), Zambia (Angus 1962), Uganda (Khan and Onim 1972), Nigeria (Williams and Allen 1976), India (Srivastava 1980), Bangla Desh (Nowsher *et al.* 1986), Malawi (Reddy *et al.* 1993), Ethiopia and

Zimbabwe (Subramanyam 1993). It has also been reported from Columbia, Fiji, Haiti, Jamaica, Nepal, Sierra Leone, Sri Lanka, Sudan, Taiwan, Trinidad and Tobago (Nene *et al.* 1996). The disease caused by *C.cajani* has also been named as 'Floury spot' (Gupta and Srivastava 1991).

The another widespread species is *Cercospora instabilis* which has been found infecting pigeonpea in Brazil (Rangel 1915), U.S.A. (Jehle and Wood 1926), Puerto Rico (Cook 1939), India and Philippines (Nene *et al.* 1996).

The disease is reported to assume economic importance in Nigeria and in Caribbean region (Spence 1975), Puerto Rico (Abrams *et al.* 1978) and several other African countries specially Kenya, Malawi, Tanzania, Uganda, Zambia and Ethiopia (Kaiser 1976, Kannaiyan 1981, Kannaiyan *et al.* 1981, Subramanyam 1993). In India, the disease is a potential problem of pigeonpea in the states of Gujarat (Desai *et al.* 1987), Bihar, Uttar Pradesh and parts of Rajasthan.

The disease causes substantial losses in yields of susceptible varieties by early leaf shedding, flower abortion and poor pod filling (Rachie and Wurster 1971). The losses are high if defoliation occurs before flowering and pod setting. Very high incidence of the disease in areas with wet and humid climate has been reported to exhibit negative correlation between severity of *C. cajani* and grain yield of pigeonpea (Rubaihayo and Onim 1975, Onim and Rubaihayo 1976). As high as 85% reduction in yield has been observed due to this disease (Onim 1980). Such correlation between the disease severity and yield losses has not been observed in dry areas.

3.2.1 Symptoms

In general *Cercospora* spp. produce lesions on pigeonpea leaves similar to *Colletotrichum cajani* which results in premature leaf shedding. However, the symptoms produced by different species of the pathogen have been described separately as follows:

C. cajani : According to Pavgi and Singh (1965), the infection appears late, when plants are in pre-blossom stage. Infected leaflets with small, irregular light brown spots surrounded by a diffuse chlorotic tissue soon wither or drop on ground. It produces round or angular brown spots often pale in the middle with a dark border. The spots are apparent on the lower side of the leaves. The disease starts with the appearance of small circular halos on the upper surface of leaves under which fungal mycelium develops on lower side (Srivastava 1980). This disease has been described by the name 'Floury spot' from northern hill region including Sikkim in India (Gupta and Srivastava 1991). It is characterized by irregular, yellowish, 5 mm wide spots on upper surface of leaves with corresponding lower area of spot covered with a white floury aggregations. The floury growth is more conspicuous on the lower surface of fallen leaves. Floury spots also appear on stem and branches ultimately resulting in premature defoliation with considerable reduction in yield.

C. instabilis : First symptoms appear on 5-6 weeks old plants as irregular, necrotic spots on leaves and petioles. The spots increase in size, reach up to new branches and become blotches after coalescing with each other. Initially, spots are dull - reddish brown but later become dark covering both the surfaces of leaves. They are 2-8 × 1.5-5 mm in size. The spots are dark on veins and petioles but light coloured on leaf blades (Pavgi & Singh 1965).

C. indica : The first symptoms appear in October on mature leaves, petioles and even young twigs. The small velvety hypophyllous stromata expand into coalescent patches, while the corresponding upper leaf surface turns yellowish to brown (Pavgi and Singh 1965). The spots are irregular in outline and raised above the surface of the leaf. Very rarely, the upper surface is infected. The spots are discrete usually but occasionally, several spots may coalesce forming diseased areas up to 15 × 5 mm in size. In early stage, the spots are brownish drab in colour. Petioles and stems are sometimes attacked. The diseased areas arising from the single spot does not cross the midrib or the primary veins of the leaflets.

C. thirumalachari : This fungus is reported to produce extensive spots on pigeonpea leaves often covering entire lower leaf surface (Sharma and Mishra 1977). The spots are bound by the veins.

3.2.2 Causal Organisms

1. *Mycovellosiella cajani* (Henn) Rangel Ex Trotter
   Synonyms : *Cercospora cajani* Henn
   Vellosiella cajani
2. *Cercospora instabilis* Rangel
3. *Mycovellosiella cajani* var. *indica* (Singh) Deighton
   Synonym : *Cercospora indica* Singh

4. *Cercospora thirumalachari* Sharma and Mishra
5. *Mycovellosiella cajani* var. *trichophila* (curzi) Deighton
   Synonym : *Cercospora trichophila* Curzi
6. *Cercospora canescens* Ellis and Morten

Mycovellosiella cajani (=Cercospora cajani) occurs very widely on pigeonpea. According to Pavgi and Singh (1965), the spots are mostly indefinite, epiphyllous, dark brown varying from small specks to 10 mm. Hypostroma hypophyllous. Conidiophores on leaf surface as well as on epidermal hairs, nonfasciculate and in pseudofascicles, some times in procumbent coremoid fascicles with branches extending outward, rarely geniculate, often with spore scars, multiseptate, pale olivaceous, 20-80 μ × 3-7 μ, branches mostly curved, with bluntly round apices, often catenulate, light olevaceous brown but subhyaline when immature; 10-50 μ × 3-7 μ, rarely upto 80 μ long, 1-9 septate. The fungus has been described as colonies hypophyllous, olivaceous brown with *conidiophores* much branched climbing leaf hairs, variable in length (28 μ to 168 μ), 1-3 μ thick near the base but broadening above to 4-7 μ, pale or mid-pale olivaceous brown. *Conidia* mostly cylindrical, rounded at the distal ends, hyaline to mid-pale, olivaceous brown, 1-3 septate, 20-30 4-6 μ in size with conspicuous scars (Srivastava 1980).

Cercospora instabilis has been reported on pigeonpea causing leaf spots mostly on Indian varieties in Brazil (Wutke and Ito 1990). The fungus produces *mycelium* septate, light brown forming substomatal stroma of 12-28 μ. *Conidiophores* in groups of 3-8, light brown, geniculate, 2-6 septate, 56-112 × 4-4.6 μ in size. *Conidia* sub-hyaline, straight or slightly curved, clavate with flat base, 3-11 septate, 26.4-145 × 2.6-4.0 μ (68 × 2 μ) in size (Pavgi & Singh 1965, Rathi and Nene 1984). The fungus reported from Brazil by Wukte and Ito (1996) was similar to *C. instabilis* but had larger fruiting bodies.

Cercospora indica, now considered as synonym to *Mycovellosiella cajani* var. *indica* was described on pigeonpea from India by Singh (1934). It has *conidiophores* branched, brancing alternate, mostly bent, arising from stroma in clusters, light brown to dark brown with prominent geniculation, 28-168 × 3.4-7 μ in size, 2-13 septate; *stromata* prominent in air spaces protruding out of stomata; *conidia* hyaline or slightly greenish yellow, multiseptate, abruptly obclavate, sometimes vermiform with distinct scars less that 2 μ in diameter, often constricted near the septa, 6.8-129 × 3-5 μ in diameter (average 37 × 4 μ), 0-9 septate. It was considered as a species different from *C. cajani* and *C. instabilis* (Singh

1934) but Chupp considered it identical with *C. cajani*. Pavgi and Singh (1965) described the fungus as the mycelium intracellular, septate and olive brown accumulated in the substomatal cavities but the stroma remains relatively poor. Branches light brown conidiophores emerge in cluster of 2-4 through the stomata which are geniculate and measure 30-120 μ × 3-4.6 μ. Conidia are tinted light brown, multiseptate (0-7), obclavate with constrictions at the septa and measuring 14-105 μ × 3.3-5.3 μ (40.6 × 4.0 μ). McRae (1932) studied *Cercospora indica* from pigeonpea and reported that the fungus grows well at a temperature of 6-37°C with optimum of 27-28°C in alternate light and darkness. Development occurred at RH above 47% but best at 100 per cent. It grew at *p*H range of 2-9.7 with an optimum of 6-7.

Cercospora thirumalacharii has been reported from India only (Sharma and Mishra 1977) who described the fungus as : *conidiophores* abundant, hypophyllous, rarely amphigenous; *stroma* when present, small, blackish brown, fasciculate or single; *conidiophores* olivaceous brown with paler tips, uniform in colour, multiseptate, unbranched, variously curved, geniculate with prominent scar of attachment to conidia, up to 16 septate, tips sub-truncate, mostly uniform in width except at the geniculations, up to 375 μ long and 3-6.5 μ wide, *conidia* hyaline, broader below and tapering upwards, straight or curved, distinctly septate 3-26 septa, prominent scar at the base, base truncate or sub-truncate, apex acute, 33-275 × 2.2-3.3 μ in size. *C. thirumalacharii* differs from *C. cajani*, *C. indica* and *C. instabilis* in that the last three have dense, unbranched, very long conidiophores with distinct scars and longer, hyaline, distinctly multiseptate conidia.

Cercodeuterospora trichophilla Curzi was reported to infect leaves of pigeonpea from Somaliland (Curzi 1932). The fungus was later considered as synonym to *Mycovellosiella cajani* var. *trichophilla* (Curzi) Deighton. The fungus causes leaf spot of pigeonpea and has been reported from Kenya and Taiwan also (Nene *et al.* 1996).

Cercospora canescens is reported to cause leaf spot symptom on pigeonpea in Philippines (Nene *et al.* 1996). In addition to these species of *Cercospora, Mycosphaerella* spp. have been found infecting pigeonpea and causing leaf spot symptoms in India (Saksena 1976) which is the first record in the world. *Mycosphaerella* has been found to have the perfect stage of some species of *Cercospora* and *Phyllosticta*.

3.2.3 Disease Cycle and Epidemiology

Not much work has been done on survival of the pathogens and the epidemiological aspects of the disease. However, the fungi are considered to survive in the field on infected leaves in the form of stroma. The time of the infection in India is reported to be flowering time in November-December for *C. cajani*; 5-6 weeks old plants, i.e. in August for *C. instabilis* and beginning of October for *C. indica* (Rathi and Nene 1984). Infection by *C. indica* takes place between 20-25°C (Singh 1934).

The disease caused by *C. cajani* appears late in the season at pre-blossom stage and spreads in patches in sole crop but uniformly in crop sown with sorghum or Bajra.

According to Reddy *et al.* (1933) cool temperature (25°C) and humid weather favours the disease, which normally appears when plants are at flowering and podding. Cyclonic rains in southern and north-eastern peninsular India result in sudden outbreaks of the disease in certain years. The disease is more common in the long duration and perennial pigeonpeas grown in eastern Africa.

3.2.4 Host Resistance

Sources of resistance against *Cercospora* species have been identified in African countries specially Uganda. According to Khan and Rachie (1972) the disease is most serious in Uganda under wet conditions. They did not find any pigeonpea line immune to *Mycovellosiella cajani*. However, Onim (1974) reported resistance in pigeonpea against Cercospora leaf spot disease. Onim and Rubaihayo (1976) screened 15000 plants of 2107 cultivars of pigeonpea against *M. cajani* in Uganda and Kenya of which 314 were selected. Out of these 11 selections were grown at different locations where UC 2515/2, UC 796/1, UC 2113/1 and UC 2568/1 were found resistant with high yield. In Kenya, 197 lines of pigeonpea were screened against the disease of which 15 lines including 657/1, ALPL 6-2, 66 and 666 showed some resistance with 4-4.5 score out of 9.0 (Songa 1991). In Brazil, Wutke and Ito (1990) tested several cultivars of pigeonpea and reported that only Indian lines were affected by *Cercospora* spp. Kannaiyan and Haciwa (1990) found ICP 8869, ICP 12792 and ICP 12165 to be least affected in Zambia. In Malawi, Reddy *et al.* (1992b) observed severe disease incidence on many pigeonpea lines but ICP 9145 was free from the disease.

Mayee and Datar (1986) proposed 0-9 point scale to score pigeonpea entries for leaf spot intensity caused by *C. indica* at seedling, flowering and pod formation stages of crop growth as follows :

Numerical grade	Description
0	No symptoms on the leaf
1	Lesions small, pinhead size covering less than 1% of the leaf area
3	Lesions 1-2 mm in diameter covering 1-10 % of the leaf area
5	Lesions enlarged but not coalescing, covering 11-25% of the leaf area
7	Lesions coalescing covering 26-50% leaf area
9	51% or more leaf area covered by large and coalescing lesions; defoliation of leaves

3.2.5 Control

Selection of seed from healthy crop and the fields away from perennial pigeonpea helps in reducing the disease as the perennial pigeonpea helps in survival of the inoculum.

The desease caused by *M. cajani* can be controlled effectively by spraying Dithane M 45 and Benlate at an interval of 7-24 and 14-21 days respectively with increase in yield (Khan and Onim 1972; Onim 1980). However, Benlate and Bavistin depressed the yield significantly when sprayed weekly. Reddy *et al.* (1993) recommended spray of Indofil M 45 @ 3 g/l of water for control of cercospora leaf spot of pigeonpea.

3.3 Powdery Mildew

The first report of powdery mildew of pigeonpea is from Ceylon (Park 1929) and simultaneously from Tanzania (Wallace 1930). The disease was later reported from India (Uppal 1937). The disease has been reported to occur in many of the African countries specially Uganda (Khan and Rachie 1972), Nigeria (Williams and Allen 1976), Kenya, Malawi, Tanzania and Zambia (Kannaiyan *et al.* 1981). In India, the disease occurs commonly in some districts of Uttar Pradesh (Kumar *et al.* 1991), Maharashtra (Patel *et al.* 1949 and Gohokar and Peshney 1985) and Tamil Nadu where it may cause serious losses while in Bihar,

Karnataka, Madhya Pradesh, Orissa and Rajasthan it is considered as a minor disease (Kannaiyan *et al.* 1981). It is an economically important disease causing serious losses in Nigeria, Kenya, Tanzania and Zambia. The disease is widespread in most of the pigeonpea growing areas of the Indian subcontinent and eastern Africa and becomes severe late in the season when crop reaches the maturity. Occasionally it causes severe defoliation adversely affecting pod setting and grain filling (Reddy *et al.* 1993). The losses in grain yield of pigeonpea are significantly correlated with the severity scores of the powdery mildew (Kannaiyan and Haciwa 1990).

3.3.1 Symptoms

The powdery mildew symptoms appear more oftenly on older leaves but younger ones and even flower buds and pods may also be infected specially under favourable weather conditions. Dull red spots, limited by veins, appear on upper surface of leaves and later white powdery patches develop on both the surfaces (Grewal *et al.* 1988). The entire lower leaf surface is covered with white powdery growth on sporulation of the fungus. Severe infection results in heavy defoliation (Rachie and Wurster 1971). The disease causes stunting of young plants and significant reduction in nodule numbers, nodule weight, shoot weight and root weight (Prameela *et al.* 1990b).

The disease starts as small white patches on the lower surface of leaves which later increase and cover the entire lamina on both the surfaces as well as petioles, stems etc. (Fig. 3.1). In severe cases, affected leaves turn yellow with crinkling and sometimes defoliation (Narayanaswamy and Jaganathan 1975).

3.3.2 Causal Organisms

1. *Oidiopsis taurica* (Lev.) Salmon
   Teleomorph : *Leveillula taurica* (Lev.) Arnaud
2. *Oidiopsis clitoriae*
3. *Erysiphe polygoni* DC

The fungus *O. taurica* has been reported to attack several hosts and described in detail by Butler (1918) and Subramanian (1971) as *mycelium* endophytic, *conidiophores* hypophyllous, emerging through stomata, solitary or fasciculate, simple, sometimes sparsely branched, septate, about

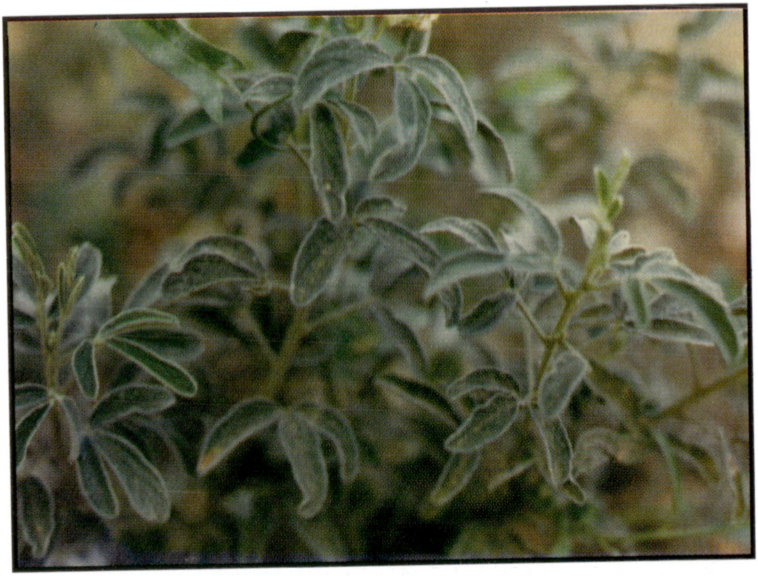

Fig. 3.1: Powdery mildew of pigeonpea.

7 μ wide. *Conidia* hyaline, produced singly at the apex of the conidiophore, one-celled, of irregular form, 40-80 μ long, 12-16 μ wide. Kamat and Patel (1949) studied isolates of the pathogen from 12 different hosts and described them as mycelium endophytic, conidia from all the hosts within a range of 39-87 μ in length and 4-28 μ in width. These figures were 39-87 μ and 10-28 μ respectively in case of isolate from pigeonpea. These isolates were found to be highly host specific. However, such a high level of specificity in different isolates of this pathogen was not observed by later workers (Pawar *et al.* 1985, Wankhede and Peshney 1992).

The isolate of the pathogen studied by Narayanaswamy and Jaganathan (1975) from pigeonpea in Tamil Nadu was found to resemble with *Oidiopsis clitoriae*. It was described as *Mycelium* septate, branched, hyaline; *conidiophores* bearing mature conidia terminally on pedicillate cell; *conidia* hyaline, single celled, smooth, thin walled, ovate to barrel shaped, uninucleate, 24.96-56.1 × 12.48-21.48 μ in size. It did not produce any perfect state. Pigeonpea was reported as new host of *O.clitoriae*.

The pigeonpea was reported to be infected by *Erysiphe polygoni* from pea (Bhardwaj and Singh 1984). The conidial state of *Erysiphe* occurring on various genera of leguminosae including *Cajanus cajan* were indistinguishable and hence they were assigned to a single species

Euoidium leguminosarum sp. Nov. by Paul and Kapoor (1987) with the characters as mycelium epiphyllous, hyaline, inconspicuous; *conidiophores* erect, cylindrical 22-29 × 10-13 μm. The mean number of developing and developed *conidia* in a chain of 6-10. Mature *conidia* ellipsoid to barrel shaped, 24-49 × 11-21 μm. Fibrosin bodies present. Germ tubes simple, short, occasionally branching dichotomously.

In addition to above mentioned fungi, pigeonpea has been found to be infected by *Ovulariopsis ellipsospora* Gorter in South Africa (Nene *et al.* 1996) and *Phyllactenia* sp. in India (Rao 1990).

3.3.3 Host Parasite Interaction

Infection of pigeonpea varieties BDN 1, Hy 3C and TTB 7 by the powedery mildew fungus caused reduction in the thickness of leaves and size of epidermal and palisade cells, number of plastids and size of starch grains. These effects were much more increased in plants with combined infection of powdery mildew and SMV (Prameela *et al.* 1990a). It also reduced the nucleic acid and protein content in leaves greatly.

Infection by powdery mildew pathogen *O. taurica* also altered cell permeability resulting in an increased leakage of electrolyte, loss in chlorophyll, sugar and phenol contents. The effect was much more increased in dual infections of powdery mildew and SMV (Prameela *et al.* 1989a).

Infection of pigeonpea plants by powdery mildew pathogen signals the future infections by *Alternaria* sp. and *Fusarium* sp. (Rao 1990).

3.3.4 Epidemiology and Disease Cycle

The isolates of *Oidiopsis taurica* from different hosts specially pigeonpea, chillies, Guar, merigold etc. have been found to be non-host specific and that the pathogen occurs in anamorphic state only (Pawar *et al.* 1985, Wankhede and Peshney 1992 and Rao 1990). It is also observed that the conidia stored in the laboratory loose germination capacity gradually. Hence, it has been concluded that the pathogen perpetuates by way of collateral hosts during off season or by dormant mycelium. The pathogen is reported to survive on perennial pigeonpea and volunteer plants growing in the shade and on the ratoon growth or as dormant mycelium on infected plant parts like axillary buds (Reddy *et al.* 1993).

The disease is polycyclic resulting in initial infection and secondary spread and the infection is directly proportional to the quantity of inoculum available in the form of conidia. The severity of the disease is influenced by environmental factors. It develops well at 20 to 35°C with an optimum of 25°C. The cool and humid climate is congineal for infection and colonization by the pathogen while warm and humid climate is good for sporulation and spore dispersal.

The host factors also influence the disease development. The varieties with thin and succulent leaves are easily colonized by the pathogen than with thicker ones. The sporulation is more on young leaves than older ones. The higher severity of powdery mildew with increased sporulation has been reported on pigeonpea leaves infected with sterility mosaic as compared to healthy ones (Prameela *et al.* 1989). Such predisposing effect has been shown in plants infected with phyllody also. Since the plants infected by sterlity mosaic and phyllody remains green for longer period, they serve good source of inoculum of powdery mildew.

The disease severity is reported to increase due to early sowing and supply of irrigation than the rainfed crop in India.

3.3.5 Host Resistance

Sources of Resistance: Screening for resistance to powdery mildew has not been done very systematically. There are few reports (Table 3.2) on the sources of the resistance identified by various workers.

Table 3.2: Sources of resistance against powdery mildew of pigeonpea

Number of entries tested	*Entries found resistant*	*Reference*
10	*Atylosia albicans, A. grandifolia, A. rugosa*	Kanniayan & Nene (1979)
182	ICP 7345-2-S10, JM 2498	Anonymous (1982)
—	ICP 7035, ICP 12792, LRG 30	Kannaiyan & Haciwa (1990)
—	ICP 9150, 13107, 13156, 13232	Reddy (1993)
—	ICP 9150, 9177, 7867, 7035, Hy 3c	Reddy *et al.* (1993)
97	PT 25, RA 4, ICP 8862, 7035, BWR 23, BDN 699, MVT 2, BSMR 736	Perane *et al.* (1997)

Prasad *et al.* (1990) screened 48 entries but none was found resistant. It has been reported that local land races of African countries specially Kenya, Malawi, Zambia suffer less due to powdery mildew as compared to Indian lines (Reddy 1993). It is important that African lines are usually late maturing with large thick and dark green leaves. It has been observed in Malawi that the disease is more serious and damaging on short duration varieties than medium and long duration ones (Subramanyam *et al.* 1995). In some varieties/genotypes multiple disease resistance has been identified. The line ICP 7867 is resistant to wilt + SMD + powdery mildew while Hy 3C and ICP 7035 to SMD + powdery mildew + halo blight (Reddy *et al.* 1993).

Technique of Screening: The technique of screening pigeonpea against powdery mildew used at ICRISAT (Anonymous 1982) is as given below.

The disease is created by dusting the conidia of the pathogen collected from the infected material on 15 days old seedlings. The disease develops 15 days after inoculation in the greenhouse. The powdery mildew severity is scored on a 9-point scale of rating as follows :

Grade	*Category*	*Symptoms*
1	Resistant	No visible symptoms
2-3	Moderately resistant	Symptoms on lower surface of few older leaves
4-5	Tolerant	Symptoms on lower surface of most of older and few younger leaves
6-7	Moderately susceptible	Symptoms on all plant parts
8-9	Susceptible	Severe symptoms on all plant parts including deformation of growing shoots and defoliation of infected leaves.

A susceptible check ICP 11293 is suggested for use to monitor the disease occurrence on the test entries.

Another scale of scoring for resistance against powdery mildew used by Prasad *et al.* (1990) is as follows :

0 = No infection
1 = Trace (5% infection)
3 = 10-25% infection
5 = 25-50% infection
7 = 50-75% infection
9 = >75% infection

The lines showing 1-3 score are considered as resistant, and 5 and above as susceptible.

3.3.6 Control

Patel *et al.* (1992) recommended 0.07% spray of thiophanate methyl twice or 0.04% dinocap for control of powdery mildew and increase in grain yield with a cost benefit ratios of 1 : 4.36 and 1 : 2.16 respectively. It checked damage due to powdery mildew and improved quantity and quality of green pods of pigeonpea. Reddy *et al.* (1993) suggested some control measures against powdery mildew of pigeonpea.

* Select field away from perennial pigeonpea affected by disease
* Late sowing of pigeonpea (after July)
* Spray wettable sulpher @ 1 g/l or triadimefon (Bayletan 25 EC) @ 0.03 per cent.

3.4 Rust

Rust of pigeonpea was reported for the first time from India (Sydow and Butler 1906). The disease has so far been reported from several other countries specially Australia, Bermuda, Colombia, Cote d'Ivoire, Guatemala, Jamaica, Kenya, Nigeria, Philippines, Puerto Rico, Siera Leone, South Africa, Sri Lanka, Tanzania, Trinidad and Tobago, Uganda, Venezuela, Vietnam and Zambia (Nene *et al.* 1996). The disease also occurs in China, Ghana, Guiana, Japan, Malaysia, Mauritius, Sudan and Taiwan (CMI Map No. 236). The disease is potentially important in some areas specially Caribbean region (Spence 1975), Puerto Rico (Cook 1939), Africa (Kannaiyan *et al.* 1981) etc. where it is widespread, although in most of the other countries it is not considered to be a serious one. The disease has been reported to cause no adverse effects on the yield of peas in Trinidad (Ariyanayagam and Spence 1978). The rust of pigeonpea is caused by different fungi in different areas.

3.4.1 Symptoms

The typical symptoms of rust are dark brown raised pustules developing on the lower surface of leaves. According to Brathwaite (1980) the disease is characterized by the development of rust coloured spots on the lower surface of leaves. The infected leaves quickly turn yellow and fall. The heavy leaf falling would cause high yield losses in the crop.

3.4.2 Causal Organisms

Uredo cajani Sydow
Uromyces dolicholi Arthur
Phakopsora pachyrhizi Sydow

The rust of pigeonpea is caused mainly by *Uredo cajani* which has been reported from Puerto Rico (Barrett 1925), Sierra Leone (Deighton 1929), Jamaica (Naylor 1974), Caribbean region (Spence 1975), Nigeria (Williams and Allen 1976), Trinidad (Rampersad 1976) and U.S.A. (Kaiser 1981). In some countries/regions, the disease is reported to be caused by *Uromyces dolicholi* specially in Trinidad and Puerto Rico (Stevenson 1917, Nowell 1923, Abrams *et al.* 1978), U.S.A. (Jehle and Wood 1926), South Africa (Doidge 1941), Kenya (Nattrass 1958), Guatemala (Muller 1950), Columbia (Kern and Thurston 1954), Ivory Coast (Viennot-Bourgin 1959) and Uganda (Mukiibi 1976). However, some confusion existed concerning the proper identification of these two fungi on pigeonpea foliage (Briant and Martyn 1929). The *U. dolicholi* is found mostly on *Rhynchosia*, a wild legume, whereas *U. cajani* occurs mostly on pigeonpea. The differentiation is possible on the basis of telial stage only which is formed in *U. dolicholi* but not in *U. cajani*. At ICRISAT (Anonymous 1978), microscopic studies revealed the presence of only *uredospores* which measured 17.5 to 22.5 (20.35) μ × 15.0 to 20.0 (18.8) μ. These measurements tallied with 20-28 × 18-24 μ reported by Sydow and Butler (1906). The uredospores germinate on slide in moist chamber within 12 h by producing germ tubes and appressoria.

The fungus *Phakopsora pachyrhizi* has been reported to cause pigeonpea rust in Australia and Philippines (Nene *et al.* 1996).The fungus causes rust of soybean but teliospores of this fungus were formed on pigeonpea when inoculated and grown in 12 h photoperiod at 60-100 % RH and a maximum day temperature of 24 +1°C and a minimum night temperature of 15 ± 1°C (Yeh *et al.* 1981). The fungus has been described as follows:

Spermogonia and aecia unknown; uredinia folicolous, hypophyllous, subepidermal, erumpent, pulverulent, scattered, often coalescent, buckthorn brown to dresden brown (ridgway), round to oval, 100-25 μm in diameter covered with a basket of paraphysis united at the base forming a dome like covering over the uredinium. *Paraphyses* is curved, inwardly slanting at the centre of the raised uredinium, clavate or clavate capitate, hyaline to sub-hyaline with a narrow lumen, 8-13 µm broad at the head and up to 45 µm long; *urediniospores* Naples yellow (ridgway), obovoid, sub-globose or pyriform, (20-) 24-30 (-32) × 16-22 (-24) µm, wall uniformly upto 1.5 µm thick, finely echinulate, germpores 7-8, scattered. *Telia* so far not observed in the Sudian material.

3.4.3 Disease Cycle and Epidemiology

The disease affects determinate as well as indeterminate cultures of pigeonpea but less disease is observed on those grown under dry conditions (Jackson 1976). The disease occurs widely in the Caribbean region and increases with the onset of flowering (Mohammed 1978). Dense planting and formation of the closing canopy seem to provide a favourable microclimate for development of the disease. The pathogen *U. cajani* is photosensitive and sporulates with diurnal periodicity. The light, rain, wind and overcast skies enhance the spore release, dispersal of the pathogen and development of the disease. It is reported that spores of *U. cajani* can germinate as long as water is present (McKie 1976). After the germination, germtubes form appressoria and penetrate the leaf within 8 h after inoculation (Rampersad 1976). Barnes (1973) observed minute white spots on leaves 7 days after inoculation and first uredosorus opened on 12th day and all opened on 14th day.

The early maturing varieties are reported to escape the severe infection (Mohammed 1978). It is expected that the varieties with narrow leaves as in Indian lines possibly may increase the light infiltration minimizing fall of lower leaves ultimately checking the disease development. Determination of spore concentration daily, identifying sources of inoculum and observing weather conditions can assist in the prediction of rust incidence.

3.4.4 Host Resistance

Resistance has been reported in pigeonpea varieties Blanco and Todo Tempo in Puerto Rico (Barrett 1925), No. 17 in Jamaica (Jackson 1976) and some germplasm lines in Trinidad (Ariyanayagam and Spence 1978). Late maturing genotypes like 1156, 113 and 158-32 and early maturing 158-1 showed some resistance to *U. cajani* in Puerto Rico (Echavez-Badel and Bosgus-Vega 1998).

3.4.5 Control

Spray of manab is reported to check development of the disease and to delay the leaf fall during the reproductive phase (Naylor 1974, Barnes 1973). In Jamaica, spray of growth regulator (ethephone) at 250-500 ppm minimized the effect of rust in susceptible variety by inducing leaf fall and second flowering but such effect was not observed in resistant variety (Hammerton 1975). It ultimately increased number of pods.

The rust of pigeonpea can be minimized by avoiding pigeonpea crop close to bean fields and rotating the crop to reduce chance of survival of the pathogen (Reddy *et al.* 1993). In Puerto Rico, the disease was found less serious in crops sown in February than in other period (Echavez-Badel and Bosgus-Vega 1998).

3.5 Synchytrium Orange Gall

This disease was first reported from Sri Lanka under the name rust caused by *Woroninella umblicata* (Park 1934 and 1935). It is a minor disease and has so far been reported from India and Sri Lanka only (Nene *et al.* 1996).

The main symptoms of the disease are formation of numerous, reddish orange galls on leaves, stems and pods. The galls are isolated or crowded together becoming cupulate on dehiscence. According to Ramakrishnan and Sundaram (1954), one or more bright reddish orange sori are found in each gall and these measure 230 to 500 μ in size.

The disease is caused by *Synchytrium umblicatum* (Berk & Broome) Karling. The pathogen was first described on *Cajanus cajan* from Ceylon under the name *Aecidium cajani* (Petch 1909) but it was considered identical to *Aecidium umblicatum* (Petch 1912). Later, it was revised as *Woroninella umblicata* by Petch (1918). However, Gaumann did not consider it right and accepted it as synonymous with *Synchytrium* which is now accepted. Ramakrishnan and Sundaram (1954) described the pathogen in India as *sporangia* thin-walled and 22 × 19 μ (15-25 × 12-22 μ) in size.

The disease being minor, no control measures are suggested.

3.6 Synchytrium Brown Gall and Wilt

The brown gall of pigeonpea caused by *Synchytrium phaseoli radiati* was first reported from India by Gupta and Sinha (1951). The disease is of rare occurrence and has not been reported from any other country. Later, Singh and Pavgi (1972) observed a wilt disease of pigeonpea in Uttar Pradesh with which a *Synchytrium* species resembling to *S. phaseoli radiati* was found associated.

The symptoms of the disease are in form of galls on leaves and stems. They are scattered uniformly, mostly single, rarely compound, spherical, cupulate, 0.4-0.6 mm in diameter. The wilting symptoms have been observed by Singh and Pavgi (1972).

The causal organism is *Synchytrium phaseoli radiati* Sinha and Gupta. The resting *sporangia* are solitary in epidermal host cells, spherical, smooth, dark brown, measuring 165-200 μ (mean 184 μ) in diameter with an epispore of 13-16.5 μ thickness. The pathogen has been reported to infect *Phaseolus radiatus, P. mungo* and *Crotalaria juncea* also (Gupta and Sinha 1951).

The disease is minor and no control measures are suggested.

3.7 Phyllosticta Leaf Spot

The first report of infection of pigeonpea by *Phyllostica cajani* seems to be from Brazil by Rangel (1915) and simultaneously the disease was reported from Bihar, India (Sydow and Butler 1916). Later, the disease was found to occur under natural conditions in United States (Jehle and Wood 1926), Antilles region of Caribbean (Cook 1939), Brazil (Batista and Vital 1952). Jamaica (Leather 1967) and Sri Lanka (Reddy *et al.* 1992a). In Jamaica and Trinidad it has been reported under the name 'Frog Eyespot' disease. The disease has been studied in detail in India by Quiyum (1965) and has been found occurring in the states of Andhra Pradesh, Gujarat, Madhya Pradesh, Maharashtra, Rajasthan, Tamil Nadu and Uttar Pradesh (Kannaiyan *et al.* 1981). The disease is the minor one but it has been occurring in increasing proportions in the state of Uttar Pradesh (Saksena and Kumar 1971).

3.7.1 Symptoms

Light brown to dark brown, small dot like spots appear on leaves after commencement of rains in July to August. The spots enlarge in size and reach up to a diameter of 12 mm. They are circular, with wavy dark brown margins and grey centres containing typical concentric rings of black pin head like pycnidial bodies. The spots become pale and brittle in the centre which later blown off forming shot holes. In severe infections spots may coalesce ultimately resulting in desiccation and defoliation.

3.7.2 Causal Organism

Phyllosticta cajani Sydow

While studying the genus *Phyllosticta* in Maharashtra India, Rao (1964) described *P. cajani* from pigeonpea. According to Pavgi and Singh (1965), the pycnidia of the fungus are amphigenous (Mostly epiphyllous) partly immersed in the mesophyll, ostiolate, flask-shapped, measuring 40-155 μ and ostioles 12.5 to 21.5 μ in diameter. Conidia are abundant and borne singly on simple, short conidiophores, usually filling the pycnidial cavity, hyaline, oval to ovate and measure 2.6 to 5.3 × 2.2 to 2.6 μ (average 4.0 × 2.0 μ).

3.7.3 Disease Cycle and Epidemiology

The pathogen *P. cajani* survives in its infective stage in diseased plant residues in soil for more than 15 months which serves as primary source of inoculum (Saksena and Kumar 1971). The secondary spread takes place by pycniospores produced on leaves. The spores germinate in 6-8 h and penetrate leaves through stomata or infect leaf surface by the infection peg produced from the appressorium. The leaves are susceptible to infection from 12-57 days after emergence. Maximum susceptibility is at age of 45 days. The lower most leaves are infected first and then the disease spreads on the upper leaves of the plant.

The disease generally appears after commencement of rains in July and persists through out the cropping season. Saksena and Kumar (1971) observed high disease intensity in the period of July to October when mean temperature range and RH were 20-30°C and 73-89 per cent. The disease reached the peak in August after which it declined with minimum during cool months of December and January. The disease can assume serious epidemic in October in north-eastern plains of India (Reddy *et al.* 1993).

3.7.4 Host Resistance

Out of 139 pigeonpea varieties screened, only one, namely 3/23-36/1 was found resistant (Saksena and Kumar 1971). The varieties ICPL

161, ICPL 87, EMC and Pusa 33 have been reported to be resistant from Tamil Nadu (Arjunan *et al.* 1986). Gupta *et al.* (1989) evaluated 195 lines of pigeonpea of which Pusa 85, ICPL 335, ICPL 269 and Pusa 5 A were resistant while 20 lines were moderately resistant. They used the rating scale as follows :

Rating	*Leaf area affected (%)*	*Description*
1	0	No infection
3	1-10	Slight infection, few small necrotic spots (Resistant)
5	11-25	Moderate infection, enlarged necrotic spots but not coalescing (Moderately resistant)
7	26-50	Heavy infection, lesions coalescing with blighting almost whole leaf surface, slight defoliation (Moderately susceptible)
9	More than 50	Severe infection, large coalescing lesions and blighting of all leaves leading to pronounced defoliation (Susceptible)

Arjunan *et al.* (1986) used a simple scale for scoring on the basis of per cent leaf area covered by the disease and appearance of the disease on leaves as follows :

Leaf area affected (%)	*Description*
0	Healthy
0.1-5.0	Infection in traces
5.1-25.0	Few small necrotic spots
25.1-50.0	Nearly 50% leaf area covered
50.1-75.0	Whole leaf is almost covered with necrotic spots
More than 75	All the leaves completely covered with necrotic spots and blighting.

However, this scale was not categorized in different reaction grades. Patil and Sapkal (1981) also screened 91 cultivars of pigeonpea under artificial inoculation and reported 19 lines to be resistant.

3.7.5 Control

The inoculum of the pathogen can be reduced by destruction of diseased crop residues. Saksena and Kumar (1971) reported Bisdithane, Dithane Z 78, Captan, Miltox and Cuman sprays to be effective in checking the secondary spread of the disease. Reddy *et al.* (1993) recommended spray of Indofil M 45 @ 3 g/l of water for control of this disease.

3.8 Web Blight

The web blight of pigeonpea was first reported from Uttar Pradesh, India (Dwivedi and Saksena 1975) although, a Rhizoctonia blight showing large, light brown sclerotia on leaves of dead plants was observed earlier on pigeonpea plants which were used as temporary shade for coffee transplants in Philippines (Orillo and Valdez 1958). However, the disease observed in Philippines seems to be different from the web blight recorded in India as symptoms of both do not agree with each other. Web blight has also been reported from Trinidad (Leather 1974 as surmised by Brathwaite 1981), Africa (Kaiser 1976), Sri Lanka (Reddy *et al.* 1992a) and Zambia (Kannaiyan and Haciwa 1992). The disease is minor but it is capable to cause serious losses under favourable conditions specially during rains.

3.8.1 Symptoms

The symptoms of the disease appear as small, irregular, water-soaked spots on leaves and stems. These spots increase in size rapidly during high humidity covering greater part of the leaf blade and stem. This is the conspicuous destructive phase of the disease. The spider web like tan coloured mycelial growth and abundant white and clearly visible microsclerotia develop on the affected parts. The sclerotia later turn brown to chestnut brown. The affected parts dry finally resulting in premature defoliation. The leaves may remain attached for few days under dry weather condition. The severely affected plants may be killed.

3.8.2. Causal Organism

Thanatephorus cucumeris (Frank) Donk
(Anamorph : *Rhizoctonia solani* Kuhn)
Synonyms : *Hypochnus cucumeris* Frank
Pellicularia filamentosa (Pat) Rogers

Corticium solani (Prill. & Delaer) Pilot
Corticium sasaki
and several others

The isolations from the diseased plant parts consistantly produced a pathogenic culture of *Rhizoctonia solani,* the imperfect state of the fungus. On the basis of host range and cross inoculation tests, the pigeonpea web blight pathogen was found to be similar to that causing web blight in mung bean and urd bean. The fungus formed the perfect state (*T.cucumeris*) in culture (Dwivedi and Saksena 1975) and on affected plant parts in the nature under warm and humid conditions with heavy dew formation in the night. The perfect state is described as follows:

The fructifications are resupinate, creamy to greyish white, loosely attached to the substratum, composed of archnoid, repent hyphae giving rise to thin hypochnoid or sub-membranous fertile patches. *Basidia* are produced in clusters terminally in discontinuous hymenium. *Hyphae* 4.5-17 μ wide, often anastomosed and without clamp connections; basal hyphae widest with branching at wide angles while median and subhymenial hyphae are narrow, thin-walled and hyaline. *Basidia* are 9-25 × 5-12 μ but sometimes short, widened, barrel shaped to sub-cylindrical without median constriction. *Sterigmeta* are straight, attenuate towards the apex, usually 4 per basidium, rarely 2, 3 or up to 7 in numbers. *Basidiospores* are hyaline, smooth, thin-walled, oblong to ellipsoid and dorsally flattened or broad, ovoid and widest towards distal end. They form secondary basidiospores (Talbot 1970). The isolates causing web blight in mung bean, urd bean and pigeonpea do not have any remarkable difference (Saksena 1980). On isolation from host in culture the imperfect stage *R.solani* is obtained which is described as follows :

Colonies white and effused, becoming light brown to buff, with frequent sectoring on agar media. *Mycelium* septate, hyaline when young but turning brown, 4.5-8.5 μ wide, lateral branches constricted at point of origin with septum near the junction. Branching of older hyphae at wider angle but in younger one it is at acute angle, cells multi-nucleate with dolipore septa and no clamp connections. *Sclerotia* whitish but later turning brown/chestnut brown, globose to sub-globose, oval or cushion shaped, 2-3 mm but may aggregate to form masses up to 1.2 cm. They are superficial and not differentiated into rind and medula. It produces large sclerotia during active parasitic phase and small light weight during saprophytic phase on dead or near to dead leaves.

3.8.3 Disease Cycle and Epidemiology

The pathogen has been isolated from seeds of pigeonpea (Kamal and Verma 1979) but it is primarily soil borne and the initial inoculum comes on leaves mainly from the soil splashed during rains. The fungus can grow in the soil very fast to a longer distance and can survive there in mycelial or sclerotial form (Saksena 1980). The highest inoculum potential is in the top 10 cm soil and none below 40 cm. The fungus is reported to penetrate through stomata by means of growing hyphal tips without formation of any swelling, mycelial cushions or appressoria. The hyphal branches grow rapidly inter- and intra-cellularly in host tissues. The involved mesophyll cells collapse and become discoloured after sometimes (Dwivedi and Saksena 1975).

The disease develops fast at mean temperature of 20.5-30.5°C and 86-100% RH. The most suited temperature is 26-28°C and 100% RH. Maximum basidiospore production and their discharge occurs after mid-night till early morning. The spore production is favoured by night temperature below 24°C, RH 95% and the evaporation rate of 1.5 mm per day. The Basidiospores germinate within two hours and infect the host if free moisture is given.

The pathogen has very wide host range and is reported to infect 30 common weeds belonging to 8 families which play important role in the initiation and early spread of the disease in main host (Saksena 1985). The disease has been observed in pigeonpea when grown mixed with urd bean and not in sole crop of pigeonpea (Naimuddin *et al.* 1998).

3.8.4 Control

Fungicidal use has not been tested on pigeonpea but blight of mung bean caused by *Corticium sasaki* could be controlled by spraying benomyl or carbendazim 0.05 per cent. Teis *et al.* (1957) obtained control of *Pellicularia filamentosa* with bordeaux mixture and Zineb.

3.9 Macrophomina Leaf Spot/Blight

The pathogen *Macrophomina phaseolina* is mainly soil borne in nature and causes root diseases. Besides the seedling blight, root rot and stem canker of pigeonpea, it causes leaf spot and foliar blight of pigeonpea in north India (Saksena *et al.* 1970). The disease is not widespread because of growth habits of the pathogen and the wider spacings used for planting the pigeonpea.

3.9.1 Symptoms

The symptoms of the disease include small, irregular, somewhat scorched brownish areas, generally along the leaf margins. These areas spread rapidly becoming reddish brown in colour and then drying with formation of numerous black, pin-head size pycnidia mostly on upper surface of infected leaf (Mahrshi 1986). In the beginning the spots are small and circular but later they coalesce forming irregular areas (Srivastava 1982).

3.9.2 Causal Organism

Macrophomina phaseolina (Tassi) Goid.
Sclerotial state : *Rhizoctonia bataticola*

The pathogen has strains which attack foliage of plants and has been described else where. The aerial infection spread through pycnidiospores produced by *M.phaseolina* form while *R.bataticola* form is responsible for root rot (Saksena 1980).

3.9.3 Disease Cycle and Epidemiology

The pathogen survives with seed, soil and diseased plant parts and reaches up to the foliage through splashing rains. The secondary spread on leaves is through wind and water borne inoculum. It penetrates the leaves through stomatal openings without forming any infectious structure (Saksena *et al.* 1970). Plants of 30-60 days age are more susceptible and the disease development is favoured by high RH, rains and a temperature around 30°C.

3.9.4 Control

In vitro, Brassicol, vapam, ceresan wet and Captan completely inhibited the growth of leaf isolate of *M.phaseolina* (Saksena *et al.* 1970). Resistance against the disease has not been observed.

3.10 Foliar Anthracnose

The name anthracnose is derived from the Greek word meaning 'ulcer' and is appropriate because of ulcer like lesions produced on pods specially in common bean. The typical symptoms are sunken spots due to drying up and collapse of the cells in the centre and with the presence of pink sticky spore masses that develop during the moist weather have quite an ulcer like appearance. In general, species of *Colletotrichum* produce the Anthracnose symptoms. The disease was first reported from Brazil (Rangel 1915). It has been reported from several other countries specially Puerto Rico (Jehle and Wood 1926), India (McRae 1932), U.S.A. Venezuella and Zambia (Nene *et al.* 1996). The foliar infection of pigeonpea by *Colletotrichum* sp. has been reported from State of Uttar Pradesh in India (Pavgi and Singh 1964, Kumar *et al.* 1991). It is an important disease of pigeonpea and becomes destructive by infecting leaves, pods and seeds (Tucker 1927a and 1927b) specially during the period of heavy rain fall. Cook (1939) named the disease as 'Foliar anthracnose' and identified it as an important disease of pigeonpea pods.

The losses are mainly due to dropping of pods at young stage and discolouration and decay of some or all the seeds in the infected pods. The extent of damage increases with the age at which the crop is harvested. In a harvest of affected crop 86.25 % pods have been found to be infected yielding 36.3% unmarketable seeds. In Zambia, the disease has commonly been observed on green pods sold in the market with an incidence up to 10 per cent (Kannaiyan and Haciwa 1990).

3.10.1 Symptoms

In case of anthracnose caused by *Colletotrichum cajani,* spots are produced on pods and leaves and the seed is destroyed (Tucker 1927a). The chief symptoms include spots on pods and leaves, blackening and shrinking of veins of infected leaves and their premature fall. The infected pods become distorted, they abort and then die. Affected young pods drop and some or all the seeds in the affected pods are discoloured and decayed.

On the leaves and pods, the spots are minute with dark margins and grey centres with scattered acervuli (Reddy *et al.* 1993). The infected seeds are blackened, smaller and shrivelled. The symptoms produced by *C. gloeosporioides* are spots on pods only which are pink brown cankers delimited by reddish brown borders resulting in pod malformation, low seed numbers and death of pods (Echavez-Badel and Alameda 1998).

3.10.2 Causal Organism

Colletotrichum cajani Rangel
(Teleomorph : *Glomerella cingulata*)

The fungus was first reported from Brazil (Rangel 1915) and has been described in detail by Tucker (1927b). According to him, the *conidia* are cylindrical, broadly elliptical or irregular with rounded ends and 12-17 × 3.5-7.2 μ in size. The *setae* are numerous on old pod spots but rare on leaves, usually somewhat curved, septate and averaging 100 × 3.5 μ. *Appressoria* apparently analogous to chlamydospores and were observed after 2 months on PDA and steamed pigeonpea pods. The conidia were formed after one week on steamed pigeonpea pods only. The fungus did not infect the varieties of *Phaseolus vulgaris* susceptible to *Colletotrichum lindemuthianum.*

Pigeonpea isolate of *C.cajani* has been reported to produce ascigerous stage in culture which corresponds in general characters with *Glomerella cingulata* (McRae 1932). Echavez-Badel and Alameda (1998) reported *C. gloeosporioides* (*Glomerella cingulata*) from Puerto Rico which infected only pods of late pigeonpea.

3.10.3 Disease Cycle and Epidemiology

The pathogen has been found associated with seeds of pigeonpea. Survival of the pathogen in crop debris and other host is not reported. The pathogen was intercepted on a flight from Puerto Rico to U.S.A. The disease is favoured by high moisture and rainfall. Nirula (1980) considered *C. cajani* as the quarantine objectionable pathogen. In Puerto Rico, pod infection by *C. gloeosporioides* was observed at 864 mm precipitation and mean minimum and maximum temperature of 21 and 30°C respectively. The disease was less in crop planted in June-July than May (Echavez-Badel and Alameda 1998).

3.10.4 Control

No work has been done on control aspects but it can be controlled by avoiding fields for pigeonpea cultivation with previous disease record. The crop may be sprayed with mancozeb @ 3 g/1 of water.

3.11 Botrytis Gray Mold

Botrytis gray mold is reported from Bangladesh, India, Nepal and Sri Lanka (Nene *et al.* 1996). The disease is the minor one but under favourable conditions it is capable to cause heavy losses to pigeonpea.

3.11.1 Symptoms

The disease appears at the time of flowering (Reddy *et al.* 1993). Main symptoms of the disease are appearance of dark gray fungal growth on the tender parts specially growing tips, flowers and young pods. The infected flowers drop and pod setting is affected adversely. Pods if formed, are reduced in size with small and shrivelled seeds (Bajpai *et al.* 1995). The affected parts shed on ground and they are covered with sporulating mycelium of the fungus heavily.

3.11.2 Causal Organism

Botrytis cinerea Pers. Ex Fries

The *mycelium* of the fungus is hyaline to brown, septate, 8-10 μ wide. *Conidiophores* light brown with hyaline tips, septate, 8-24 μ wide, branched, bearing small pointed sterigmata. *Conidia* hyaline, one-celled, oval, globose or short cylindric, borne in clusters at tips and measure 4-24 μ × 4-18 μ (14.9 × 8.4μ). The fungus induces production of 3 phytoalexines by leaves of pigeonpea (Cooksay *et al.* 1982).

3.11.3 Disease Cycle and Epidemiology

The pathogen *B. cinerea* has been reported to be associated with seeds of pigeonpea (Ellis *et al.* 1977b, Kumar and Srivastava 1985). The disease has been reported to be more severe on medium to late maturing varieties which flower between 161 to 196 days under Pantnagar conditions. The varieties flowering between 83-117 days are affected less (Bajpai *et al.* 1995).

3.11.4. Control

Spray of crop with Ronilan or Daconil @ 3 g/1 at flowering is effective (Reddy *et al.* 1993). Seed treatment with carbendazim + thiram (1 : 2)

@ 200 g/quintal is effective in chickpea and may be used in pigeonpea also for controlling seed borne inoculum. Destruction of sheded leaves and flowers will reduce inoculum build up.

3.12 Wet Leaf Rot/Seedling Blight

This disease was reported from Pusa in Bihar, India in experimental areas during the month of September (Mishra and Mehra 1969). Later, it was observed in Uttar Pradesh by Singh and Pavgi (1972) who named the disease as 'Wet leaf rot'. The pathogen of this disease causes seedling blight symptoms also in pigeonpea (Naimuddin *et al.* 1999). The disease has so far been reported from India only.

3.12.1 Symptoms

According to Mishra and Mehra (1969), the disease first appears on tender unfolded young leaves later involving older leaves and tender shoots. The infected portion partly looses the green colour showing tendency of wet rot. At advanced stages, luxuriant growth of shining, silvery conidiophores develops on the surface of infected parts on the tips of which minute, greyish black conidial heads appear within 3 days. The rot then extends downwards and infected parts hang limply culminating in death of distal parts. Naimuddin *et al.* (1999) described seedling blight symptoms which resemble to phytophthora blight except that production of dark coloured conidial heads on silvery conidiophores, hanging appearance of the killed growing point and no lesion on petioles or stems of affected plants. The pathogen has been reported to cause flower blight of pigeonpea in Trinidad (Brathwaite 1981).

3.12.2 Causal Organism

Choanephora cucurbitarum (Berk & Rav.) Thext.

The fungus produces sporangia and conidia in culture. The *sporangia* are terminal, pendent with definite columella, 38.5-152 μ in diameter and release light brown, ovoid, smooth *Sporangiospores* of 14.5-23.5 × 8-14 μ size each provided with a tuft of hair like appendages at both the ends. The *conidiophores* are erect ending in capitate vesicle from which short secondary vesicles are produced bearing short sterigmata on which conidia are borne. The *conidia* are light brown to reddish brown, avoid, longitudinally striate and often provided at the base with a short hyaline appendage. Conidia measure 13.5-20.5 μ × 8.0-12.5 μ in size.

3.12.3 Disease Cycle and Epidemiology

Not much work has been done on this aspect of the disease. However, it seems to be much influenced by the environmental conditions. As per observations of Mishra and Mehra (1969), the disease appeared in September and continued to spread till end of the October after which it declined sharply showing no evidence of fresh infection towards end of November. During the period of the disease spread, the maximum temperature was 33-36°C, minimum temperature 17-24°C and RH 85-100 per cent. During the November, RH was identical but maximum and minimum temperature ranges were 26-31°C and 10-13°C respectively. Almost all the leaves affected by leaf folder were parasitized by the pathogen probably due to the fact that injury and increased moisture in the folded leaves facilitated infection of this facultative parasite (Naimuddin *et al.* 1999).

3.12.4 Host Resistance and Control

Under the natural infection conditions, Mishra and Mehra (1969) reported E 12 (R 10/ P2), E 25 (R 10 H/P 2), E 42 (R 21/P2), E 171 (S 28/P1), BR 60, E 1 (R1/P2) and E 130 (R 105/P2) to be free from the disease while several other genotypes were infected. Out of 148 genotypes, 103 including ICP 7119 (Hy 3 C), ICP 7200, ICP 8610, ICP 9252, ICPL 151, ICPL 270, Asha (ICPL 87119), BWR 370, KPBR 80-2-1 were found free from the disease (Naimuddin *et al.* 1999).

No fungicides have been tested against the disease.

3.13 Leaf Blight

A severe leaf spot and leaf blight of pigeonpea was reported from Nagaland (Singh 1988). The disease appeared in July and continued till October. It is a minor disease and not reported from other countries although, pathogen is of common occurrence.

3.13.1 Symptoms

The symptoms have been described by Singh (1988) as dark brown circular to elliptical lesions, 2-10 mm in diameter, coalescing to form dark brown patches. At advance stage of infection, the leaves turn yellow and finally discoloured and die. The white mycelial growth with abundant conidia develops on blighted leaves under humid conditions.

3.13.2 Causal Organism

Fusarium semitectum Berk and Ravenel
= *Fusarium pallidoroseum* (Cooke) Saccardo

Fusarium semitectum produces white, cottony, mycelial growth on PDA which later changes to light yellow or buff brown. The *hyphae* are septate, 3-6 µm, branched, creeping; *conidiophores* phialidic producing *macroconidia* measuring 15-35 × 3.5-4.5 µm. They are hyaline, fusoid, abundant, 3-7 septate and wedge shaped. The *chlamydospores* are thick walled, globose, intercalary, 8-12 µm in diameter formed singly or in chain.

3.13.3 Disease Cycle and Epidemiology

The fungus *F. semitectum* was found internally associated with pigeonpea seeds (Ellis *et al.* 1977a) in Puerto Rico and it was responsible for reducing germination of seed in the field (Ellis *et al.* 1978). The association of this fungus with the pigeonpea seeds has been reported in India (Kumar and Srivastava 1985 and Solanke *et al.* 1990) and Trinidad (Maximay *et al.* 1992) also. The seed infection has been found to increase in the field past maturity (Ellis *et al.* 1977b).

3.13.4 Control

No control measures are recommended. The infection of the seed can be minimized with increase in its germination by seed treatment with captan (Ellis *et al.* 1977a), spray of benomyl on the crop and timely harvest of the crop after maturity (Ellis and Paschal 1977, Ellis *et al.* 1977b).

3.14 Cercoseptoria Leaf Spot

This disease was first reported from India by Pavgi and Singh (1965) and later from Zambia (Kannaiyan and Haciwa 1990). The disease is considered as minor one.

3.14.1 Symptoms

The disease is characterized by formation of light brown, polygonal spots limited by veins which turn reddish brown surrounded by dark brown margins. The spots are 0.5 to 2.5 mm in size but may coalesce together forming large patches.

3.14.2 Causal Organism

Cercoseptoria cajaniocola Pavgi and Singh

Cercoseptoria is near to *Cercospora* and synonym to *Pseudocercospora*. The pathogen has been described on pigeonpea by Pavgi and Singh (1965). The infection spots are foliicolous, scattered, limited by veins, coalescent to form blotches, light reddish brown and 0.5-2.5 mm in size. The stromata are prominent, subepidermal, densly fasciculate, produced on both the surfaces of leaf and are 30 to 75 µ in size. The *conidiophores* arise in groups, 1-3 septate, non-geniculate, straight or slightly curved, 23.8-40.0 × 2.0-2.6 µ in size. *Conidia* are hyaline, sub-cylindrical to filamentous, slightly flattened, pointed downwards, multiseptate, 40.6-155.5 × 1.3-2.2 µ in size.

3.14.3 Disease Cycle and Epidemiology

No detailed study has been done on this aspect. The pathogen survives on diseased leaves as stroma in the field and produced conidia under favourable conditions. The inoculum thus produced infects the fresh crop and spreads through air.

3.14.4 Control

The disease is minor and no recommendations have been made to control the disease. However, crop rotation and timely weeding may help in reducing the build up of the inoculum and to control the disease.

3.15 Brown Leaf Spot

This disease was first reported from India during October to December (Pavgi and Singh 1965). The infection was sparse and sporadic. The symptoms of the disease could be confused with those of *Cercospora instabilis*. The symptoms appears as small, olive brown spots which often enlarge and become coalescent. Older lesions develop zonate rings and diffused chlorosis around the spots. No shot holes are produced and the infection is folicolous. The spots are few, brown, irregularly round to oval, scattered, some times coalescent, 5-8 × 4-6 mm with pycnidia developing in lighter areas. The effect of the disease on host was negligible. The lighter brown perithecia in the umbrinous spots can be distinguished from the brown stromata of *Cercospora* on careful examination.

The disease is caused by *Leptosphaerulina briosiana* (Poll.) Grahm and Luttrell which incites leaf spots on species of *Medicago* and is pathogenic on other legumes also. It produces 3-5 × 0-2 μ size septate ascospores (chiefly 4 septate). It is distinct from *L. arachidicola* by absence of dimorphic ascospores and larger dimensions of the ascocarp, asci and ascospores.

No work on control aspect is reported.

3.16 Pyrenochaeta Leaf Spot

This disease was reported from India in the middle of August onward (Pavgi and Singh 1965). The spots appeared usually on lower leaves and the infection gradually spread on to the upper foliage. The infection continued till diseased leaves fell down in December finally leaving no traces of the pathogen on the host plant. The symptoms appear as small olive brown spots which often enlarge and become coalescent. Older lesions develop zonate rings and diffuse chlorosis around the spots. No indications of tissue freying into shot holes is discernible at any time. The infection is foliicolous; spots few, brown, irregularly round to oval, scattered, sometimes coalescent, 5 to 8 × 4 to 6 mm showing zonate rings. Pycnidia developing in the lighter areas.

The disease is caused by *Pyrenochaeta cajani* Singh and Pavgi which has pycnidia amphigenous but mostly epiphyllous, dark brown, ostiolate, spherical to pyriform, partially burried in the mesophyll with ostioles protruding, measuring 115 to 218 μ in diameter. Pycnidiospores hyaline, ovate to cylindrical, occasionally slightly curved and measuring

2-5.5 μ × 1.3-2.3 μ. Setae mostly around the ostiole, stiff, erect, dark brown. 0-4 septate and measuring 30 to 180 μ × 6 to 8 μ.

No work has been done on other aspects of the disease.

3.17 Periconia Leaf Spot

A leaf spot disease of pigeonpea was recorded from Bihar, India on variety Bahar grown during the post-rainy season (Mehta and Sinha 1983). Symptoms of the decease include small, necrotic spots with reddish brown and silver shining appearance on leaflets.

The disease is caused by *Periconia byssoides* Pers. (Mehta and Sinha 1983). Another species reported on *Cajanus* and several other hosts is *Periconia igniaris* Mason & Ellis, a *Periconia* state of *Didymosphaeria igniaria* Booth (Ellis 1971). It is distinguished from *Periconia curta* by its longer narrower conidiophores, shorter branches, much more strongly echinulate conidia and in culture, by the production of rose madder or wine coloured pigments. *Conidiophores* are up to 550 μ long, 9-13 μ thick at the base, 6-10 μ immediately below the head. *Conidia* spherical, brown, 7-10μ in diameter with spines approximately 1 μ long.

3.18 Phoma Leaf Spot

In India, *Phoma herbarum* Westend has been reported infecting leaves of pigeonpea (Rajak and Rai 1982). The fungus form dull grey to green colonies with compact aerial mycelium exhibiting uniform growth rate and attaining 4.5 to 5 cm diameter on oat agar after 7 days. *Pycnidia* abundant, dark brown to black, globose to sub-globose, sometimes coalescing to form irregular fructifications of 72-150 μ in size. *Pycnidiospores* are hyaline, one-celled, ovoid on malt agar and rice agar but ellipsoid on oat agar media 3.7-7.4 μ × 1.5-3 μ in size. The red pigment turns violet blue on application of strong NaOH.

Kernkamp and Hemerik (1953) found pigeonpea to be infected by *Ascochyta imperfecta* Pk from alfalfa in Minnesota, U.S.A. *A. imperfecta* as well as *Phoma herbarum* have been considered as synonyms to *Phoma medicaginis* Malbr. & Roum.

3.19 Algal Leaf Gall

A parasitic alga *Cephaleuros virescens* has been reported to infect pigeonpea in Puerto Rico (Stevenson 1918). An algal leaf gall of pigeonpea has also been reported from India (Singh and Pavgi 1972). The alga is endophytic and forms numerous small solitary galls on upper surface of young leaves. Leaves near soil are more infected showing bronz appearance.

3.20 Cladosporium Leaf Spot

At Bhagalpur, India, Rizwi (1978) observed a severe leaf spot on pigeonpea during October. The disease is characterized by greyish, circular spots surrounded by a zone of yellow halo. The spots are small, chlorotic patches on the upper surface of the leaflets which later turn gray to olive green in colour and defoliation takes place. The pathogen is identified as *Cladosporium cladosporioides* (Fr.) de Vr. The disease has so far been reported from India only and no further work has been done except that the pathogen is found associated with seeds (Kumar and Srivastava 1985, Pande and Verma 1992).

A similar disease of pigeonpea has been observed in Zambia by Kannaiyan and Haciwa (1990) with the name Cladosporium leaf blight caused by *Cladosporium oxysporum* Berk and Curtis. It causes spotting of pods also in case of severe infections.

3.21 Myrothecium Leaf Spot

This is a minor disease reported from India only (Nene *et al.* 1996). The disease is reported to be caused by *Myrothecium gramineum* Lib. in Rajasthan exhibiting small, oval to irregular, brown spots on leaves. The spots enlarge, coalesce giving blighting appearance to the leaves under higher humidity. Brown to black coloured sporodochia are observed in the central part of the spot on the lower surface of leaf (Fig. 3.2). The affected portion often cracks. The conidia swarm out in a loose gelatinous mass on proving with a needle. The conidia in mass appear olivaceous in colour.

3.22 Stemphyllium Leaf Spot

A leaf spot of pigeonpea caused by *Stemphyllium* sp. has been reported on variety Mauritous from Hawaii. The pathogen produced severe spotting and caused defoliation of leaves under inoculation test in pot culture (Anonymous 1947).

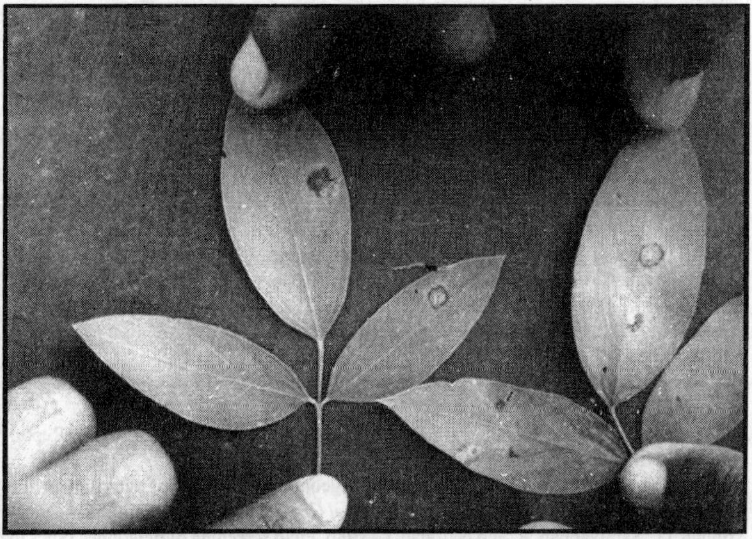

Fig. 3.2: Myrothecium leaf spots of pigeonpea.

3.23 Other Leaf Infecting Pathogens

Other fungi recorded on pigeonpea are *Pithomyces sacchari* (Speg) Ellis which has conidia of 12.25 × 15 μ in size. The fungus *Stachybotrys parvispora* Hughes has been reported on dead leaves of *Cajanus* sp. *Phaeoisariopsis griseola* (Sacc) Ferrasis has been reported from Zambia on variety Hy 3C (Kannaiyan and Haciwa 1990). The fungus *Chaetoseptoria wellmani* which causes serious infections of several legumes in Guatemala has been found to infect pigeonpea also (Muller, 1953).

3.24 Pod-Rots

A pod rot disease of pigeonpea has been reported from India by Bhargava *et al.* (1980). The disease is characterized by appearance of water-soaked lesions on pods. The lesions initially appear at the base of the pod. The infection gradually spreads to entire pod. In severe cases the entire pod gets covered by the green spore mass of the pathogen *Aspergillus flavus*. The younger pods are more susceptible than the older ones. The rainfall during the maturity or harvesting of the crop favours the spread of the disease.

REFERENCES

Abrams, R., Morales, A. and Julia, P. J. 1978. Status of research on pigeonpea in Puerto Rico. *Tropical Grain Legume Bulletin* 11:12-17.

Angus, A. 1962. Annotated list of Plant pests and diseases in Zambia Pt 1. Plant Pathologists report : Chilanga, Zambia. Mot. Makulu Research Station p. 21.

Anonymous 1947. Plant Pathology, Plant Physiology, Entomology and vegetable crops. Report, Hawaii Agricultural Experiment Station 1944-46. pp. 67-145.

Anonymous. 1973, Report of the Faculty of Agriculture, 1971-72. St. Augustine, Trinidad and Tobago : University of West Indies.

Anonymous. 1978. Pulse Pathology (Pigeonpea) Report of Work 1977-78. Progress Report 1, ICRISAT, Hyderabad, India, pp. 252.

Anonymous. 1982. Pulse pathology (Pigeonpea) Report of Work 1981-82 Progress Report 23, ICRISAT, India, pp. 1-113.

Anonymous. 1983. Pulse Pathology (Pigeonpea) Report of Work 1982-83 Progress Report 30, ICRISAT, India pp. 187.

Anonymous. 1986. Pulse Pathology (Pigeonpea) Report of Work 1985 - 86. Progress Report 48, ICRISAT, India, pp. 85.

Ariyanayagam, R.P. and Spence, J.A. 1978. Pigeonpea improvement activities at the University of West Indies, Trinidad. *Tropical Grain Legume Bulletin* 13:14-18.

Arjunan, G., Samiyappan, R. and Natrajan, C. 1986. Field screening of pigeonpea types to Phyllosticta leaf spot. *International Pigeonpea Newsletter* 5 : 36.

Bajpai, G. C., Tripathi, H. S., Singh, I. S. and Singh, A. K., 1995 Susceptibility of pigeonpea cultivars of different maturity groups to Botrytis gray mold. *International Chickpea and Pigeonpea Newsletter* 2 : 67.

Barnes, R. F. 1973. A preliminary list of literature on pigeonpea *Cajanus cajan* (L) Millsp. Department of Biological Sciences Pt. Pathology Bulletin 1. University of West Indies, Saint Augustine, Trinidad.

Barret, O.W. 1925. The food plants of Puerto Rico,1925. *Journal of the Department of Agriculture, Puerto Rico* 9 : 61-208.

Bates, G.R. 1957. Botany and Plant Pathology. Report of the Ministry of Agriculture, Rhodesia and Nyasaland, 1955-56. pp. 79-86.

Batista, A. C. and Vital, A. F. 1952. (Monograph of the species of Phyllosticta in Pernambuco.). *Boletim da Secretaria da Agricultura Pernambuco* 19 : 1-80.

Bhardwaj, C. L. and Singh, B. M. 1984. Host range of *Oidium* state of *Erysiphe pisi* from peas on some leguminous hosts in Kangra valley of Himachal Pradesh. *Indian Phytopathology* 37 : 732-733.

Bhargava, S.N., Shukla, D.N. and Dwivedi, D.K. 1980. Pod-rots of pea, red gram and Brassica. *National Academy Science Letters* (India) 3 : 287.

Briant, A. K. and Martin, E. B. 1929. Diseases of cover crops. Tropical Agriculture 6 : 258-260.

Butler, E.J. 1906. The wilt disease of pigeonpea. *Agricultural Journal of India* 1 : 25-36.

Butler, E. J. 1918. Fungi and diseases in plants. Thacker Spink & Co. Calcuttà, 547 pp.

Ciferri, R. 1927. (Report on Phytopathology. Principal diseases of cultivated plants observed during the year 1926). *Informe Annual, Estacion, Agronomica de Moca, Republica Dominicana* 2 : 36-44.

Ciferri, R. and Gonzalez, Fragoso R. 1927. (Parasitic and saprophytic fungi of the Dominican Republic (10th Series). *Boletin de la Real Sociedad Espinola de Historia Natural* 27 : 165-177.

Commonwealth Mycological Institute. 1951. Distribution maps of plant diseases. Map 236. Kew Survey, UK: CMI.

Cook, M.T. 1939. (Disease of economic plants in the Antilles) Monograph Series No. 4 Rio Pidras, Puerto Rico: University of Puerto Rico, 530 pp.

Cooksey, C. J., Dahiya, J. S., Garratt, P. J. and Strange, R. N. 1982. Two novel stilbene-2-carboxylic acid phytoalexins from *Cajanus cajan. Phytochemistry* 21 : 2935-2938.

Curzi, M. 1932. (Of African fungi and diseases. I. Concerning certain parasitic Hyphomycetes from Italian Somaliland). *Bolletino della R. Stazione di Patologia Vegetale di Romans* 12: 149-168.

Deighton, F.C. 1929. Report of the Mycological Section. Report, Lands and Forest Department, Sierra Leone, 1928. pp. 14-19.

Desai, B. G., Vora, M. S. and Patel, J. C. 1981. A note on survey of pigeonpea diseases in Gujarat state. *Pulse Crop Newsletter* 1 (3) : 54.

Doidge, E. M. 1941. South African rust fungi. 4. *Bothalia* 4 : 229-236.

Dwivedi, R. P. and Saksena, H. K. 1975. Web blight diseases of arhar (*Cajanus cajan* (L) Millsp.) caused by *Thanatephorus cucumeris. Indian Journal of Farm Sciences* 3 : 113-114.

Echavez-Badel, R. and Alameda, M. 1998. Incidence of anthracnose in long day pigeonpea trials. *Journal of Agriculture of the University of Puerto Rico* 82 : 209-211.

Echavez-Badel and Bosques-Vega, A. 1998. Reaction of the new long day pigeonpea genotypes to rust *Uredo cajani. Journal of Agriculture of the University of Puerto Rico* 82 : 201-208.

Ellis, M. B. 1971. Dematiaceous Hyphomycetes. Commonwealth Mycological Institute, Kew Surrey, UK. 608 pp.

Ellis, M.A. and Paschal, E.H. II. 1977. Method of controlling internally seed born fungi of pigeonpea (*Cajanus cajan*). *Proceedings of the America Phytopathological Society* 4 : 176 (Abstr.).

Ellis, M. A., Paschal, E. H. II and Powell P. 1977a. The effect of maturity and foliar fungicides on pigeonpea seed quality. *Plant Disease Reporter* 61 : 1006-1009.

Ellis, M. A., Paschal, E. H. II and Rosario, E. 1777b. Similarities in seed borne fungi of four leguminous crops. *Proceedings of American Phytopathological Society* 4: 176 (Abstr.).

Ellis, M. A., Paschal, E. H. II, Ravalo, E. J. and Rosario, E. 1978. Effect of growing locations on internally seed borne fungi, seed germination and field emergence of pigeonpea in Puerto Rico. *Journal of Agriculture of the University of Puerto Rico* 62 : 355-360.

Gohokar, R. T. and Peshne, N. L. 1985. Powdery mildew of pigeonpea new to Vidarbha. *PKV Research Journal* 9 (1) : 98.

Grewal, J. S., Mahendra Pal and Kulshreshtha, D. D. 1988. Fungal diseases of pulse crops. Pages 259-315 in Pulse Crops (Eds. B. Baldev, S. Ramanujam and H. K. Jain). Oxford & IBH Publishing Co. Pvt. Ltd., New Delhi, India.

Gupta, D. K. and Srivastava, L. S. 1991. Floury spot of arhar, a new disease from NEH region. *Plant Disease Research* 6 : 103.

Gupta, R. P., Singh, D. P., Singh, B. B. and Singh, S. P. 1989. Field screening of pigeonpea germplasm for resistance to phyllosticta leaf spot. *International Pigeonpea Newsletter* 10 : 25.

Gupta, S.C. and Sinha, S. 1951. Further additions to the *Synchytria* of India. *Indian Phytopathology* 4 : 7-10.

Gurjar, R. B. S. 1988. Screening of certain pigeonpea cultivars/germplasm accessions against alternaria blight in Rajasthan. *Indian Phytopathology* 41 : 281 (Abstr.).

Hammerton, J.L. 1975. Effects of growth regulators on pigeonpea (*Cajanus cajan*). *Experimental Agriculture* 11 : 241-245.

Hasija, S. K. 1964. Additions to the fungi of Jabalpur IV. *Mycopathologia et Mycologia Applicata* 23 : 234-239.

Jackson, P. E. 1976. Gungo peas (*Cajanus cajan*). *Bulletin Ministry of Agriculture and Fisheries*, Jamaica, New Series 64 : 164-166.

Jehle, R. A. and Wood, J. I. 1926. Diseases of field and vegetable crops in the United States in 1925. *Plant Disease Reporter* 45 (Suppl.): 152.

Kaiser, W. J. 1976. Important diseases and pests of bean (*Phaseolus vulgaris),* lima bean (*Phaseolus lunatus)* and pigeonpea (*Cajanus cajan*) in Africa. *African Journal of Plant Protection* 1 : 97-102.

Kaiser, W. J. 1981. Diseases of chickpea, lentil, pigeonpea and tepary bean in continental United States and Puerto Rico. *Economic Botany* 35 : 300-320.

Kamal and Verma, A. K. 1979. Seed borne mycoflora of arhar (T 21) effect of culture filtrate of some isolates on seed germination and fungicidal seed treatment. *Indian Journal of Mycology and Plant Pathology* 9: 41-45.

Kamat, M. N. and Patel, M. K. 1948. Some new hosts of *Oidiopsis taurica* (Lev.) Salmon in Bombay. *Indian Phytopathology* 1:153-158.

Kannaiyan, J. 1981. Diseases observed on pigeonpea in East Africa. *International Pigeonpea Newsletter* 1 : 27-28.

Kannaiyan, J. and Haciwa, H. C. 1990. Diseases of pigeonpea in Zambia. *International Pigeonpea Newsletter* 12 : 22-23.

Kannaiyan, J. and Haciwa, H. C. 1992. New record of fusarium wilt and web blight of pigeonpea in Zambia. *International Pigeonpea Newsletter* 15 : 18.

Kannaiyan, J. and Nene, Y. L. 1977. Alternaria leaf spot of pigeonpea. *Tropical Grain Legume Bullettin* 9 : 34.

Kannaiyan, J. and Nene, Y. L. 1979. Occurrence of powdery mildew on *Atylosia* species. *Tropical Grain Legume Bulletin* 15 : 22-23.

Kannaiyan, J. and Nene, Y. L. 1986. Screening pigeonpea for resistance to alternaria blight. *Indian Phytopathology* 39 : 547-549.

Kannaiyan, J., Nene, Y. L., Reddy, M. V. and Raju, T. N. 1981. International survey of pigeonpea diseases. Pulse Pathology Progress Report No. 12. Patancheru, A.P., India : ICRISAT, 82 pp.

Kern, D. and Thurston, H. W. 1954. Additional species of Uredinales from Columbia. *Mycologia* 46 : 354-357.

Kernkamp, M. F. and Hemerik, G. A. 1953. The relation of *Ascochyta imperfecta* to alfalfa seed production in Minnesota. *Phytopathology* 43 : 378-383.

Khan, T. N. and Onim, J. F. M. 1972. Breeding and genetic improvement of pigeonpea (*Cajanus cajan* (L.) Millsp.). Annual Project Report, National Research Council, Uganda.

Khan, T. N. and Rachie, K.O. 1972. Preliminary evaluation and utilization of pigeonpea germplasm in Uganda. *East African Agricultural and Forestry Journal* 38 : 78-82.

Kumar, J., Dutta, M. and Prasad, Rajendra. 1991. Pigeonpea diseases at different altitudes in Garhwal hills, India. *International Pigeonpea Newsletter* 14:17.

Kumar, K. and Patnaik, P. 1985. Seed borne nature of *Alternaria alternata* in pigeonpea, its deterioration and control. *Indian Journal of Plant Pathology* 3 (1) : 69-73.

Kumar, K. and Patnaik, P. 1986. Effect of fungicidal treatment of *Alternaria alternata* infected pigeonpea seeds on germination. *Pesticides* 20 (3) : 17-18.

Kumar, K. and Srivastava, S. S. L. 1985. Fungi associated with pigeonpea seeds, their effect and control. *Indian Journal of Plant Pathology* 3 (1) : 53-56.

Lal, H.C., Upadhyay, J.P. and Ojha, K.L. 1998. Management of alternaria leaf blight of pigeonpea through plant extracts and chemicals of plant origin. *Journal of Applied Biology* 8 : 80-85.

Lal, H.C., Upadhyay, J.P. and Ojha, K.L. 1999. Evaluation of homeo-drugs against alternaria leaf blight of pigeonpea. *Journal of Applied Biology* 9 : 81-83.

Leather, R. I. 1967. A catalogue of some plant disease and fungi in Jamaica. *Bulletin, Ministry of Agriculture*, Jamaica, New Series No. 61.

Mahmood, M., Sinha, B. K., Kumar, S., Chowdhury, S. K., Singh, C.P. and Murtaza, M. 1983. *Rajendra Agriculture University Journal* 4:89-90.

Mahrshi, R. P. 1986. A report on three pigeonpea diseases in Rajasthan. *International Pigeonpea Newsletter* 5 : 32-34.

Maximay, S., Duncan, E. J. and Brathwaite, C. W. D. 1992. Internally seed borne fungi of pigeonpea (*Cajanus cajan* (L.) Mill sp.) in Trinidad, isolation and occurrence. *Tropical Agriculture* 69 (3) : 260-262.

Mayee, C. D. and Datar, V. V. 1986. Phytopathometry. *Technical Bulletin No. 1*.Marathwada Agricultural University Parbhani, Pages 146.

Mckie, M. O. P. 1976. A study of the germination of uredospores of *Uredo cajani* in the water, distilled water and 0.5 % glucose. B. Sc. Agriculture Project, University of West Indies, St. Augustine, Trinidad, Trinidad and Tobago.

McRae, W. 1932. Report of the Imperial Mycologist. Scientific Reports of the Imperial Institute of Agricultural Research, Pusa, 1930-31. pp. 73-86.

Mehta, P.P. and Sinha, R.K.P. 1982. A new leaf spot disease of arhar from India. *Science and Culture* 48 :44.

Mehta, P.P. and Sinha, R.K.P. 1983. A leaf spot caused by *Periconia byssoides,* new to post-rainy season pigeonpea. *International Pigeonpea Newsletter* 2 : 59-60.

Mishra, D.P. and Mehra, R. C. S. 1969. *Choanephora cucurbitarum* on *Cajanus cajan* in India. *Indian Phytopathology* 22: 515-517.

Mohammed, Caroline, L. 1978. Preliminary investigation in pigeonpea rust, *Uredo cajani* Syd. M.Sc. thesis, University of West Indies, St. Augustine, Trinidad, Trinidad and Tobago. 190 pp.

Mukiibi, J. 1976. Possible relationship between intercropping and plant disease problems in Uganda. Paper presented at the Symposium on Intercropping for Semi-Arid Areas, University of Dar-es-Salam, Tanzania.

Muller, A. S. 1950. A preliminary survey of plant disease in Guatemala. *Plant Disease Reporter* 34 : 161-164.

Muller, A. S. and Chupp, C. 1945. (The Cercosporae of Venezuela). *Boletin de la Sociedad Venezolana de Ciencias Naturales* 8: 35-39.

Naimuddin, Chaudhary, R. G. and Vishwadhar. 1998. Role of mixed cropping in the development of web blight of pigeonpea. Page 59 in Abstracts National Symposium on Management of Biotic and Abiotic Stresses in Pulse crops, 26th to 28th June 1998, Indian Institute of Pulses Research, Kanpur, India.

Naimuddin, Chaudhary, R. G. and Vishwadhar. 1999. A note on the seedling blight of pigeonpea caused by *Choanephora cucurbiterum* (Berk &Rao) Thaxt. *Annals of Plant Protection Society* 7:107-109.

Narayanaswamy, P. and Jaganathan, T. 1975. A note on powdery mildew disease of pigeonpea (*Cajanus cajan* (L.) Millsp.). *Science and Culture* 41 : 133-134.

Narula, P. N. 1983. Short duration pigeonpea escape leaf blight disease in late seedling in Bihar. *International Pigeonpea Newsletter* 2: 50-51.

Nattrass, R. M. 1958. Report of the Senior Plant Pathologist. Report Department of Agriculture, Kenya 1956. Pt. 2, pp. 9-14.

Naylor, A. G. 1974. Diseases of Plants in Jamaica. Kingston, Jamaica Ministry of Agriculture, Agricultural Information Services, 129 pp.

Nene, Y. L., Sheila, V. K. and Sharma, S. B. 1996. A world list of chickpea and pigeonpea pathogens. 5th edn. Patancheru, Andhra Pradesh, India : ICRISAT, pp. 27.

Nirula, K.K. 1980. Quarantine to seed exchange at the ICRISAT. *Seed Pathology News* 13 : 11-12.

Nowell, W. 1923. Diseases of crop plants in lesser Antilles. London, UK West Indian Comm. 383 pp.

Nowsher, A.Z. M., Khan, A. and Shamin Shamsi. 1986. Hyphomycetes from Bangladesh. *Bangladesh Journal of Botany* 15 : 111-121.

Nutsugah, S. K., Kodama, M., Otani, H., Nakajima, H. and Kohmoto, K. 1993a. Tennazonic acid production of *Alternaria tenuissima* and its phytotoxicity to pigeonpea. *Journal of Faculty of Agriculture*, Tottory University 29 : 1-14.

Nutsugah, S. K., Kohmoto, K., Otani, H., Kodama, M. and Sunkeswari, R. R. 1994. Production of a host specific toxin by germinating spores of *Alternaria tenuissima* causing leaf spot of pigeonpea. *Journal of Phytopathology* 140 : 19-30.

Nutsugah, S. K. Otani, H. Kodama, M., Akimitsu, K. and Kohmoto, K. 1993b. Suppressive effect of light on necrosis development of pigeonpea leaves elicited by *Alternaria tenuissima* toxin. *Journal of the Faculty of Agriculture*, Tottory University 29 : 15-23.

Nutsugah, S. K., Park, P., Otani, H., Kodama, M. and Kohmoto, K. 1993c. Ultrastructural changes in pigeonpea cells caused by a host specific toxin from *Alternaria tenuissima*. *Annals Phytophathological Society of Japan* 59 (4): 407-415.

Ojha, C. B., Choudhary, S. K. and Singh, N. B. 1993. Inheritence of resistence to alternaria leaf blight in pigeonpea (*Cajanus cajan* (L.) Millsp.). *Indian Journal of Genetics and Plant Breeding* 53 : 115-117.

Onim, J. F. M. 1974. Improvement of pigeonpea. Development of resistance to *Mycovellosiella cajani*. M.Sc. thesis, Makerere University, Uganda.

Onim, J. F. M. 1980. Foliar fungicides for the control of *Mycovellosiella cajani* causing the leaf spot of pigeonpea. *Indian Journal of Agricultural Sciences* 50 : 615-619.

Onim, J. F. M. and Rubaihayo, P. R. 1976. Screening of pigeonpea for resistance to *Mycovellosiella cajani*. *SABRAO Journal* 8 : 121-125.

Orillo, F. T. and Valdez, R. B. 1958. Four diseases of coffee hitherto undescribed in the Philippines. *Philippine Agriculturist* 42 : 292-302.

Pal, M. 1984. Control of seed borne *Alternaria tenuissima* in pigeonpea. *Indian Phytopathology* 37 : 548-550.

Pande, Alka and Varma, K. V. R. 1992. Seed borne fungi of pigeonpea, their pathogenicity and fungicidal control. *Biovigyanam* 18:33-38.

Park, M. 1929. Report of the Mycological Division. Technical Report, Department of Agriculture, Ceylon, 1928, pp. 1-6.

Park, M. 1935. Report of the work of the Mycological Division. Report of the Directorate of Agriculture, Ceylon, 1934.pp. D 124-34.

Patel, M.K., Kamat M.N. and Bhide, V.P. 1949. Fungi of Bombay, *Supplement I. Indian Phytopathology* 2 : 149.

Patel, P. K., Lakhtaria, R. P., Andani, V.P. and Vaishnav, M. U. 1992. Control of powdery mildew of pigeonpea by different fungicides. *Indian Journal of Mycology and Plant Pathology* 22 : 106 (Abst.).

Pathak, A. K. and Gurjar, R. B. S. 1989. Field reaction of pigeonpea varieties and lines in a natural out break of alternaria blight. *Indian Journal of Mycology and Plant Pathology* 19 : 198-199.

Patil, B. G. and Sapkal, R. C. 1981. Reaction of tur varieties to Phyllosticta leaf blight. *Indian Journal of Mycology and Plant Pathology* 11 : 117.

Paul, Y. S. and Kapoor, J. N. 1987. Taxonomy of anamorphs of Erysiphaceae-II. *Indian Journal of Mycology and Plant Pathology* 17: 298-304.

Pavgi, M. S. and Singh, U. P. 1964. Parasitic fungi from northern India. III. *Mycopathologia et Mycologia Applicata* 24 : 347-354.

Pangi, M.S. and Singh, R.A. 1965. Some parasitic fungi on pigeonpea from India. *Mycopathologia et Mycologia Applicata* 27 : 97-106.

Pagji, M. S. and Singh, R. A. 1971. Parasitic fungi from north India. VIII. *Mycopathologia et Mycologia Applicata* 43 : 117-125.

Pawar, R. N., Utikar, P. G. and Shinde, P. A. 1985. A study of powdery mildew of chilli. *Journal of Maharashtra Agricultural Universities* 10 (2): 218.

Perane, R. R., Bendre, N.J., Aher, R.P. and Mhase, L.B. 1997. Evaluation of pigeonpea genotypes against powdery mildew (*Oidiopsis taurica* (Lev.) Salmon). *Legume Research* 20 (1):67.

Petch, T. 1909. Revision of Ceylone fungi. *Annals of Royal Botanical Garden, Peradoniya.* 4: 302.

Petch, T. 1912. Ustilagineae and Uredineae of Ceylon. *Annals of Royal Botanical Garden Peradoniya* 5 : 256.

Petch, T. 1918. *Tropical Agriculturist* I: 262.

Prameela, H.A., Joshi, S.S., Vishwanath, S. and Anilkumar, T.B. 1990a. Histological and Histochemical changes in pigeonpea due to single and dual infections by powdery mildew and sterility mosaic virus. *Biochem. Physiol. Pflanzen* 186 : 55-61.

Prameela, H.A., Vishwanath, S. and Anilkumar, T.B. 1989a. Physiological and biochemical changes in pigeonpea (*Cajanus cajan* (L) Millsp.) due to single and dual infection with powdery mildew and sterility mosaic. *Biochem. Physiol. Pflanzen*. 184 : 439-445.

Prameela, H.A., Vishwanath, S. and Anilkumar, T. B. 1989b. The predisposing effect of sterility mosaic to powdery mildew infection in pigeonpea. *Zentralblatt fur Mikrobiologie* 144 (2): 111-114.

Prameela, H.A., Vishwanath, S. and Anilkumar, T.B. 1990b. Effect of single and combined infections of powdery mildew and sterility mosaic on nodulation and biomass of pigeonpea. *Zentralblatt fur Mikrobiologie* 145 : 37-39.

Prasad, M., Rajendra, Dutta, G.C., Saini and Gautam, P.L. 1990. Occurrence of pigeonpea powdery mildew in the hills of Garhwal, Himalaya. *International Pigeonpea Newsletter* 12 : 21-22.

Qaiyum, A. 1965. Studies of Phyllosticta leaf spot of arhar (*Cajanus cajan*). M.Sc. thesis, Agra University, Agra, India.

Rachie, K.O. and Wurster, R.T. 1971. Potential of Pigeonpea (*Cajanus cajan* (L.) Millsp.) as a horticultural crop in east Africa. *Acta Horticulturae* 21 : 172-178.

Rajak, R.C. and Rai, M.K. 1982. Species of *Phoma* from legumes. *Indian Phytopathology* 35 : 609-612.

Ramakrishnan, T.S. and Sundaram, N.V. 1954. Notes on some fungi from south India. IV. *Indian Phytopathology* 7 : 140-151.

Rampersad, M. 1976. Determination of uredospore germination in pigeonpea. Applied Botany Study Project, University of West Indies, St. Augustine, Trinidad, Trinidad and Tobago.

Rangel, E. 1925. Fungus parasites of Pigeonpea (*Cajanus indicus* Spreng.). *Boletim de Agricultura,* Sao Paulo 16: 145-156.

Rao, V. G. 1964. The genus *Phyllosticta* in Bombay, Maharashtra. IV. *Mycopathologia* 22 : 157-166.

Rao. V. 1990. Powdery mildew of pigeonpea and their host range. *Indian Phytopathology* 43 : 262 (Abstr.).

Rathi, Y.P.S. and Nene, Y.L. 1984. Diseases of Pigeonpea (Hindi). Pages 190-204 in "Faslon ke Rog" (eds. Ram Krishna Parashar and Rajendra Kumar). Directorate of Translation and Publication, G.B. Pant University of Agriculture and Technology, Pantnagar, Nainital, U.P. India.

Reddy, A.R., Chauhan, V.B., Venkateswarlu, S., Singh, O.N., Singh, H.N. and Singh, R.M. 1984. Reaction of pigeonpea cultivars to alternaria blight in post-rainy planting. *Madras Agricultural Journal* 71 : 34-135.

Reddy, M.V. 1993. Is African pigeonpea germplasm a source of resistance to powdery mildew. *International Pigeonpea Newsletter* 17:27.

Reddy, M. V. and Jain, K.C. 1992. Recent advances in breeding for resistance to disease inpigeonpea. Pages 77-83 in New Frontiers in Pulses Research and Development : Proceedings of National Symposium, 10-12 November 1989 (Eds. J.N Sachan), Directorate of Pulses Research, Kanpur, India.

Reddy, M.V., Raju, T.N., Sharma, S.B., Nene, Y.L. and McDonald, D. 1993. Handbook of Pigeonpea diseases, Patancheru, India : *ICRISAT Information Bulletin* No. 42, pp. 61.

Reddy, M.V., Saxena, K.B., Jayasekara, S.J.B.A. and Faris, D.G. 1992a. Assessment of diseases on short duration pigeonpea in Sri Lanka. *International Pigeonpea Newsletter* 15 : 15-27.

Reddy., M.V., Subramanyam, P., Linkoswe, A.A., Saka, V.W., and Muku, W.A.B. 1992b. Survey of pigeonpea diseases in Malawi. *International Pigeonpea Newsletter* 15 : 24-25.

Rizwi, M.A. 1978. A new leaf spot disease of pigeonpea. *Indian Phytopathology* 31 : 235.

Rubaihayo, P.R. and Onim, J.F.M. 1975. A study of some characters of pigeonpea. *SABARAO Journal* 7 : 183-187.

Saksena, H.K. 1980. Epidemiology of diseases caused by *Rhizoctonia* species. Pages 59-64 in Proceedings of the Consultants Group Discussion on the Resistance to Soil-borne Diseases of Legumes, 8-11 January 1979, Patancheru : ICRISAT, Patancheru, India.

Saksena, H.K. 1985. Relationship of environment and Rhizoctonia aerial blights. *Indian Phytopathology* 38 : 584-585.

Saksena, H.K. and Kumar, K. 1971. Some aspects of epidemiology and control of phyllosticta leaf spot of arhar (*Cajanus cajan* (L.) Millsp.). *Proceedings of the Indian National Science Academy* 37 : 399-406.

Saksena, H.K., Singh, S.B. and Kumar, K. 1970. Leaf spot and blight disease of arhar caused by *Rhizoctonia.* Pages 241-247 in Recent Advances in Crop Production : Proceedings of the Symposium, February 1970, U.P. Institute of Agricultural Sciences, Kanpur, India.

Saksena, H.K., Singh, U.N. and Singh, R.R. 1976. *Mycosphaerella* from a leaf spot of arhar (*Cajanus cajan* (L.) Millsp.). *Indian Journal of Farm Sciences* 4 : 124-125.

Sen Gupta, P. K. 1974. Diseases of major pulse crops. PANS 20:409-15.

Sharma, D., Kannaiyan, J. and Saxena, K.B. 1987. Sources of resistance and inheritance of resistance to alternaria blight of pigeonpea. *SABRAO Journal* 19 : 109-114.

Sharma, N.D. and Mishra, R.P. 1977. Some additions to fungi of India. II. *Journal of the Indian Botanical Society* 56 : 130-141.

Singh, H.B. 1988. Leaf blight of pigeonpea by *Fusarium semitectum. International Pigeonpea Newsletter* 7 : 29-30.

Singh, R.A. and Pavgi, M.S. 1972. Some diseases of pigeonpea in Uttar Pradesh, India. *FAO Plant Protection Bulletin* 20: 116-118.

Singh, U.B. 1931. Studies in the genus *Cercospora. Journal of the Indian Botanical Society* 10 : 73-91.

Singh, U.B. 1934. Studies on *Cercospora indica,* new species parasitic on *Cajanus cajan* Spreng. *Indian Journal of Agricultural Sciences* 4 : 343-360.

Singh, U.P., Chauhan, V.B. and Reddy, P.R 1984. Field Screening of pigeonpea and *Atylosia* for resistance to *Alternaria tenuissima. International Pigeonpea Newsletter* 3 : 38-39.

Singh, U.P. and Fazili, M.A. 1988. Survival of *Alternaria tenuissima* in soil. *Indian Phytopathology* 41 : 251-253.

Singh, U.P., Fazili, M.A., and Zargar, G.H. 1986. The relationship among plant stature, flowering period and susceptibility of pigeonpea varieties to *Alternaria tenuissima. Indian Phytopathology* 39 : 532-535.

Singh, U.P., Singh, P. and Singh, R.M. 1988. Inheritance of field resistance to alternaria blight in pigeonpea. *International Pigeonpea Newsletter* 7 : 4-5.

Singh , U.P., Zargar, G.H. and Fazili, M.A. 1986. Growth of foliage of pigeonpea (*Cajanus cajan* (L.) Millsp.) and disease progress of alternaria blight. *Journal of Phytopathology* 115 : 147-151.

Sinha, B.K. and Mahmood, M. 1993. Epidemiology of alternaria leaf blight of pre-rabi pigeonpea ir Bihar caused by *Alternaria tenuissima* (Kunze ex Pers.) Wiltshire. *Journal of Applied Biology* 3 : 52-55.

Solanke, R.B., Choulwar, S.B. and Kore, S.S. 1990. Efficacy of some fungicides on seed mycoflora, seed germination and seedling vigour of pigeonpea. *Research Bulletin of Punjab University of Sciences* 41 (1-4) : 109-111.

Songa, W.A. 1991. Evaluation of pigeonpeas for cercospora leaf spot resistance in Kenya. *International Pigeonpea Newsletter* 13 : 24 - 26.

Spence, J.A. 1975. The importance of diseases in relation to the grain legume research programme in the eastern Caribbean. Pages 151-155 in Tropical diseases of legumes (Eds. J. Bird, and Marmorosch, K.). New York, U.S.A., Academic Press.

Srivastava, R.C. 1980. Fungi causing plant diseases at Jaunpur (U.P.) IV. *Indian Phytopathology* 33 : 221-224.

Srivastava, R.C. 1982. Fungi causing plant disease at Jaunpur (U.P.). V. *Indian Journal of Mycology and Plant Pathology* 12 : 244 - 246.

Stevenson, J.A. 1917. Diseases of vegetable and garden crops. *Journal Department of Agriculture, Puerto Rico* 1 : 93-117.

Stevenson, J.A. 1918. A check list of Puerto Rican fungi and host index. *Journal Department of Agriculture, Puerto Rico* 2 : 125-164.

Subramanian, C.V. 1971. Hyphomycetes. Indian Council of Agricultural Research, New Delhi, India, pp. 930.

Subramanyam, P. 1994. Pigeonpea diseases in eastern and southern Africa. Pages 32-36 in Improvement of Pigeonpea in Eastern and Southern Africa : Annual Research Planning Meeting 1993, Bulawayo, Zimbabwe, 25-27 October 1993 (eds. S.N. Slim, S. Tuwafe and L. Singh). Patancheru, India : ICRISAT.

Subramanyam, P., Reddy, M.V., Linkoswe, A.A., Saka, V.W. and Muku, W.A.B. 1995. Diseases of pigeonpea in Malawi. *International Pigeonpea Newsletter* 16 : 75.

Sydow, H. and Butler, E.J. 1906. Fungi Indiae orientalis. Part I. *Annals of Mycology* 4 : 424-445.

Sydow, H. and Butler, E.J. 1916. Fungi Indiae orietalis. Part V. *Annals of Mycology* 14 : 177-220.

Talbot, P.H.B. 1970. Principles of fungal taxonomy. McMillan, London.

Telix, S. 1960. A list of *Cercospora* occurring in Mauritius, with short notes on the newly recorded species of some economic importance. *Revue Agricole et Sucriere de l'Ile Maurice* 39:9-14.

Theis., T., Freyre, R.H. and Kennard, W.C 1957. *Pellicularia filamentosa* on *Tephrosia vogelli* and *Cajanus indicus* in Puerto Rico. *FAO Plant Protection Bulletin* 5 : 159-160.

Tucker, C.M. 1927a. Pigeonpea anthracnose. *Journal of Agricultural Research* 34 : 589-596.

Tucker, C.M. 1927b. Report of the Plant Pathologist. Report of the Puerto Rico Agricultural Experiment Station 1926. pp. 28-30.

Uppal, B.N. 1937. Summary of work done under the Plant Pathologist to the Government, Bombay Presidency, Poona. Report of the Department of Agriculture, Bombay, 1935-36. pp. 203-207.

Venkateswarlu, S., Reddy, A.R., Singh, O.N. and Chauhan, V.B. 1981. Alternaria blight : the most serious disease of post-rainy season (rabi) pigeonpeas. *International Pigeonpea Newsletter* 1 : 28-29.

Viennt-Bourgin, G. 1959. (Uredinales of Africa-Uredinales of Ivory Coast). *Encyclopedie Mycologique* 31 : 137-248.

Wallace, G.B. 1930. Mycological work. Report, Department of Agriculture Tanganyika 1928-29. Pt 2. pp. 35-36.

Wankhade, Shalini V. and Peshney, N.L. 1992. Conidial survival and cross infectivity of certain powdery mildew fungi prevalent in Vidarbha. *Indian Journal of Mycology and Plant Pathology* 22 : 195-196.

Williams, F.J. and Allen, D.J. 1976. Pigeonpea diseases. Page 58 in Pathology : Grain Legume Training Course, 16 August to 26 November 1976. Ibadan, Nigeria: International Institute of Tropical Agriculture.

Wutke, E.B. and Ito, M.F. 1990. Occurrence of *Cercospora* spp. in pigeonpea. *Summa Phytopathologica* 16 : 178-183.

Yeh, C.C., Tschanz, A.T. and Sinclair, J.B. 1981. Induced teleospore formation by *Phakopsora pachyrhizi* on soybeans and other hosts. *Phytopathology* 71 : 111-112.

4

Diseases Caused by Bacteria

Pigeonpea is not damaged much by bacterial pathogens. There are a few diseases caused by bacteria attacking pigeonpea of which bacterial leaf spot and stem canker is important. It occurs commonly and may become serious under favourable weather conditions. The literature on bacterial diseases of pigeonpea/legumes has been reviewed by Rangaswami (1962), Patel and Jindal (1970), Chand (1986) and Jindal and Patel (1988).

4.1 Bacterial Leaf Spot and Stem Canker

This disease was first reported from India in the states of Maharashtra by Kulkarni *et al.* (1950). The disease has also been reported from several other pigeonpea growing countries specially Sudan (Sabet 1959, Sabet *et al.* 1969), China (Fang *et al.* 1964), Puerto Rico (Corter-Monllor and Ruiz 1987), Fizi (Davis *et al.* 1988), Zambia (Kannaiyan and Haciwa 1990), Sri Lanka (Reddy *et al.* 1992a) and Malawi (Reddy *et al.* 1992b). In addition to these countries, the bacterial leaf spot and stem canker either or both the diseases occur in Australia, Myanmar and Panama (Nene *et al.* 1996). In no case the disease has been found severe although, it has potential to damage the crop extensively under favourable weather conditions. In india, the disease has been found to occur in the states of Tamil Nadu (Rangaswami 1962), Punjab, Haryana, Delhi (Patel and Jindal 1970), Uttar Pradesh (Singh and Pavgi 1972), Gujarat (Desai *et al.* 1981), Rajasthan (Mahrshi 1986), Madhya Pradesh (Agrawal and Prasad 1990), Andhra Pradesh, Orissa and Bihar (Kannaiyan *et al.* 1981).

The disease occurs widely in Malawi but may not cause more damage as cankers on stem are mostly superficial (Reddy *et al.* 1992b). The disease is considered as the serious one in Fiji (Davis *et al.* 1988).

Gaikwad and Kore (1981) observed up to 40% disease incidence at Parbhani, Maharashtra and found 10-15% affected grains in the diseased plants.

4.1.1 Symptoms

Symptoms of the disease have been described as small (0.5 mm), round, water soaked spots on leaves. With the development, the spots become quadrilateral surrounded by 0.5 mm halo on upper surface. The spots are light brown initially, become dark brown later and are raised due to drying of the exudation. They are present all over the leaf and may coalesce to form large lesions of 2 mm in severe cases. The infection extends to main and lateral veins of leaf, its edges and petioles resulting in general yellowing of leaf and cracking of petioles and finally their shedding (Kulkarni *et al.* 1952).

In the seedlings, characteristic cankerous lesions develop on the stem just above the primary leaves usually causing breakage. The broken shoot remains attached to plant until it is detached by wind or other means (Reddy *et al.* 1987). The lesions on the main stem and side branches are dark brown and upto 12.5 mm long and 2.5 mm broad. When numerous in number, they cause pealing of bark. A gummy bacterial exude is also formed by the side of these cankers (Kulkarni *et al.* 1952). The cankers on the stem are generally not deep and do not cause girdling but severe infection which is established early, may cause mortality of the seedlings (Jindal and Patel 1988). Severe infection of stem may cause death of even full grown plant (Anonymous 1982). Desai *et al.* (1983) described the symptoms as 'rough stem canker' and 'smooth stem canker' as follows:

Rough Stem Canker : The disease starts and advances as minute specks from the stem base. The cankerous, ocher brown growth develops on stems, branches, twigs, petioles and peduncles (Fig. 4.1R). The patches are common in the form of rings on stem at junctions of branches. The infection may extend to the top of the branches and twigs in the form of distinct lines or bands. It results in heavy flower drop and formation of under-developed pods. The lesions are irregular in shape surrounded by marked yellow green halos which on rupturing secrete light pink to brownish-black gummy material.

Smooth Stem Canker : Desai *et al.* (1983) suspected these symtoms to be produced due to *Pseudomonas* spp. The affected areas on the stem, branches, twigs, petioles and peduncles become slightly raised, smooth

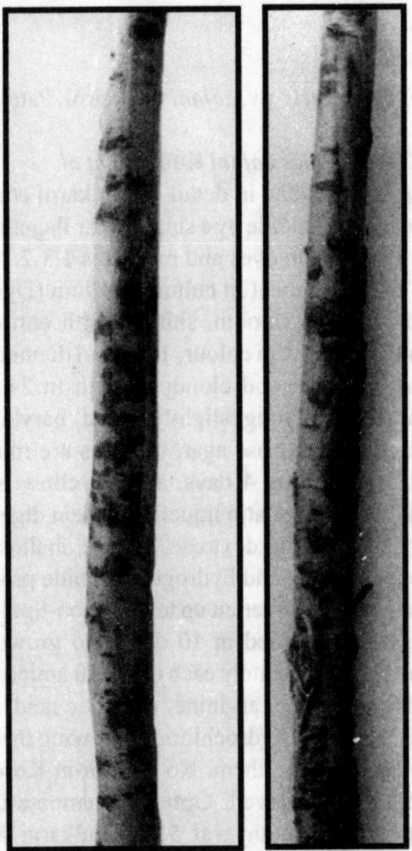

Fig. 4.1: Smooth (S) and rought (R) bacterial stem canker of pigeonpea.

and light to dark purplish-black (Fig. 4.1S) and involve larger areas than in rough stem canker. The patches are typically surrounded by broad, light brown halos. The lesions become cankerous due to excessive longitudinal rupturing of the surface tissues and secret light pink to brownish-black gummy material. These symptoms have also been observed in Madhya Pradesh (Agrawal and Prasad 1990) but its etiology needs confirmation.

These two symptoms of stem cankers are distinguishable at later stage only when characteristic cankerous growth develops on coalesced spots.

4.1.2 Causal Bacterium

Xanthomonas campestris pv. *cajani* (Kulkarni, Patel & Abhyanker) Dye.

Synonym : *Xanthomonas cajani* Kulkarni *et al.*

The bacterium was studied in detail by Kulkarni *et al.* (1952). It is a short rod, gram negative, motile by a single polar flagellum, capsulated, readily stained with common dyes and measures 1.3-2.2 × 0.9-1.4 μ in size. It produces brown pigment in culture medium (Dye 1962).

On PDA, colonies are smooth, shining with entire margins and pulvinate, naphthaline yellow in colour, 1.5 cm in diameter after 7 days; in nutrient dextrose broth, good cloudy growth in 24 h; on nutrient agar, colonies are round, shining, slightly raised, baryta yellow, 7 mm after 4 days; on nutrient dextrose agar, colonies are round with entire margins, convex, 1.2 cm after 4 days, amber yellow in colour. Milk peptonized, litmus reduced, gelatin liquefied, casein digested and starch hydrolyzed; acid but no gas in dextrose, lactose, maltose and sucrose; salicin not utilized; ammonia and hydrogen sulphide produced; nitrates not reduced, sodium chloride tolerant up to 3 % ; non-lipolytic; Loeffler's solidified blood serum liquefied in 10 days. No growth in inorganic basal medium containing separately each of the 10 amino acids (glycine, lyrosine, tryptophane, cystine, arginine, asparatic acid, glutamic acid, creatine, histidine, guanidine hydrochloride) showing that the bacterium cannot derive its carbon from them. No growth in Koser's liquid and solid citrate media was observed. Optimum temperature for growth 26-32°C and thermal death point was 51°C (Kulkarni *et al.* 1950 and 1952). The pathogen survived for one year with high virulence at 6-8°C in culture under paraffin oil but frequent sub-culturing reduced the virulence of the pathogen (Rai and Singh 1986a).

According to Cortes-Monller and Ruiz (1987), this bacterium forms butter yellow, mucoid and shiny colonies. It hydrolyses gelatin, starch, fats, casein and esculin; acidifies glucose, sucrose and maltose but not salicin and uses citrate and matonate.

Host Range : Large number of plant species belonging to diversified groups have been tested by artificial inoculation but the bacterium is reported to be host specific (Kulkarni *et al.* 1952, Sabet 1959, Gaikwad and Kore 1981, Rai and Singh 1986b, Mahrshi 1986 and Cortes-Monller and Ruiz 1987). Studies on several strains of *X. phaseoli* and *X.cajani* isolated from pigeonpea (Sabet 1959), and several species of *Xanthomonas* infecting leguminous hosts (Bhatt and Patel 1954) showed that they are indistinguishable by the usual bacteriological procedures except their host ranges. The *X. cajani* was host specific. Hence, species under study including *X.cajani* were considered as formae speciales of *Xanthomonas phaseoli*. The leaf and stem isolates of the pathogen from pigeonpea also showed similar characters (Mahrshi 1986).

4.1.3 Host Parasite Interaction

The histopathological studies of infected pigeonpea leaf were conducted by Rai and Singh (1985). The vertical sections through leaves exhibited the presence of bacteria in intercellular spaces. It caused destruction and granulation of protoplast in spongy and palisade parenchyma which ultimately resulted in cell destruction, collapse and formation of bacterial pockets. The mesophyll cells around these pockets enlarged to form round, elliptical or retort-like abcission cells. With the advancement in the disease severity, large cavities full of bacteria were formed in the mesophy11 affecting cellular organization of leaf. The leaf tissues towards lower epidermis appeared to be macerated in which bacterial pockets were formed frequently. The physiology and biochemistry of the infected plant has not been studied.

In stem, the cortical cells, phloem parenchyma, cambium and sclerenchymatous xylem parenchyma become meristematic. Intercellular tanin, starch as well as lignin of cell walls disappear. A large mass of undifferentiated and unorganized tissues is produced due to hypertrophy and hypoplasia (Jindal and Patel 1988).

4.1.4 Disease Cycle and Epidemiology

The pathogen *Xanthomonas campestris* pv. *cajani* has been found to be seed borne in nature (Patel and Jindal 1970). The bacterium survives in the infected pigeonpea seeds from harvest until the next sowing season and is located in seed coat only (Rai and Singh 1986a). Artificially and naturally infected seeds have been reported to produce 15 and 10% infected plants respectively. On seed, the pathogen has been considered as quarantine objectionable pathogen (Nirula 1980). Survival of the pathogen on other host is not possible as this is reported to be host specific. No information is available on its survival in the plant debris.

The pathogen is active during the monsoon from July to September when the RH ranges from 80 to 90%, temperature 24 to 31°C and plants are succulent (Kulkarni *et al.* 1952). The disease is also favoured by shade which happens specially due to rapid growth of inter-mixed crops like Sorghum. The plant age also plays important role in the infection. According to Gaikwad and Kore (1981), the leaves and stems are attacked up to the plant age of 135 to 145 days. However, Rai and Singh (1986b) reported that pigeonpea plants are most susceptible to *X. campestris* pv. *cajani* at the age of 1-5 weeks showing maximum disease intensity (45%) and shortest incubation period of 2 days. The susceptibility declines with the age up to 10 weeks after which infection does not take place.

4.1.5 Host Resistance

Resistance to bacterial leaf spot and stem canker has been identified in several germ plasm lines and cultivars (Table 4.1). In a screening test of large number of pigeonpea lines received from Kenya, India, Tanzania, the Philippines and Mozambique, a large proportion of the germplasm from countries other than India proved to be highly susceptible to this disease (Reddy *et al.* 1987). Amongst the Indian genotypes, BDN 1 had very small stem lesions as compared to very large galls produced on stems of susceptible lines from other countries which resulted in breakage of stem and drying of plant. Davis *et al.* (1988) reported that resistance to bacterial stem canker exists in pigeonpea lines in Fiji.

Table 4.1: Sources of resistance to bacterial leaf spot and stem canker of pigeonpea

Number of entries tested	*Entries found resistant*	*Reference*
2065	None was free but 148 were moderately resistant	Anonymous (1978)
—	C 49, C 60, C 69, E 200, E !75, JA 8, Pant A 2	Gaikwad & Kore (1981)
249	ICP 8863	Anonymous (1982)
587	ICP 6524 (free), ICP Nos. 6933, 7217, 7445, 7490, 7585, 7980, 8860, 8863, PR 5490, and 5341-3 had less disease	Anonymous (1983)
—	AS 71-37 (free)	Desai *et al.* (1983)
15	S 80	Mahrshi (1986)
235	ICP Nos. 12807, 12848, 12849, 12937, 13051, 13116 and 13148	Reddy *et al.* (1987)
21	Bahar, AS 71-37 (JA 4), ICP 4070 and 5 were MR	Agrawal and Prasad (1990)
35	ICPL 85049 was resistant to both and 6 lines to leaf spot	Arjunan *et al.* (1991)
46	ICPL 270 and 21 lines MR	Sriniwasulu *et al.* (1991)
8	Basant	Bordoloi and Rathaiah (1997)

The resistance to bacterial stem canker is probably linked with colour of the stem. In general, the lines with green stem show higher susceptibility than the lines with purple or sun-red stem (Reddy *et al.* 1987). Even the green coloured stem segregant from the resistance purple stemed genotypes show susceptibility to the disease. Such type of observation has been made by Agrawal and Prasad (1990) also. In the same way, Arjunan *et al.* (1991) observed red flowered lines to be more susceptible than yellow flowered lines.

Scoring Technique : For rating the reaction of this disease, a 9-point scale was used at ICRISAT (Anonymous 1978) as follows:

1 = No infection
3 = Lesions few, seen after careful examination
5 = Lesions common but not destructive
7 = Lesions very common causing some damage
9 = Lesions large causing severe damage

Other scales used for scoring the pigeonpea genotypes against bacterial stem canker are as described below :

(1) A 0-4 point scale used by Mahrshi (1986) is as follows :

0 = Free from disease = Resistant
1 = 5 % disease intensity = Moderately resistant
2 = 25 % disease intensity = Moderately susceptible
3 = 50 % disease intensity = Susceptible
4 = 51 % or more disease intensity = Highly susceptible

(2) The scale used by Reddy *et al.* (1987) was based on size of the lesion on stem as : R = Stem lesion up to 2 mm, MR = Stem lesion 2-20 mm and S = Stem lesions more than 20 mm in size.

(3) Agrawal and Prasad (1990) used the criteria of per cent incidence for scoring as : R = Up to 10% incidence, Moderately resistant = More thn 10% and up to 20% canker, Susceptible = More than 20% to 50% disease incidence and Highly suscepible = More than 50% incidence of stem canker.

For creating artificial epiphytotic of the disease, no method has been standardized. However, Mahrshi (1986) could inoculate leaves. stems of pigeonpea using cotton swabs absorbed with 48 h old culture of the bacterium and by exposing plants to high humidity before and after inoculations.

4.1.6 Control

Growth of 32 species of *Xanthomonas* including *X.cajani* have been found to be reduced by certain antibiotics (Thirumalachar *et al.* 1956). The disease could be controlled by three sprays of Streptocycline 100 ppm at an interval of 10 days (Singh *et al.* 1978). Gaikwad and Kore (1981) have also found Streptocycline 100 ppm or Agrimycine 150 ppm or Agallol 200 ppm to inhibit growth of the pathogen completely *in vitro*. In the same way Rai and Singh (1986c) reported that out of 35 fungicides/antibiotics tested, 22 inhibited growth of the bacterium. They found 0.01% Agrimycine 100 (Streptomycin) to be the best for seed treatment followed by 0.2 % thiram. In the field, spray of Agrimycin 100 was best for control of the disease with significant increase in the yield. Next were Miltox 0.2 %, Streptocycline 0.01 % and blue copper 0.3 per cent.

4.2 Halo Blight

Costa *et al.* (1957) first reported that halo blight pathogen (*Pseudomonas* sp.) of coffee in Brazil was able to infect pigeonpea during the host range studies. However, first record of the disease is from Ethiopia (Allen 1979). The disease is considered as minor one and is reported from Australia (Hayward *et al.* 1983) and Zambia also (Kannaiyan and Haciwa 1988). In India, *Pseudomonas* sp. is suspected to cause a smooth stem canker of pigeonpea (Desai *et al.* 1983).

4.2.1 Symptoms

The symptoms on leaves include angular dark brown spots of about one mm diameter often surrounded by a chlorotic zone of up to 10 mm width (Hayward *et al.* 1983). The symptoms are occasionally seen on the primary leaves of the seedlings and on younger leaves of old plants. It is more prevalent on soft, young growth of old plants. The lesions on pods are rare. Abundant bacterial ooze is observed when infected plant tissues are placed in a drop of water on glass slide. The disease is characterized mainly by localized infection of the foliage and systemic chlorosis is the rare phenomenon. Kannaiyan and Haciwa (1988) described symptoms on leaves in Zambia as pinhead size, dark brown spots surrounded by a large chlorotic halo. The spots coalesce causing blight during rainy period. The disease may cause defoliation in case of susceptible cultivars.

4.2.2 Causal Bacterium

Pseudomonas syringae pv. *phaseolicola* (Burkholder) Young, Dye & Wilkie

Synonym : *Pseudomonas phaseolicola*

Allen (1979) reported *P. phaseolicola* on pigeonpea from Ethiopia. This isolate infected groundnut but not *Phaseolus* spp. However, Hayward *et al.* (1983) isolated the pathogen on sucrose peptone agar and found it pathogenic to *Phaseolus vulgaris.* The pathogen was observed on some weeds like *Macroptilium atropurpureum* and *Neonotonia wightii*. In Zambia, it causes severe halo blight of *P. vulgaris.* Isolates of the pathogen from different hosts exhibit different host range which indicate existence of strains in the pathogen as surmised by Jindal and Patel (1988).

4.2.3 Disease Cycle and Epidemiology

The bacterium is possibly seed borne in pigeonpea either internally or extenrnally (Hayward *et al.* 1983). The pathogen is able to infect certain crops and weed plants on which survival of the pathogen is possible. The disease severity increases during the rainy period and ends with cessation of rains.

4.2.4 Host Resistance and Control

Kannaiyan and Haciwa (1988) scored 57 genotypes of pigeonpea in Zambia of which 22 were free from the disease. In some demonstration plots, the lines ICPL 81, ICPL 87, ICPL 362, ICPL 7035, BDN 1, Hy 3C, C 11, GW 3, 81/3/3 and 576/3 showed least disease severity as compared to several other lines.

4.3 Leaf Curl Syndrome

An abnormal shoot development in pigeonpea was reported to be induced by a nodulating *Rhizobium* strain IC 3342 (Upadhyay *et al.* 1991). The affected plants exhibited typical leaf curl symptoms. The xylem exudates and leaf extract from affected pigeonpea plant had high concentration of cytokinin. The zitin ribiside and dihydrozitin ribiside were 7-9 times more than in normal plant samples. The culture filtrate of curl inducing strain of bacterium also had 26 and 8 times higher zitin and N^6-isopentenyl-adenine than in the normal strain. However, the sap from symptomless plants nodulated by curl inducing strain of *Rhizobium* had ZR and DZR as in normal plant.

4.4 Other Bacterial Infections

Besides the above described bacterial diseases of pigeonpea, some other bacterial infections have been mentioned in the literature (Nene *et al.* 1996).

(1) *Xanthomonas campestris* pv. *cassiae* is reported to cause bacterial blight of pigeonpea.
(2) *Pseudomonas andropogonis* is mentioned as the cause of bacterial leaf spot of pigeonpea.

4.5 Improvement by Genetic Engineering

Improvement in pigeonpea is possible by adopting genetic engineering. For genetic manipulations, successful transformation protocols are a prerequisite. This has been done by using *Agrobacterium tumefaciense* based vectors in many leguminous plants. Rathore and Chand (1997) reported induction of tumours in pigeonpea cultivars Bahar, Pant A 106, H 82-1, UPAS 120, and ICPL 151 by a wild stain A 281 of *A. tumefaciense.* The strain T 37 and A 6 did not induce tumours in ICPL 151 and UPAS 120. The study indicated that Bahar and Pant A 106 can be used for *Agrobacterium* Ti plasmid mediated gene transfer. An efficient regeneration system and optimization of parameters for transformation can lead production of tanasgenic pigeonpea plants.

REFERENCES

Agrawal, S.C. and Prasad, K.V.V. 1990. Bacterial stem canker of pigeonpea in Madhya Pradesh. *Indian Journal of Pulses Research* 3 : 92-93.

Allen, D.J. 1979. New disease records from grain legumes. *FAO plant Protection Bulletin* 27 : 134-136.

Anonymous. 1978. Pulse Pathology (Pigeonpea). Report of Work 1977-78, Pulse Pathology No. 1. ICRISAT Patancheru, India, pages 252.

Anonymous. 1982. Pulse Pathology (Pigeonpea). Report of Work 1981-82, Pulse Pathology No. 23, ICRISAT, Patancheru, India, pp. 113.

Anonymous, 1983. Pulse Pathology (Pigeonpea). Report of Work 1982-83, Pulse Pathology No. 30, ICRISAT, Patancheru, India, pp. 187.

Arjunan, G., Samiyappan, R. and Thiyagarajan, K. 1991. Field screening of short duration pigeonpea lines for resistance to bacterial leaf spot and stem canker (*Xanthomonas campestris* pv. *cajani*). *Madras Agricultural Journal* 78 : 78.

Bhatt, V.V. and Patel, M.K. 1954. Comparative study of species of *Xanthomonas* parasitizing leguminous plants in India. *Indian Phytopathology* 7 : 160-180.

Bordoloi, D.K. and Rathaiah, Y. 1997. Field screening of pigeonpea varieties for resistance to bacterial leaf spot and fusarium wilt grown in the lower Brahmaputra valley zone of Assam. *PKV Research Journal* 21 : 101-102.

Chand, J.N. 1986. Bacterial diseases of legumes and their management. *Indian Journal of Mycology and Plant Pathology* 16 : 1-15.

Cortes-Monllor A. and Ruiz, H. 1987. Bacterial leaf spot of pigeonpea in Puerto Rico. *Journal of Agricultural University of Puerto Rico* 7 ; 177-184.

Costa, A.S., Franco Do Amaral, J., Viegas, A.P., Silva, D.M., Teixeira, C.G. and Pinheiro, E.D. 1957. Bacterial halo blight of coffee in Brazil. *Phytopathologische Zeitschrift*. 28 : 427-444.

Davis, R., Ogle, H., Hayward, C., Irwin, J. and Kumar, J. 1988. Etiology of stem canker disease of pigeonpea in Fiji. *ACIAR Food Legume Newsletter* No. 8 : 5-6.

Desai, B.G., Patel, J.C., Patel, J.A., Sharma, A.N. and Shah, R.M. 1983. Uncommon bacterial cankers on pigeonpea in north Gujarat, India. *International Pigeonpea Newsletter* 2 : 53-54.

Desai, B.G., Vora, M.S. and Patel, J.C. 1981. A note on survey of pigeonpea diseases in Gujarat state, *Pulse Crop Newsletter* 1(3) : 54.

Dye, W.E. 1962. The inadequacy of the usual determinative tools for the identification of *Xanthomonas* spp. *NZJ Science* 5 : 393-416.

Fang, C.T., Chen, H.Y. and Chu, C.L. 1964. A comparative study of the species of the genus *Xanthomonas* from leguminous plants. *Sinica* 7 : 21-31.

Gaikwad, B.M. and Kore, S.S. 1981. Bacterial leaf spot and stem canker of pigeonpea (*Cajanus cajan*) caused by *Xanthomonas cajani*. *Indian Journal of Mycology and Plant Pathology* 11 : 50-56.

Hayward, A.C., Teakle, D.S., Saxena, K.B., Wallis, E.S. and Moffett., M.L. 1983. Report of halo blight of pigeonpea from Australia. *International Pigeonpea Newsletter* 2 : 54-55.

Jindal, J.K. and Patel, P.N. 1988. Bacterial diseases of pulse crops. pp. 316-337. In Pulse Crops (Eds. B. Baldev, S. Ramanujam and H.K. Jain). Oxford and IBH Publishing Co. Pvt. Ltd., New Delhi, India.

Kannaiyan, J. and Haciwa, H.C. 1988. Halo blight - a new bacterial disease of pigeonpea in Zambia. *International Pigeonpea Newsletter* 7 : 25-26.

Kannaiyan, J. and Haciwa, H.C. 1990. Diseases of pigeonpea in Zambia. *International Pigeonpea Newsletter* 12 : 22-23.

Kannaiyan, J., Nene, Y.L., Reddy, M.V. and Raju, T.N. 1981. International survey of pigeonpea disease. Pulse Pathology Progress Report No. 12. Patancheru, A.P., India : ICRISAT, 82 pp.

Kulkarni, Y.S., Patel, M.K. and Abhyankar, S.G. 1950. A new bacterial leaf spot and stem canker on pigeonpea. *Current Science* 19 : 384.

Kulkarni, Y.S., Patel, M.K. and Abhyankar, S.G. 1952. A new bacterial leaf spot and stem canker of pigeonpea. *Indian Phytopathology* 5 : 21-22.

Mahrshi, R.P. 1986. A report on three pigeonpea diseases in Rajasthan. *International Pigeonpea Newsletter* 5 : 32-34.

Nene, Y.L., Sheila, V.K. and Sharma, S.B. 1996. World list of chickpea and pigeonpea pathogens. 5th edn. Patancheru, A.P., India : ICRISAT, pp. 27.

Nirula, K.K. 1980. Quarantine to seed exchange at the ICRISAT. *Seed Pathology News* 13 : 11-12.

Patel, P.N. and Jindal, J.K. 1970. Bacterial diseases in seed legumes in 1968 and 1969. Paper presented at the Fourth Workshop Conference on Pulse Crops held at PAU, Ludhiana, India in April 1970.

Rai, M. and Singh, D.V. 1985. Histopathological investigations on bacterial leaf spot of pigeonpea caused by *Xanthomonas campestris* pv. *cajani*. *Indian Phytopathology* 38 : 596 (Abst.).

Rai, M. and Singh, D.V. 1986a. Survival and virulence of *Xanthomonas campestris* pv. *cajani* in debris, seed and soil and *in vitro*. *Indian Phytopathology* 39 : 467-469.

Rai, M. and Singh, D.V. 1986b. Investigations on age of maximum ontogenic susceptibility of pigeonpea plants to *Xanthomonas campestris* pv. *cajani* and its host range. *Farm Science Journal* 1 (1-2) : 63-64.

Rai, M., Singh, D.V. 1986c. Evaluation of chemicals for control of bacterial leaf spot and stem canker disease of pigeonpeas. *Pesticides* 20 (12) : 38-40.

Rangaswami, G. 1962. Bacterial plant diseases in India. Asia Publishing House, Bombay, pp. 163.

Rathore, R.S. and Chand, L. 1997. *In vitro* transformation of pigeonpea genotypes by wild strain of *Agrobacterium tumefaciens*. *International Pigeonpea Newsletter* 4 : 38-39.

Reddy, M.V., Raju, T.N. and Nene, Y.L. 1987. Field screening of pigeonpea germplasm for resistance to bacterial leaf spot and stem canker. *International Pigeonpea Newsletter* 6 : 62-65.

Reddy, M.V., Saxena, K.B., Jayasekara, S.J.B.A. and Faris, D.G. 1992a. Assessment of diseases on short duration pigeonpea in Sri Lanka. *International Pigeonpea Newsletter* 15 : 15-17.

Reddy, M.V., Subramanyam, P., Likoswe, A.A., Saka, V.W. and Msuko, W.A.B. 1992b. Survey of Pigeonpea diseases in Malawi. *International Pigeonpea Newsletter* 15 : 24-25.

Sabet, K.A. 1959. Studies in the bacterial diseases of Sudan crops III. On the occurrence, host range and taxonomy of bacteria causing leaf blight disease of certain leguminous plants. *Annals of Applied Biology* 47 : 318-331.

Sabet, K.A., Ishag, F. and Khalil, O. 1969. Studies on the bacterial diseases of Sudan Crops. vii. New Records. *Annals of Applied Biology* 63 : 357-369.

Singh, D.V., Nath, L. and Kishun, R. 1978. Chemical control of bacterial leaf spot on pigeonpea. *Pesticides* 12 : 29-30.

Singh, R.A. and Pavgi, M.S. 1972. Some diseases of pigeonpea in Uttar Pradesh, India. *FAO Plant Protection Bulletin* 20 : 116-18.

Srinivasulu, B., Radhakrishnan, K.V. and Reddy, M.V. 1991. Reaction of some pigeonpea lines to bacterial leaf spot and stem canker in Andhra Pradesh, India. *Legume Research* 14 : 155-156.

Thirumalachar, M.J., Patel, M.K., Kulkarni, N.B. and Dhande, G.W. 1956. Effect *in vitro* of some antibiotics on thirty-two *Xanthomonas* species occurring in India. *Phytopathology* 46 : 486-488.

Upadhyay, N.M., Parker, C.W., Latham, D.S., Scott, K.F. and Dart, P.J. 1991. Evidence for cytokinin involvement in *Rhizobium* (IC 3342) induced leaf curl syndrome of pigeonpea (*Cajanus cajan* Millsp.). *Plant Physiology* 95 (4) : 1019-1025.

5

Diseases Caused by Viruses, Mycoplasma and Viroids

Pigeonpea is not infected by large number of viruses, mycoplasma or viroids and only few diseases are important. The most important is sterility mosaic which has all the characters of being a virus disease. Yellow mosaic and Arhar mosaic are of minor importance. The witches broom and phyllody are important in some areas only and are caused by mycoplasma like organisms. There is only one disease, the mosaic mottle which is caused by viroid.

Many of the other viruses have been reported to infect the pigeonpea but mostly under greenhouse inoculation test only. However, some have potential to become a serious problem for pigeonpea cultivation under certain environmental conditions. It has been seen that the viruses infecting a crop are not described properly after systematic study. Sometimes they are described on the basis of symptoms only which is very confusing. Different strains of the same virus may induce widely different symptoms on the same cultivars of a crop; a virus may cause different symptoms in different cultivars and unrelated viruses may cause similar symptoms in a common host. The yellow mosaic symptoms are produced by several related or unrelated strains/viruses. Identification of a virus therefore requires great caution and should be confirmed after studying maximum properties particularly the particle morphology, transmission, biophysical properties, serology, host range and the reaction of diagnostic species to infection, purification and the properties of particles which require sufficient laboratory facilities and the technical know-how, Important virus diseases of pigeonpea have been reviewed suitably by some workers (Ramakrishnan and Kandaswamy 1972, Nene 1973, Haque 1979, Reddy *et al* 1990b and Rishi and Sharma 1999).

5.1 Sterility Mosaic Disease

The sterility mosaic of pigeonpea was first reported from Bihar in India (Mitra 1931, Su 1931). The disease was described in detail by Alam (1933). However, the infectious nature of the disease was established by Capoor (1952). The disease appears to be restricted in Asian countries mainly India, Bangladesh, Thailand, Nepal, Myanmar and Sri Lanka (Nene *et al.* 1996). The disease has been reported to occur in most of the pigeonpea growing states of India including Bihar, Uttar Pradesh, Tamil Nadu, Gujarat, Karnataka, Rajasthan, Madhya Pradesh, Orissa, Andhra Pradesh, Maharashtra and West Bengal (Kannaiyan *et al.* 1981a, 1981b). The incidence of the disease was higher in Bihar, Uttar Pradesh (21.4 & 15.4 % respectively). In Tamil Nadu, the incidence varied from stray to 30% and in few places 75-100 per cent (Ramakrishnan and Kandaswamy 1972) suggesting heavy losses (Janarthanan *et al.* 1973). The disease is a major problem in Gujarat also (Desai *et al.* 1981). The disease incidence has increased greatly in Maharashtra exhibiting a range of 3-71 % with an average of 42% (Zote *et al.* 1991). The disease is increasing in many of the states specially Gujarat, Maharashtra, Andhra Pradesh, Tamil Nadu and Karnataka (Reddy and Raju 1993). In Karnataka, it is increasing due to large scale adoption of wilt resistant but sterility mosaic susceptible variety ICP 8863 (Mahalinga *et al.* 1998). The disease is widespread in Sri Lanka but not in Myanmar probably due to use of tolerant varieties (Anonymous 1990).

A negative correlation has been observed between the degree of sterility and the yield of pigeonpea (Alam 1933). The sterility may be up to 100% in plants of suspectible variety infected at the age of 45 days or less (Reddy and Nene 1981a). Thus yield reduction in case of early infection is related with percentage of plants infected but it is not so in case of late infections. The early infection increases number of secondary branches, prolong crop duration causing up to 95% losses. The yield losses are the result of reduction in plant height, branching/plant and reduction in flowering etc. (Dahal and Neupane 1991). The reduction in all the growth components as well as the yield components has been reported due to the disease but it differs from variety to variety (Singh and Rathi 1994). The annual yield losses in pigeonpea due to sterility mosaic disease in India have been estimated to be 205000 tonnes which comes to about 76 million US dollars (Kannaiyan *et al.* 1984). The disease has been considered to be a serious problem for pigeonpea cultivation in India and Nepal causing annual pigeonpea grain losses worth of US dollars 82 million.

Lot of information has been generated on this disease and has been reviewed suitably from time to time (Chaubey 1968, Chenulu 1984, Reddy *et al.* 1990b, Ghanekar *et al.* 1992, Lal and Rathore 1994, Nene 1995, Vishwadhar *et al.* 1996 and Singh *et al.* 1999b)

5.1.1 Symptoms

The symptoms of the disease were initially described as dwarfing of leaves, bushy habit of plant, yellowish green leaves and sterility due to suppression of flowering (Alam 1933). The diseased plants can be seen in patches in the field and are easily spotted from a distance due to their pale green and bushy appearance without flowers and pods (Fig. 5.1). The structure of lamina remains smooth and in many cases from the apparently healthy looking plant may throw an erect branch with pale green small leaves bearing no flowers while side branches may bear flowers and pods (Capoor 1952, Nene 1972). Sometimes plant may not show any symptom in first flush but on ratooning, the new growth shows clear symptoms which include serious reduction in leaf size, increased number of secondary and tertiary branches arising from the leaf axils and complete or partial cessation of reproductive structures (Nene 1972).

On inoculation of seedlings, the initial symptoms appear as vein clearing in younger leaves (Fig. 5.2) and in localized areas on leaves of older plant while primary leaves do not show any symptom. Late infection causes partial cessation of the reproductive structures in few branches.

According to Ramakrishnan and Kandaswamy (1972) the mild form of the disease is associated with a faint mosaic mottling and yellowing of leaves while the severe form is accompanied by mosaic with dark and light green patched blisters on leaves. The lamina is reduced, narrow and linear and leaflets become crowded at the apex of branches which may be partially or completely without flowers. While screening the pigeonpea genotypes, Reddy and Nene (1979) observed three types of symptoms of this disease:

(i) Severe mosaic on leaflets, reduction in leaf size, profuse

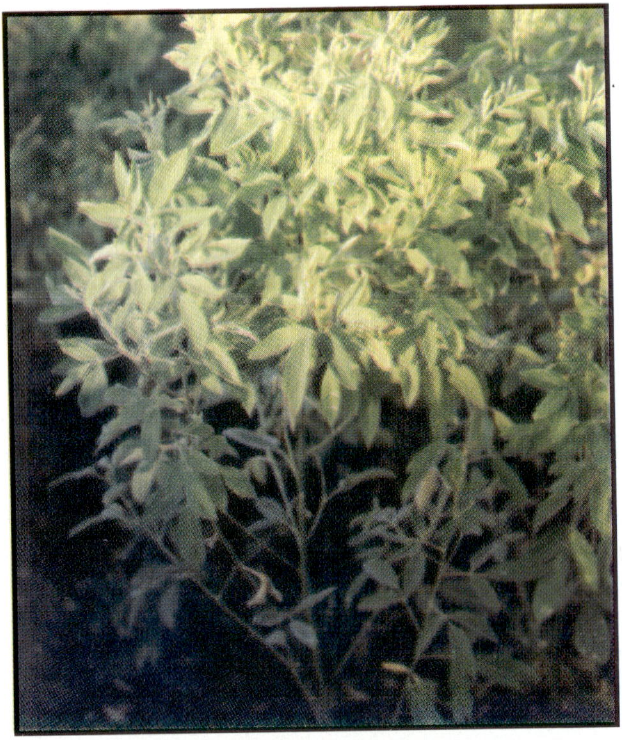

Fig. 5.1: Sterility mosaic of pigeonpea.

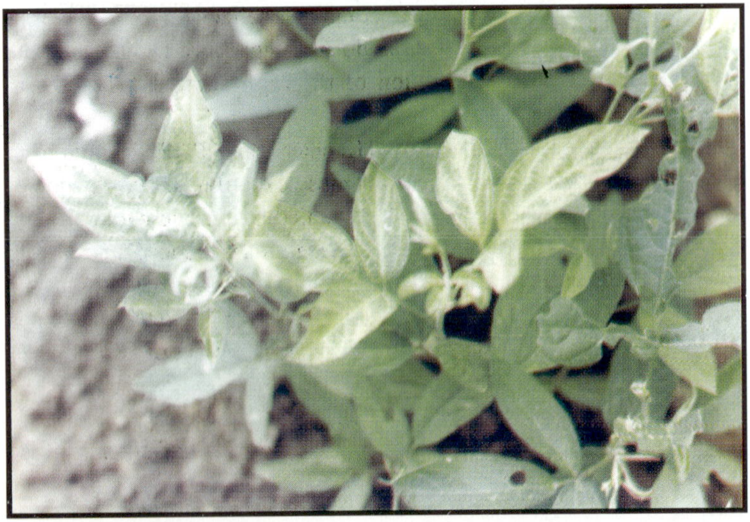

Fig. 5.2: Sterility mosaic of pigeonpea at early stage showing vein yellowing.

branching without flowers and pods. Sometimes leaf becoming filiform.

(ii) Mild mosaic on leaflets with partial sterility.

(iii) Ring spots characterized by green islands surrounded by chloratic haloes on leaflets. The symptoms may disappear with maturity. No sterility is observed as in case of variety ICP 2376. It is considered as the tolerant reaction of the variety.

Since, the disease is characterized by the mosaic symptoms on the leaflets and sterility of plants, the disease is named as 'Sterility mosaic'. In the infected plant, the symptoms may disappear during the hot summer but may reappear with the commencement of the monsoon as soon as the new growth in plant takes place. The symptoms of the disease and its severity also depend on the stage of the crop at infection. The plants inoculated at the age of 16 days to 45 days showed severe stunting reduced leaf size, bushy appearance and no flowering but later inoculations caused less severe symptoms. The plants inoculated at age of 9 weeks flowered in normal ways (Rathi 1983).

5.1.2 Causal Agent/Pathogen

Many of the reports indicate the cause of the sterility mosaic disease of pigeonpea to be a virus or virus like organism. On the basis of experimental results, Capoor (1950 and 1952) described it as a virus disease and proposed the name of cause as "pigeonpea sterility mosaic virus". However, there are conflicting reports and the nature of the cause of this disease has not yet been confirmed, although, some useful information has been generated (Seth 1962, Nene 1972, Rathi 1983, Ghanekar *et al.* 1992, Reddy *et al.* 1994) with regard to etiology of this disease.

Transmission: The infectious nature of the disease was established by Capoor (1952) who successfully transmitted the disease from the diseased to healthy plants of pigeonpea through grafting. It was later confirmed by several workers (Janarthanan *et al.* 1972a, Nene 1972, Mali *et al.* 1977) but union of graft was successful only in few cases. A tissue implantation method of graft inoculation was developed at ICRISAT in which infected stem pieces about 1 cm long are used as scion after treating them with 0.3% metasystox. They are implanted below the growing point of healthy pigeonpea plant by making a vertical slit in the stem. It estimates the mites associated with the diseased scion if any (Reddy *et al.* 1990b). The symptoms appear within a month of grafting.

Capoor (1952) reported mechanical transmission of the disease using juice extracted from the diseased leaves but it could not be confirmed by the later workers (Kandaswamy and Ramakrishnan 1960, Narayanaswamy and Ramakrishnan 1965a, Nene 1972 and Mali *et al.* 1977). However, Rathi (1983) reported the mechanical transmission of the disease in few plants when the inoculum was prepared in M/15 phosphate buffer (*p*H 8.0) containing 4% polyethylene glycol (PEG).

The efforts of transmitting the disease through seed, soil, dodder, white flies, leaf hopper, thrips and aphids were not successful (McRae 1932, Nene 1972, Rathi 1983, Ghanekar *et al.* 1992). Possibilities of transmission of the disease through the soil nematodes specially *Rotylenchulus reinformis* and *Tylenchorhynchus* spp. was reported (Narayanaswamy and Ramakrishnan 1965a, Narayanaswamy *et al.* 1963) but it could not be confirmed.

Thus the disease is transmitted in nature by eriophyid mites, *Aceria cajani* Channabasavanna (Seth 1962). The results have been confirmed by several workers (Oldfield 1970, Nene 1972, Janarthanan *et al.* 1972a, Ramakrishnan and Kandaswamy 1972, Nene and Reddy 1976a, Mali *et al.* 1977 and Rathi 1983).

Electron Microscopy: The electron microscopy of the partially purified preparations or ultra thin sections of diseased leaves did not give any evidence of presence of any virus like particles, mycoplasma like bodies or inclusion bodies (Rathi 1983, Reddy *et al.* 1994). Ghanekar *et al.* (1992) reported long flexuous rods often associated in purified preparations but such particles were observed in preparations from apparently healthy plants also.

Effect of Tetracycline : Application of tetracycline as spray or root dip and penicilline as foliar spray on the inoculated plants did not affect the appearance of symptoms of the pigeonpea sterility mosaic. Hence, the possibility of the mycoplasma associated with the disease has been rejected (Rathi 1983 and Ghanekar *et al.* 1992).

Mite Toxaemia : The pigeonpea sterility mosaic was considered probably caused by mites without an infectious agent (Slykhuis 1980). There is evidence to preclude the mite toxaemia as a likely cause of the disease. Constant association of large population of mites with diseased plants has often lead the possibility of mite toxaemia in certain crops. In case of pigeonpea also high population of mites on diseased plants and negligible on healthy plants of resistant as well as susceptible varieties has been reported (Vishwadhar and Rathore 1994). However, it has been demonstrated that only those mites fed on diseased plants are able to transmit the disease and not those fed on healthy plants. This observation rules out the possibility of mite toxaemia (Reddy *et al.* 1989). There are some genotypes of pigeonpea like ICP 8136 which favours multiplication of mites but are resistant to the disease.

Pathogenic Variability: The pigeonpea genotypes have shown differential reaction against the sterility mosaic disease when tested over locations indicating the variability existing in the isolates of pathogen (Reddy *et al.* 1990b). The variety ICP 2376 shows ring spot reaction but a variant of SMD from fields of farmers could cause severe mosaic on this variety (Reddy *et al.* 1991) indicating it as different from already identified strain. Thus a set of 7 genotypes, namely ICP 2376, 7035, 8862, 8863, 10976, 11164 and Bahar has been recommended as differentials for identifying the variants/strains of SMD. Based on the reaction on these genotypes at 9 locations, 5 variants have been identified as Variant-1 (from Gwalior), Variant-2 (from Badnapur and Patancheru), Variant-3 (from Coimbatore, Kumarganj, Pudukkottai), Variant-4 (from Bangalore, Delhi) and Variant-5 (from Kanpur) by Reddy *et al.* (1933a). The pathogen from Nepal has been found different from that of occurring at ICRISAT Centre in India (Chaurasia 1993). Looking to the variability of sterility mosaic pathogen, a well planned programme has been formulated to work on this aspect in India (Reddy *et al.* 1996). More efforts are needed to study the extent of variability, categorization of the pathotypes, their distribution, occurrence and severity in different cropping zones and the disease endemic areas.

Thus, the cause of the sterility mosaic of pigeonpea still remains a challenge but the evidences of infectious nature of the disease through transmission experiments, variability existing in the pathogen and availability of stable host resistance indicate the cause to be a virus or alike organism.

5.1.3 Vector Mite

The vector of pigeonpea sterility mosaic is an eriophyid mite *Aceria cajani* belonging to order Acarina and family Eriophydeae.

Habitat and Population Dynamics: These mites are light shy in nature and hence, feed on the lower side of the leaves preferably on the terminal tender parts of the plant. They can be seen under steriomicroscope and hand lense partially or totally burried in the thick mass of the leaf hairs. Their presence on plant goes unnoticed as they do not cause any visible injury to leaves. The diseased plants harbour much larger population than the healthy one. In a full grown plant, about 45-75% mite population is concentrated in the lower stratum while middle and upper strata share remaining population (Vishwadhar and Rathore 1994). The population in the diseased plant is evenly distributed on leaves of all ages but in healthy plant it is concentrated in young leaves. More than 90% of the population is observed on the lower surface of leaves irrespective of diseased or healthy plants. The mites are evenly distributed on the entire surface of the leaf in the case of diseased plant while they are concentrated at the pedicel end in leaves of healthy plant. In both the cases, vegetative buds had larger population than leaves. Multiplication of mites is reported to be fast on susceptible genotypes but resistant ones do not support the multiplication (Reddy and Nene 1980, Muniyappa and Nangia 1982). The wild relatives of pigeonpea, namely *Atylosia volubilis, A. albicans, A. lineata* and *A. sericea* are apparently resistant and do not support multiplication of mites while *A. cajanifolia*, a susceptible line support good population of mites.

Method for Studying the Mite: Vishwadhar and Rathore (1994) suggested a technique for quicker and uniform estimation of *Aceria cajani* population on standing pigeonpea crop in the field as follows:

(i) Draw 50% vegetative bud samples from lower stratum and 25% each from middle and upper strata of plant. It is sufficient for diseased as well as healthy plants.

(ii) For estimation of mite population on leaves of diseased plants, draw 15 trifoliates of all ages (50% from lower and remaining from middle and upper strata) while for healthy plant sample at least 5 younger leaves each from lower and middle strata.

(iii) Count mites under steriobinocular on squares or discs of 5 mm area from any part in case of diseased leaves but from the pedicel end in case of healthy sample.

(iv) Examine only the lower surface of the leaflets/squares/discs.

A method has been described to estimate the exact number of mites harbouring in the pigeonpea leaves (Janarthanan *et al.* 1972b). The sample leaves are immersed in methanol, ethanol or acetone mixed with glycerol in proportion of 10 : 1. The leaves are taken out after 3-4 hours, spread gently over a clean glass slides and examined under a steriobinocular under proper illumination so that all mites are seen clearly.

Morphology: The mite, *Aceria cajani* is worm like 200-250 µ long with two pairs of legs attached one behind the other at the anterior end near its mouth parts. There are two cirri located at the posterior end which act as a hold-fast for attachment of mite with the host. The scanning electronic microscopic study revealed the presence of striated dorsal shield setae at the anterior end which are directed posteriorly in adult but anteriorly in nymphs (Sheila *et al.* 1988). Small, rounded structures called as microtubercles are embaded in the transverse rings on the dorsal and ventral surfaces of the elongated abdomen (Keifer 1952). The striated genital coverflap is present on the ventral side of adult female. The males are slightly smaller than the females. The adults do not possess wings and eyes and hence there dispersal is passive. They feed with puncturing and sucking type mouth parts that consist of slender stylet.

The spermatophores released by adult male may be found attached to the leaf surface, trichomes etc. and each of them consists of a stalk with an expanded head having a sperm sac.

Life Cycle: The mites have the life cycle of less than 2 weeks and comprises of egg, 2 nymphal stages and adults. The information on the life cycle and reproduction has been furnished by Oldfield *et al.* (1981). The female lays 1-3 eggs daily which are 30 × 40 µ in size, oval, milky white, translucent and are found loosely attached to a filamentous trichome of the vegetative tips of plant. They are slightly smaller than the glandular trichomes, milky white and translucent as compared to pale yellowish glands of trichomes. The eggs hatch after 4-5 days releasing the first nymphal stage and subsequently develop into second nymphal stage. The nymphal stage lasts for 2-5 days after which they develop into adults. The males are smaller than females. The adults do not possess wings and eyes therefore their dispersal is passive mainly through the wind current.

Pathogen Vector Relationship: The results show that even a single mite is sufficient to transmit the disease. The nymphs and adults are equally efficient in transmitting the disease (Janarthanan *et al.* 1972a). However, the extent of transmission depends on population of mites (Reddy *et al.* 1989) being 35% with one viruliferous mite/plant and 100% with 20 mites/plant. The acquisition access period is between

5-10 minutes while the inoculation access period ranges from 20-30 minutes. The incubation period in the host plant varies from 11-27 days which depends on levels of mites used for inoculation (Rathi 1983). The transmission of the pathogen is of persistent type. Once the pathogen is acquired by the mite, it is retained for whole of its life provided they are fed on susceptible pigeonpea variety. The transmission is not transovarial (Ghanekar *et al.* 1992).

5.1.4 Host Pathogen Interaction

Infection of the pigeonpea plant with sterility mosaic brings the histological and biochemical changes which may be different in resistant and susceptible varieties.

Histological Changes: The infection of plant by SMD pathogen reduces the thickness of leaf, size of palisade and epidermal cells, number of palisade and protein positive plastids in palisade and spongy cells (Prameela *et al.* 1990a). The reduction was more due to combined infection of sterility mosaic and powdery mildew. The infection by sterility mosaic exhibited absence of fibres and hypertrophied phloem cells in mid-veins with larger cellular spaces (Singh and Rathi 1996a). The phloem cells of diseased mid-vein also showed presence of foreign ribonucleoprotein and inclusions in the nucleus of phloem cells (Singh and Rathi 1996b).

Biochemical Changes: Infection of Plant by sterility mosaic causes drastic decrease in chlorophyll contents, total carbohydrate, carotine and xanthophyll. These changes are due to increased activity of chlorophyllase, decreased synthesis of sucrose which decreases photosynthetic activity (Narayanaswamy and Ramakrishnan 1965b). Nambiar and Ramakrishnan (1969b) reported significant reduction in photosynthesis and rate of Hill reaction in diseased plant. The reducing sugars increased but starch and resin decreased (Nambiar and Ramakrishnan 1968). The size of starch grains is reduced in plants with combined infection of sterility mosaic and powdery mildew (Prameela *et al.* 1990a).

The diseased leaves exhibited decrease in chloroplastic protein. The amino acid contents of protein does not change but free amino acids change in quantity as well as in quality. The total nitrogen showed progressive increase during the day with decrease in C : N ratio (Narayanaswamy and Ramakrishnan 1966a). The high concentration of amino acids in the bound form in the diseased leaves suggested their probable incorporation into the virus protein (Nambiar and

Ramakrishnan 1969c). The nucleic acid and protein were reduced due to infection (Prameela *et al.* 1990a). The RNA and DNA contents were more in diseased leaves and the RNA fractions presumably contained viral as well as plant RNA (Nambiar and Ramakrishnan 1969b). The infection causes increase in RNAse activity and rapid accumulation of RNA in BDN 1 (Rao *et al.* 1985). The diastic activity in the infected pigeonpea leaves is increased but peroxidase activity is lowered. The activity of catalase, nitrate reductase and proteolytic enzymes are increased (Narayanaswamy and Ramakrishnan 1966b).

The infection by SMD is reported to decrease Ca, K, Na, and Mn content of pigeonpea leaves (Nambiar and Ramakrishnan 1969a). It also reduced to different organic acid contents variably in leaf, petiole, stem and buds and increased the rate of respiration (Narayanaswamy and Ramakrishnan 1966c). The infection increased the leakage of electrolytes from cells which was more in dual infection of sterility mosaic and powdery mildew (Prameela *et al.* 1989a).

The infection reduced the phenol contents in pigeonpea plants (Prameela *et al.* 1990b) and the effect was different in resistant (Hy 3C) and susceptible (T- 21) varieties of pigeonpea (Bhatt 1980 and Rathi 1983). The healthy leaves of resistant variety exhibited greater activity of peroxidase, polyphenol-oxidase with more total polyphenol contents than the leaves of susceptible variety. The peroxidase activity increased after inoculation in both cases but later it decreased and the decrease was more in susceptible variety. The phenolic contents increased after inoculation but later they decreased in resistant variety but continued to increase in susceptible one. Ultimately the phenol contents decreased in both the varieties. In healthy leaves of resistant variety, an isozyme of peroxidase and a few proteins specific to resistant variety were detected while in susceptible variety higher amount of soluble protein and the proteins specific to susceptible variety were observed. After inoculation, the isozymes of peroxidase were altered in susceptible variety but not in resistant one. The soluble protein increased in both the varieties being more in susceptible than in resistant variety. The proteins of susceptible variety showed alteration in their electrophoretic pattern but such changes did not occur in the resistant variety.

5.1.5 Disease Cycle and Epidemiology

The sterility mosaic disease of pigeonpea is not seed born and it seems to be introduced by the mite vector in rainy season crop from the external sources. Reddy *et al.* (1988) observed the disease with living mite population on pigeonpea plants growing on bunds around sugarcane fields, along the irrigation channels, in kitchen gardens and on plants left unharvested from the previous crop in Uttar Pradesh. Such plants with mites were observed in last week of June and are considered the link for recurrence of the disease in rainy season crop. In Karnataka and Tamil Nadu, plants of pigeonpea as ratooned or perennial have been observed infected with the disease and harbouring the mite population in April in the irrigated tract (Reddy *et al.* 1989a). The pathogen and the vector can survive on pigeonpea plants maintained along the sugarcane fields on bunds, around vineyard and mulberry fields and in some areas their cultivation in turmeric fields for providing shade (Reddy *et al.* 1990a). Such types of widely spread off season pigeonpea plants are responsible for increasing the spread of the disease in states of Gujarat, Andhra Pradesh, Maharashtra, Tamil Nadu and Karnataka although, the disease was traditionally endemic in Uttar Pradesh and Bihar only (Reddy and Raju 1993). The vector mite has been found to survive on diseased plants of certain wild relatives of pigeonpea like *Cajanus scarabaeoides* var. *scarabaeoides. C. platycarpa* and *C. cajanicola* of which the first one occurs widely in some semi-arid tropics. It is considered as an alternative host for survival of the vectors and the pathogen of sterility mosaic in the areas where off-season pigeonpea plants do not exist specially in Andhra Pradesh around Hyderabad (Reddy *et al.* 1993b). Eriophyid mites have been found on the lower surface of leaves of *Oxalis corniculata,* a perinnial weed occurring in pigeonpea fields (Rathi 1983).

Once the plants are infected, the mites multiply fast on diseased plant increasing the disease severity. A minimum and maximum temperature range of 10-25°C and 25-35°C respectively and minimum RH of 60% is conginial for built up of the vector population on leaves (Vishwadhar *et al.* 1995). According to Zote *et al.* (1997), the heavy outbreak of sterility mosaic seems to be due to heavy precipitation during early May and the early stage of crop growth which results due to differential sowing dates and the duration of genotypes under cultivation. The irrigated crop of pigeonpea or that grown near any irrigated crop have been found to show high incidence of the disease probably due to increased vector population (Padule *et al.* 1982).

Sowing time is also important. In Karnataka, high incidence of the disease has been observed on crops of varieties ICP 8863 and TTB7 sown in May-June as compared to sown in or after July (Lakshmikantha *et al.* 1997).

It has also been observed that pigeonpea sown late (September) near the Kharif planting develop more disease which is due to spread of the disease from already infected plants of early plantings to the late sown crop. It has also been observed that the mid-late or late varieties of pigeonpea suffer more due to secondary disease cycles repeated several times in such varieties while the early ones are generally escaped (Zote *et al.* 1991).

In a particuiar area, the disease may increase faster by using susceptible variety as happened in Karnataka State due to large scale cultivation of SMD susceptible but wilt resistant variety ICP 8863 (Mahalinga *et al.* 1998).

The spread of the mite vector from diseased plants takes place in a passive manner through the wind current up to 2 km down wind from the source of inoculum. The spread in the upwind direction is less than 200 metres only (Reddy *et al.* 1989). There is no information on the influence of the wind velocity on extent of vector dispersal.

In Uttar Pradesh, the greatest population of mites was observed on NPWR 15 in May and smallest in January and positive correlation existed with the maximum and minimum temperature and negative with maximum RH. The correlation was non-significant with minimum RH and rainfall (Singh and Rathi 1997).

5.1.6 Interaction with Other Diseases

There are reports which indicate interaction between sterility mosaic and other diseases of pigeonpea. The extract from the diseased plant inhibited the spore germination of *F. udum* (Chadha and Raychaudhury 1965). The diseased plants are less vulnerable to infection of wilt and other root diseases (Ghanekar *et al.* 1992).

On the other hand, plants infected by Sterility mosaic are more susceptible to attack of *Leveillula taurica* (Reddy *et al.* 1984). The extract from SM diseased plants enhances the conidial germination of *L. taurica* and the infected leaves support high conidial production (Prameela *et al.* 1989b).

The pigeonpea plants carrying the sterility mosaic pathogen are protected from the attack of mungbean yellow mosaic virus and *vice versa* (Rathi 1983). In case of simultaneous inoculations by both the pathogens, sterility mosaic dominates.

The pigeonpea plants infected by sterility mosaic are preferred more by leaf hoppers, *Empoasca kerri* Pruthi probably due to reduced C : N ratio (Jayraj and Seshadri 1967).

5.1.7 Host Resistance

Resistance to sterility mosaic in pigeonpea was reported as early as 1931 by Alam who reported Sabour 2 E to be resistant.

Sources of Resistance: The earlier reports indicated no variety resistant to sterility mosaic in pigeonpea (Kandaswamy and Ramakrishnan 1960, Prasad 1965). These reports probably were based on general field observations without any systematic screening due to lack of standardized screening techniques. The systematic screening started after development of screening techniques at ICRISAT (Nene *et al.* 1981a). The screening of pigeonpea for resistance to sterility mosaic was undertaken at Coimbatore, ICRISAT (Patancheru), Badnapur (Maharashtra), Pantnagar, Kanpur, Faizabad and Varanasi in India and a good number of resistant genotpes were identified (Table 5.1). The work was undertaken at various centres of All India Coordianted Project on Improvement of Pulses and based on these results of multilocation tests, resistant donor for national breeding programme have been identified and recommended as ICPL 83027, 88024, 83024, 87119, 85047; ICP 8860, PDA 85-1, 85-14, PR 5149, PS 397430 Sel, DPPA 85-7, 84-12, 85-13, 85-15 (Anonymous 1992). The resistance of the lines ICP 7867, 10976 and 10977 was confirmed by multilocation testing (Nene *et al.* 1989).

As a result of these efforts, a few high yielding varieties with resistance to sterility mosaic have been identified/developed and recommended for commercial cultivation like ICPL 151, ICPL 87119, ICPL 371, Bahar, DA 11, Hy 3C.

Techniques of Screening: Screening of pigeonpea against sterility mosaic under inoculated conditions was first reported by Ramakrishanan and Kandaswamy (1972). They adopted the twig-tying technique in which twig of the diseased plant was tied with the test plant. This technique was not practical for large scale screening. The scientists at ICRISAT developed efficient techniques and recommended for large scale screening (Nene *et al.* 1981a):

(i) *Leaf Stapling Technique* : The leaf stapling technique (Nene and Reddy 1976b) is a very effective method for screening the material in pots as well as in field. The inoculum is maintained as diseased plants in pots kept in partial shed so that population of mites is multiplied. A diseased leaflet with 50-139 mites is folded on primary leaf of 10-15 days old test seedlings and

Table 5.1: Sources of resistance to pigeonpea sterility mosaic disease

Entries tested	*Entries found resistant*	*Reference*
—	NP (WR) 15, P 4835, 1178, 1289, 1100, 2621	Ramakrishnan & Kandaswamy (1972)
549	None	Subramanian *et al.* (1973)
34	L 3, P 4785	Singh *et al.* (1975)
2804	ICP 3783, 6986, 6997, 7035 and 7119	Nene & Reddy (1976a)
—	ICP 4782	Gangadharan *et al.* (1980)
116	15 genotypes	Gupta *et al.* (1981)
Many thousand	68 lines and *Atylosia volubilis*	Nene *et al.* (1981b)
21	Few were resistant	Muniyappa and Nangia (1982)
143	P 961	Sivaprakasam and Ambalagan (1983)
120	Malkapur B, Mahud A, Yeotmal	Zote *et al.* (1983a)
164	ICP 8847 to 8857, C 11, Hy 3c, Pant A 2, Pant A 3, 6, 7, 8, 76, 77, 1234, ICP 3783, 6997, 7035 and 5444 and several others	Rathi (1983)
—	ICP 8858, 7875-2, 6997	Zote *et al.* (1983b)
19	ICP 10976, 10984, 7353	Samiyappan & Sivaprakasam (1985)
1500	ICP 10976 & 8862	Samiyappan and Arjunan (1986)
22	ICP 7336, 8861, 6997, 8869, 8854, 7201	Zote & Dandnaik (1986)
20	3203, 3211 and 3212	Dwivedi & Shukla (1986)
48	ICPL 269 (as donor)	Thiyagarajan *et al.* (1987)
591	43 lines from different maturity groups	Singh *et al.* (1987)
—	BSMR 520, 615, 731, 732, 242, 243, 294, 493, 528, BWR 175	Zote & Dandnaik (1987)
—	250 BSMR series	Zote *et al.* (1987)
150	24 lines	Gupta *et al.* (1988a)
162	ICP 7035, 8862, 11049, 11204, 11206, 11207, 11231, LRG 36, DA 13 were immune	Gupta *et al.* (1988b)
88	ICP 7867, 10976, 10977	Nene *et al.* (1989)
568	MA 165, 166, ICPL 86, 146, PDA 2, DA 11, DA 13, DA 15, MA 97, Bahar	Reddy *et al.* (1989b)
14	BSMR 165, 225, 285, 294, 311	Zote & Dandnaik (1989)
Many	Pant A 3, 8505, 8508, 86-1, 86-2	Rathi and Tripathi (1989)
43	6 lines of long duration	Mishra & Prasad (1989)
172	PR 5114, ICP 7035, ICPL 366, Bahar, ICPL 86012, Rampur local	Singh *et al.* (1989)
61	Pant A 8505, 8508	Pal *et al.* (1989)
271	ICPL 84024, 83006, BSMR 146, 198, 736, 253 & Co 5	Shirsikar *et al.* (1990)
240	134 B, 24 B2 and 19 others	Chauhan *et al.* (1991)

Table 5.1: *contd...*

Entries tested	*Entries found resistant*	*Reference*
—	ICPL 371 with good yield	Saxena *et al.* (1992)
—	ICPL 87119 with good yield	Reddy *et al.* (1995)
120	23 lines	Das and Gupta (1992)
Many selections	BSMR 136, 146, 175, 205, 108, 65, 595, 251, 275, 217	Zote *et al.* (1993)
200	ICP 7035, 7119, 8861, 11289, Phule T 25, Bahar, ICP 2376, 7234, 7898, 8860, 8862, 8867, 8869, 10976, ICPL 366, 85063	Pawar *et al.* (1993)
Many	DA 35, KA 32-1, ICPL 227, 305, 335, 83024, 85059, ICP 8862	Rathi & Tripathi (1993)
866	ICP 7035, 6997, 7197, 7234, 7867, 8094, 8862, 10976, 10979, 10996, 11049, 11204, 11206, ICPL 335, 342, 366, 83024, BSMR 235	Amin *et al.* (1993)
347	ICPL 83024, Bahar, DA 11, DA 33, KA 32-1	Vishwadhar *et al.* (1994)
295	ICPL 366, ICP 7035, 10976	Raguchander *et al.* (1995)
153	ICP 2630, 3782, 3783, 4725, 7035, 7239, 7281, 7403, 7867, 8116, 8117, 8859, 8853, 8861 11278	Srinivas *et al.* (1997a)
450	36 lines with ICP & NDA numbers	Singh *et al.* (1995)
—	13 line extra short duration	Singh *et al.* (1996)
60	None from Extra short duration	Garg *et al.* (1996)
81	ICPL 88046, Bahar, DA35, K32-1, Pusa 19, Pusa 14, DA11, 32, 33 & GAUT 9005	Singh *et al.* (1999a)

stapled in such a way so that both the surfaces of test leaf remain in contact of lower surface of primary leaf of test seedling. If the diseased leaflets are small in size, two such leaflets may be stapled in such a way so that their lower surfaces remain in contact of both the surfaces of test leaflets. The infected leaf used for inoculation of seedling dries and the mites move on to healthy inoculated leaf and transmit the pathogen. The symptoms of the disease appear mostly on the freshly emerged trifoliate leaf within 5-7 days and not on the inoculated leaf. The plants showing doubtful symptoms are pruned so that fresh growth appears with clear symptoms. The infection percentage is directly proportional to the number of diseased leaflets used as inoculum and it is negatively correlated with the age of seedlings (Nene and Reddy 1977). Pinning the leaf in place of stapling has been found to be more effective probably due to less injury caused to test seedling (Rathi 1983). Observations are recorded on disease incidence and severity as described later. The leaf stapling technique requires more inoculum and labour and hence, more easy methods were developed.

(ii) *Infector Row/Spreader Row Technique*: This technique was developed to overcome the problem of large amount of inoculum and labour required for inoculation of all the test seedlings (Nene *et al.* 1981a, 1981b and Reddy and Nene 1981b). This method consists of planting the sterility mosaic susceptible variety of pigeonpea like BDN 1 or NPWR 15 all over the field in rows at a distance of 10-20 m about 4 months in advance of sowing of test material. These plants are inoculated artificially by leaf stapling technique and maintained. The mite vecor multiply on these infector rows and inoculum is ready for spread through wind on test lines to be planted later. The spread of the disease is satisfactory and uniform by this technique but a few precautions are to be taken as follows:

(a) Save the test crop from the spray or drift of insecticides.
(b) Select plot downwind to avoid spread of the diseases in other pigeonpea fields.
(c) Plant the infector rows across wind direction that prevails for first 2-3 months after planting.
(d) Provide sufficient irrigation to infector rows specially in summer months.
(e) Prune the infector rows at regular interval to keep their growth under check and encourage the new growth.

The infector row method works very well but it requires more work for sowing and maintenance and inoculation of the infector rows throughout the field. It also needs more irrigation water. Hence this method was modified as "Infector Hedge Technique."

(iii) *Infector Hedge Technique*: This technique is similar to infector rows technique except that in place of infector rows sown in whole of the field, 4-8 infector rows are sown as hedge on the western border of the field as the wind mostly flows from the western side (Nene *et al.* 1981c). A line of the susceptible variety is sown after every 10 rows of the test material for monitoring the uniform spread of the disease. The severity of the disease may be less on lines away from the hedge due to late infection but it does not interfere with effective screening as disease incidence rather than the disease severity is recorded/ considered. One hedge is sufficient to spread the disease in field at least up to 200 m down the wind (Ghanekar *et al.* 1992).

Method of Observations: The observations of the disease are recorded on incubation period, number of plants infected and the type of symptom severity like ring spot, mild mosaic, severe mosaic, partial or complete sterility. Observations on the incidence of the disease are recorded at 30-45 days and finally at maturity. Early observations are essential as some of the plants with mild mosaic or ring spot symptoms may recover later. For the critical studies such as inheritance of resistance, it is necessary to observe plants at frequent intervals from the early stages of infection, record the symptoms as and when they show and uproot the plants. In case of late infection, it is possible that the symptoms may not appear in the first growth or may not be very clear. In such cases de-topping the plants helps in better expression of symptoms on the regrowth and thus better evaluation (Reddy and Nene 1981b).

Nene *et al.* (1981a) recommended a nine-point scale for easy scoring of plants as follows:

Rating	*Description*	*Interpretation*
1	No symptoms in any plant	Resistant
2	Symptoms on 10% or fewer plants	Moderately resistant
5	Ring spot symptoms on most plants but disappearing with age, no sterility	Tolerant
7	Mild mosaic symptoms on most plants causing partial sterility	Moderately susceptible
9	Severe mosaic on most plants with almost complete sterility	Susceptible

In this scale, the ratings 1-3 are acceptable for selection for breeding programme; 5 is acceptable if lines with 1-3 are not available while ratings 7-9 are not acceptable. The scale adopted under All India

Coordinated Pulses Improvement Project Programme is based on per cent incidence of the disease as Resistant up to 10%, Tolerant 10-20 %, Moderately resistant 20-30 % and Susceptible above 30 per cent (Amin *et al.* 1993).

Maintenance of Inoculum: Sufficient amount of the inoculum in the form of diseased pigeonpea leaves with large number of living mites is necessary for successful inoculation to develop the disease in test entries. After harvest of the crop, the mites do not survive easily due to increasing temperature in the summer months. During the off season, the viruliferous mites are maintained on diseased pigeonpea plants grown in pots under partial shade (Reddy and Nene 1981b, Nene *et al.* 1981a). One should not depend on infected plants in the field for source of inoculum as number of mites associated with such plants may be less to transmit the disease. Nene and Sheila (1992) could induce the callus in leaves of ICP 7182 and ICP 8863 infected as well as un-infected by SMD. In both the cases, colour of the callus was different but the presence of virus was not ascertained in callus. If it is confirmed, it will be helpful for maintaining the pathogen by tissue culture.

Genetics of Resistance: Resistance to sterility mosaic in pigeonpea is reported to be controlled by 4 independent non-allelic genes of which two are dominant and two recessive (Singh *et al.* 1983). At least one dominant and one recessive genes are necessary for expression of resistance. The symbols Sv 1, Sv 2, are assigned. Sharma *et al.* (1983, 1984) found susceptibility to be dominant over resistance. Two loci and more than 2 allels at each locus were the suggested explanations in F_1 and F_2 generations in different cross combinations. In crosses involving ICP 7035, ICP 7349, ICP 8850 with susceptible line, resistance was dominant in some while susceptibility in others. The disease reaction was governed by two independent non-allelic genes with at least 3 multiple allels at one of the loci (Srinivas *et al.* 1997b). For less virulent isolate of sterility mosaic, the inheritance was explained by two independent non-allelic recessive genes in crosses involving ICP 7035, ICP 7349, ICP 8850 resistant and ICP 8863 susceptible lines. On the other hand, the resistance was dominant in crosses ICP 7035 × ICP 8863 and ICP 7349 × ICP 8863 while susceptibility was dominant in case of ICP 8850 × ICP 8863 when more virulent isolate was used (Srinivas *et al.* 1997c). It indicates that the reaction is governed by single gene with 3 allels, one exhibiting dominance of resistance and the other being recessive over the allel for susceptibility. According to Murugesan *et al.* (1997) resistance to sterility mosaic is controlled monogenetically.

The sterility mosaic resistant genotypes ICP 7035, ICP 7349 and tolerant one ICP 11251 have been found to be good combiners for most of the yield component traits and appear to be promosing for use in breeding programme (Srinivas *et al.* 1998). The genotype ICP 8850, 2376 and 7994 are not good combiners.

Mechanism of Resistance: It is observed that most of the resistant varieties of pigeonpea do not favour the multiplication of *A. cajani* (Reddy and Nene 1980, Muniyappa and Nangia 1982) indicating the association of resistance of the host to disease with resistance to mite (Reddy *et al.* 1989a, Vishwadhar and Rathore 1994). However, a line ICP 8136 has been reported resistant to pathogen but not to mite vector (Ghanekar *et al.* 1992). In the same way ICP 2376 exhibits ring spot symptoms which are hypersensitive response but this genotype favours the multiplication of mites.

The cuticle and epidermal cell walls in resistant varieties are significantly thicker than in susceptible varieties which possibly plays important role in inoculation by the short stylet of infective mites (Reddy *et al.* 1994 & 1995). The disease incidence has been reported to be higher in varieties with light yellow to yellow coloured outer surface of the vexillum while those with sun red to purple colour had low disease (Chaudhary *et al.* 1995). Zote *et al.* (1991) observed midlate varieties to suffer more due to sterility mosaic while short duration varieties are escaped from the attack. The level of chlorogenic acid in leaves of 20 days old seedlings can be used to rapidly screen germ plasm for disease resistance against pigeonpea starility mosaic virus (Bhite *et al* 1997).

5.1.8 Control

The efforts to control the sterility mosaic through acaricidal spray or soil application of pesticides or the cultural practices were not very successful. The only promising way is to use resistant varieties (Rathi and Tripathi 1989).

Chemical Control: The pigeonpea plants remain protected from infection of the sterility mosaic up to maturity by seed treatment with Temic 10 G (Rathi 1979 & 1983) or by seed treatment with Carbofuran (Reddy *et al.* 1990b, De *et al.* 1996) for 45 days.

The plants could also be protected from infection up to 75 days by soil application of carbofuran 3% @ 1.2 kg a.i./ha or aldicarb @ 1.5 kg/ha at the time of sowing (Reddy *et al.* 1990b) or application of phorate @ 1 kg a.i./ha (De *et al.* 1996).

Foliar spray of Metasystox 0.1 % + Quenching oil 2% between 96 h before to 25 h after inoculation reduced the disease greatly (Rathi 1983). The spray remained effective for 2-3 days only. Effective kill of the vector and control of the disease was also obtained by spray of 0.1 % acaricide like Kelthane, Tedion, Morestan etc. (Reddy *et al.* 1990b, De *et al.* 1996). Spray of Wettable Sulphur 0.25% or Neem based insecticides have also been found effective (Natrajan and Dhahira 1992, De *et al.* 1995).

The pigeonpea plants are more susceptible to infection by the SMD and the infection decreases with advancement of the age of plant. Hence, seed treatment or soil application of insecticides may prove beneficial if genotype used is not highly susceptible.

Cultural Control: Rathi (1983) did not find any difference in the disease incidence in pigeonpea crop sown at different dates from 20th June to 5th October. On the other hand, Ghanekar *et al.* (1992) recorded low indicence of the disease in crop sown from December to February as compared to March to October. Appearance of first symptoms of the disease was observed to be delayed in UPAS 120 and T 21 varieties sown in January and February but 75 days after sowing, disease incidence reached to 100% in both the varieties (Singh and Rathi 1996c). In north India, early pigeonpea varieties are sown in middle of June in pigeonpea wheat cropping system. By the time the mite population is build up (September), the crop becomes of 75-80 days and hence, escape the incidence of complete sterility while delayed sowing results in heavy incidence (Vishwadhar *et al.* 1996).

The crop density has also been reported to influence the disease incidence considerably. The disease was reported lower in 6 varieties planted at 50 cm row spacing as compared to 150 cm. spacing (Gurha *et al.* 1983). Such effect was not observed in other 3 varieties. According to Bhatnagar *et al.* (1984) the disease is decreased by sole cropping as compared to intercrop with Sorghum. Further, the disease in the intercrop increases at low plant densities. On the other hand, Zote *et al.* (1988) did not find any effect of intercropping of pigeonpea with Sorghum or pearl millet.

5.2 Witches Broom

The witches broom symptoms on pigeonpea were first reported from New Guinea (Van Velson 1961) and were thought to be due to mealybug (*Pseudococcus citri*). The disease was later observed and studied at El

Salvador but the cause could not be identified (Wellman 1972). The diseased pigeonpea plants showing pale green foliage and witches broom symptoms were observed in Dominican Republic near Haiti (Maramorosch and Hichez 1973, Hirumi *et al.* 1973). The disease has also been reported from Jamaica (Naylor 1974), Puerto Rico (Maramorosch *et al.* 1974a, 1974b). It is important in America (Kannaiyan *et al.* 1984) and very serious in the Dominican Republic where large areas have almost 100% incidence in certain years (Reddy *et al.* 1990b). The disease also occurs in Australia, Bangladesh, Costa Rica, Panama, Taiwan and Trinidad (Nene *et al.* 1996).

5.2.1 Symptoms

The witches broom disease of pigeonpea is characterised by prolific and clustered branching of the plant at nodes. The leaves are pale green in colour and reduced in size. The flowers are produced in clusters with petioles elongated and many of them fail to develop beyond the bud stage and do not set the fruits. Sometimes the plant is affected partly (Brathwaite 1981).

5.2.2 Causal Organism

The pigeonpea plants showing pale green foliage and witches broom like symptoms in Dominican Republic exhibited presence of the mycoplasma like organism as well as bullet shaped (Rhabdo) virus in the phloem (Maramorosch and Hichez 1973). The presence of MLO was observed in diseased plants collected in Puerto Rico also but dual infection of MLO and rhabdo virus was observed in some samples only (Maramorosch *et al.* 1974a, 1974b). Later studies established that witches broom of pigeonpea is caused by the mycoplasma like organism which is found associated in phloem (Vakili and Maramorosch 1974) while rhabdo virus alone was responsible for another disease named as "pale mosaic" (Iicha-Baquero 1980). McKoy *et al.* (1983) also observed MLO of typical polymorphic morphology in sieve tubes of witches broom affected plants while rhabdovirus particles were associated with plants showing mild foliar vein yellowing but not with witches broom. The witches broom occurred when leaf hoppers of *Empoasca fabae* complex colonize the plants and the disease could be controlled by suppressing insects. Similarly *Empoasca plebeia* and *Acinopterus* sp. were also associated and may the vector of MLO causing witches broom.

5.2.3 Control

For disease control, resistant sources against MLO as well as to leaf hoppers should be searched out. Insect control may also help. Select field away from the perennial pigeonpea, destroy infected plants, avoid ratoon cropping and control leaf hoppers by spray of Metasystox (Reddy *et al.* 1993b).

5.3 Phyllody

The phyllody of pigeonpea was first reported from India (Bhatnagar *et al.* 1966) and later from Zambia (Kannaiyan and Haciwa 1990). It also occurs in Myanmar and Thailand (Nene *et al.* 1996). The disease has not so far been reported from any other country. In India, the disease has been observed in states of Maharashtra (Marekar 1980). Gujarat (Kannaiyan *et al.* 1981a) and Karnataka (Reddy *et al.* 1983). The disease is considered important in Karnataka where it was recorded with a severe outbreak with more than 10% incidence at the farm of Gandhi Krishi Vigyan Kendra. The incidence in rainy season reached up to 61% on variety Hy 3C (Rangaswamy *et al.* 1990).

5.3.1 Symptoms

Symptoms of the disease have been described in detail (Bhatnagar *et al.* 1966, Reddy and Ravi 1984, Reddy *et al.* 1983). The disease can easily be recognized at the time of flowering and the diseased plants can be spotted in the field due to their bushy appearance with axillar proliferation of phylloid flowers. The plants have excessive branching, shortened internodes, reduced leaf size and transformation of flowers into phylloid structures. On artificial inoculation through grafting, the calyx and corolla were transformed into leaf like structures, gynophores appeared like reduced pods and stemens were reduced in size while carpels were converted into small leaf like structures (Reddy and Ravi 1984). In few cases, the corolla withered and stemens enlarged into leaf like structures. Marekar (1980) observed plants having green petals instead of yellow and pod formed up to certain height but without any seed setting.

5.3.2 Causal Organism

Mycoplasma like organism (MLO)

The disease was initially considered as the natural variation by Marekar (1980). On the basis of transmission of the disease through wedge grafting and types of the symptoms, the cause of the disease was suggested to be mycoplasm like organism by Reddy *et al.* (1983). Reddy and Ravi (1984) demonstrated the transmission of disease through wedge grafting, and remission of disease symptoms by application of tetracycline giving evidence of the disease being caused by MLO which was later confirmed by Ravi and Reddy (1987) also.

The electron microscopic studies conducted by Ravi and Reddy (1987) revealed presence of mycoplasma like bodies in the sieve tubes of the phloem tissues of the affected pigeonpea plants. These bodies measured 300 nm in size. The presence of MLO and suppression of the symptoms of the disease due to application of tetracycline confirmed the cause of the disease as mycoplasma like organism.

Transmission: The disease was found to be transmitted by wedge grafting (Reddy *et al.* 1983, Reddy and Ravi 1984). The incidence of the disease was found correlated with leaf hopper *Orosius albisinctus*. Later, Suryanarayana *et al.* (1997b) confirmed *O. albisinctus* as the vector of the disease. The minimum acquisition and inoculation periods were found to be 1 day each and incubation period of 20 days. Both the sexes of the insect were equally efficient in transmitting the pathogen. They retained the infectivity through out their life span (Suryanarayana *et al.* 1997a). The transmission efficiency was high on 5-10 days old seedlings of pigeonpea.

Host Range: The weeds *Parthenium hysterophorus, Richardia scabra, Cleome monophylla, Borreria stricta, Lagesea mollis, Bidens biternata* have been considered as the potential reservoirs of the pigeonpea phyllody pathogen and also for colonization by the vector (Suryanarayana and Ravi 1994). In addition to these 6 weed plants 30 other plant species, namely *Gomphrena celosiods, Ageratum conyzoides, Collastephus chinensis, Centroptherum anthelminticum, Conyza stricta, Emilia sonchfolia, Gerbera jamaesonii, Guizotia abyssinica, Spilanuthus calva, Tagetas erecta, Heliotropium indicum, Trichodesma zeylanica, Evolvulus elsinoides, Cajanus cajan, Cicer arietinum, Crotalaria juncea, C. mucronata, Glycine max, Lupinus hartwegii. Macrotyloma. uniflorum, Medicago sativa, Phaseolus vulgaris, P. lunatus,*

Psophocorpus tetragonalobus, Vigna mungo, V. radiata, V. unguiculata, Leucus espera, Ocimum americanum, and *Sesamum orientale* have been reported to be the host of this pathogen (Suryanarayana *et al.* 1997b).

5.3.3 Disease Cycle and Epidemiology

At least 36 plant species have been reported to be the host of pigeonpea phyllody pathogen. The vector has been found to transmit the disease to pigeonpea and respective host from atleast 15 of these hosts many of which are the commen weeds. They may serve the purpose of survival of the pathogen and as a reservoir for transmission of the disease on the fresh crop of pigeonpea in the field. In Karnataka, high incidence of the disease occurs in rainy season specially on the crop sown during July-September. The incidence was found positively correlated with the population of the vector leaf hoppers (Suryanarayana and Ravi 1994).

5.3.4 Host Resistance

Rangaswamy screened 41 entries of pigeonpea against phyllody but none was free (Rangaswamy *et al.* 1990). The entries 2377, PDA 86-1, MTH 5, C 11, PT 20, Pant A 8508, MRG 66, CORG 12, 850-6 and BDN 5 exhibited 10% or less disease. Variable disease on 34 genotypes has been recorded by Rangaswamy *et al.* (1993) also. There is need to screen genotypes systematically under controlled conditions.

5.3.5 Control

In addition to use resistant varieties, it is suggested to select fields away from perinneal pigeonpea and sesamum and to control leaf hoppers by spray of metasystox (Reddy *et al.* 1993b).

5.4 Rosette Disease

This disease was reported from Andhra Pradesh, India (Maramorosch *et al.* 1976) and resembled with the witches broom.

5.4.1 Symptoms

The main symptoms of the disease are stunting of plants due to shortening of internodes, bushy appearance of plants without any significant reduction in leaf size, slight chlorosis around the base of the midrib of many young leaflets. The affected plants had smaller branches with rough brown surface and they are found scattered or in cluster in the field. The flowers and pods are produced but yield is reduced drastically.

5.4.2 Causal Organism

Mycoplasma like organism (MLO)

The MLO was detected in the phloem sieve elements of the diseased plants. It was confined to phloem and phloem paranchyma cells. The MLO is pleomorphic, 80 to 800 μm in diameter with trilaminar unit type membrane and contain ribosome particles (RNA) and fibrillar material (DNA) in the nuclear region. The unit type membrane is approximately 10 nm thick. The serial sections revealed the MLO to undergo binary fission. No virus particles were detected in the rosette affected plants. The rosette disease from India and witches broom from the Caribbean islands are suspected to be caused by different strains of the same MLO species. Its transmission is suspected by means of leaf hoppers or psyllids.

No further work has been done on this disease.

5.5 Rhynchosia Little Leaf

A weed *Rhynchosia minima* is reported for the first time to be affected by a little leaf diseases (RLL) which is caused by a mycoplasma like organism (MLO). The disease is vectored by a cicadellid leaf hopper *(Ollarianus ballo)* which infected the pigeonpea also (Dabak 1983). No work has been done on control aspect of the disease. The virus is reported from Jamaica only (Nene *et al.* 1996).

5.6 Yellow Mosaic

The yellow mosaic of pigeonpea was first found occurring at New Delhi, Uttar Pradesh and Andhra Pradesh in India by Williams *et al.* (1968). The disease has also been reported to occur in Jamaica (Naylor 1974), Puerto Rico (Bird 1962), Sri Lanka (Newton and Peiris 1953), Nepal and Philippines (Nene *et al.* 1996). The cause of the yellow mosaic of pigeonpea has been assigned as mungbean yellow mosaic virus (Nene 1972). However, the causal virus of yellow mosaic of pigeonpea seems to be different in different countries.

The disease is reported to be widespread in Sri Lanka (Reddy *et al.* 1992) while at other places it is treated as the minor disease, although, it has potential to cause serious damage to pigeonpea crop. The losses depend on the intensity of the disease and may vary from 22% in trace infections to 64.3% in heavy infected plants (Mishra and Gurha 1980). In the post-rainy season crop, the disease causes reduction in pods/plant, seeds/pod, 100 seed weight and yield/plant to the extent of 33, 14, 11 and 41% respectively (Beniwal *et al.* 1983).

5.6.1 Symptoms

The symptoms of the disease consist of bright yellow splotches on leaves without leaf distortion and sometimes the symptoms are confined to a single branch of the plant but mostly entire plant is affected (Williams *et al.* 1968). The symptoms of this disease are described in detail by Nene (1972, 1973). The first symptom appears as yellow, diffused spots scattered on leaves. The spots are not limited by veins and veinlets and expand slowly. In later stages, leaflets show broad yellow patches alternating with green colour or whole of the lamina turns yellow. In the advanced stage, irregular necrotic areas with bleached appearance can be seen. The leaf size may be reduced in cases of early infections while late infections do not cause any conspicuous reduction in leaf size. In some cases yellow mottle having very bright colour is noticed. In advanced stages, entire lamina turns bright yellow.

5.6.2 Causal Virus

Mungbean yellow mosaic virus (MYMV)

The cause of yellow mosaic disease of pigeonpea in India, has been found to be the mungbean yellow mosaic virus (Nene 1972, 1973) which is a gemini virus transmitted by white flies *Bemisia tabaci* only. The adult white fly has minimum acquisition and inoculation periods of 15-60 and 10 to less than 60 minutes and the period is longer in case of transmission in pigeonpea (Rathi and Nene 1976).

5.6.3 Control

The disease is not serious and hence, control measures have not been worked out. The disease is reported more severe in crop sown in

September than in June-July (Mishra and Gurha 1980). The disease is less at row spacing of 50 cm as compared to 150 cm (Gurha *et al.* 1983). Control of white flies will help in reducing the spread of the disease in field.

5.7 Yellow Mosaic (Sri Lanka isolate)

Yellow mosaic of pigeonpea was reported in Sri Lanka (Newton and Peiris 1953). The disease was not serious and was confined to dry farming areas.

The disease was characterized by bright yellow blotchy foliage mottle making the plant very conspicuous. This virus is transmitted by sap to *Psophocarpus tetragonolobus* and hence it differs from MYMV which is not able to infect *P. tetragonolobus*.

5.8 Yellow Mosaic (Horsegram yellow mosaic virus)

In Karnataka state of India, yellow mosaic of horsegram was reported to be transmitted by white flies to pigeonpea (Muniyappa and Veeresh 1984). They reported yellow mosaic in pigeonpea to be caused by Horsegram yellow mosaic virus (HYMV). The virus is not transmitted mechanically and has germinated particles of 15-18 × 30 nm in size (Muniyappa *et al.* 1987). The virus has been detected in naturally infected pigeonpea plants showing yellow mosaic symptoms. The white flies *Bemisia tabaci* fed on purified HYMV through a parafilm membrane, transmitted the virus to host plants including pigeonpea.

5.9 Yellow Mosaic (Rhynchosia mosaic virus)

The Rhynchosia mosaic virus was found to infect pigeonpea under inoculated condition (Bird 1962) in Puerto Rico. Later, it was reported to occur under natural conditions also (Bird and Sanchez 1971, Bird *et al.* 1975) producing yellow mosaic symptoms. The symptoms include the presence of bright yellow patches interspersed with green leaves.

The Rhynchosia virus seems to be related to whitefly transmitted bean (double) yellow mosaic virus studied by Capoor and Verma in India. The electron microscopic studies failed to reveal the presence of the causal agent in diseased pigeonpea and it was thought to be a viroid or a group of microorganisms not yet known to cause the diseases (Maramorosch *et al.* 1974a). The virus is reported on the leguminous weed *Rhynchosia minima* and is transmitted by *B. tabaci*. It has the host range including several varieties of *Nicotiana tabacum, N. glutinosa, Abelmoschus esculentus, Gossypium hirsutum, Phaseolus vulgaris, P. lathyroides, Cajanus cajan, Canavalia ensiformis, Ipomea quinquefolia* and *Spermacoce tenuior* (Bird 1962).

5.10 Yellow Mosaic (Alfalfa mosaic virus)

An Iranian isolate of alfalfa mosaic virus responsible for cowpea yellowing has been reported to induce the yellow mosaic symptoms in pigeonpea (Kaiser 1979).

5.11 Pale Mosaic

This disease was reported from Sri Lanka (Newton and Peiris 1953). It is characterized by vein banding followed by a light green mottle. Unlike yellow mosaic, it is reported from the wet zone and spreads more rapidly. Also, it was not able to infect *P. tetragonolobus* up to 20 days while yellow mosaic induced conspicuous vein banding in newly formed foliage in 10-15 days followed by yellowish mottle symptoms.

Mosaic Diseases of Pigeonpea

Several viruses have been reported to cause mosaic symptoms in pigeonpea which are different from each other in one or the other way. Hence, each of them is being described here separately.

5.12 Mosaic Disease of Pigeonpea

Mosaic of pigeonpea was reported from Uttar Pradesh, India affecting about 10% plants under natural conditions (Bisht and Banerjee 1965). The affected plants exhibited mild as well as severe symptoms which were confined to the trifoliate leaves of the upper branches. On the young leaves, faint, scattered, green and yellow spots appeared which gradually developed into severe mosaic. The leaf size was not reduced but the pods produced by the plants were small, poorly developed and green with small shrivelled seeds.

The disease was transmitted to pigeonpea by grafting but not by three common insect vectors tested. The disease could not be transmitted to mungbean and urdbean even by grafting. It was quite different from pigeonpea sterility reported earlier. The causal virus was not identified.

5.13 Arhar (Pigeonpea) Mosaic

The arhar (pigeonpea) mosaic was reported from Uttar Pradesh, India on few plants but it was different from the mosaic disease of pigeonpea reported earlier by Bisht and Banerjee (1965) and other viral diseases of pigeonpea reported so far (Mall 1975). The disease has not been reported from any other country. The diseased plants showed mild mosaic as well as severe mosaic symptoms which were found to be caused by two isolates of a single virus. The disease caused yield losses through reduction in number, weight and size of fruits as well as seeds (Singh and Mall 1978a). The reproductive capacity of plants was reduced more by the severe strain than the mild strain of the virus and losses differed in different varieties of pigeonpea. The virus affected the quality of produce greatly by altering the chemical composition (Singh and Mall 1974a, 1978b).

5.13.1 Symptoms

Two types of symptoms have been described by Singh and Mall (1976a). The mild mosaic symptoms include mild mosaic mottling and slight distortion and reduction in the size of leaflets with dwarfing of affected plants bearing smaller pods. Another types of symptoms, the severe mosaic consists of irregularly scattered, chlorotic and dark areas of varying shape and sizes. The leaflets become twisted and reduced in size with dwarfed plants bearing fewer and smaller pods.

5.13.2 Causal Virus

Arhar (Pigeonpea) mosaic virus

The isolates of virus obtained from plants showing mild and severe mosaic symptoms were named as 'Arhar mild mosaic' (AMM) and 'Arhar severe mosaic' (ASM) viruses respectively (Singh and Mall 1976a). The cross protection tests indicated that both the isolates are the related strains of a single virus different from all other viruses reported so far on pigeonpea. Hence, the virus is named as Arhar (Pigeonpea) mosaic virus.

Transmission : The virus is transmitted easily by sap but not by seed or aphids specially *Myzus persicae, Aphis craccivora, A. gossypi, A. neri, Lipophis pseudobrassicae* and *Rhopalosiphum maidis.*

Physical Properties : Both the strains have the tolerance of dilution between 10^{-5} and 10^{-6}; resistance to heat is 60-65°C in case of AMM and 80-85°C for ASM while longevity *in vitro* of these strains at 22-25°C is 16-17 days and 11-12 days respectively. Both strains are able to retain their infectivity for 735 days in desiccated pigeonpea leaves stored at 15-31°C (Singh and Mall 1976a). The infectious sap had negative reaction against yellow mosaic virus, potato virus X, red clover mosaic virus and Wisconsin pea mosaic virus.

Host Range : Both the strains showed similar host range with systemic infection of *Arachis hypogoeae, Cajanus cajan, Cassia occidentalis, Cassia tora, Cicer arietinum, Clitoria ternatea, C. juncea, C. striate, Dolichos biflorus, Indigofera hirsuta, Lathyrus odoratus, L. sativus, Lens esculenta, Lupinus albus, Medicago denticulata, Melilotus alba, M. indica, M. parviflora, Phaseolus aureus, P. calcaratus, P.mungo, Pisum sativum, Taphrosia purpurea, T. pratense, Trigonella foenum-graceum* and *Vigna sinensis.* However, isolate AMM showed mild reaction to host plants as compared to ASM isolate.

5.13.3 Host Pathogen Interaction

The virus, after infection remarkably influences the host and its activities in various ways as follows :

Nodulation : The nodule number and size along with their dry weight are reduced greatly in the infected plants. This reduction is more in early infected plants than the late infected ones and the severe strain caused more reduction than the mild strain (Singh and Mall 1975). The virus thus adversely affected the nitrogen fixing capacity of plants. Such adverse effects on nodulation and nitrogen fixation were observed in cowpea, mungbean and urdbean also (Singh and Mall 1974b).

Host Physiology : The virus infection caused reduction in the rate of hill reaction and increased the respiratory loss at all the stages of infection and thus reduced the capacity of gross productivity per unit area (Singh and Mall 1976b).

Chemical Contents : The virus infection resulted in reduced chlorophyll, carbohydrate (Water soluble, total, reducing and non-reducing sugars and starch). Such reductions due to the viral infection were recorded in other leguminous plants also (Singh and Mall 1979a).

The chemical composition of fruits and seeds of pigeonpea is also affected greatly by the infection. The total nitrogen and protein increased in fruit coats but decreased in other parts of fruits. The nitrite, nitrate and total free amino acids increased in all parts of fruits. The total organic P fractions were less in fruits affected by mild strain than by the severe strain but reverse was true with the inorganic phosphorus contents. The infection also reduced various carbohydrate fractions (Singh and Mall 1978b). These parameters were reduced greatly in other crops, namely lentil, Kasuri methi (*Trifolium cerniculata)* and methi (*Trigonella foenum-graceum*) also (Singh and Mall 1974a).

Rhizosphere Fungi : The arhar (Pigeonpea) mosaic virus was able to infect the pea variety Bonville and altered the rhizosphere fungal flora of the same. At least 8 fungi were specific to rhizosphere of diseased pea plant. Infection increased the R/S ratio, peroxidase activity and total nitrogen of plant but reduced total carbohydrate and catalase activity of the plant (Srivastava and Singh 1978).

5.13.4 Control

The pigeonpea varieties respond differently to the virus showing possibility of resistance. The variety Sharda suffers more than Prabhat and T 17 (Singh and Mall 1978a).

Copper sulphate (2%), mercuric chloride (1%) and the nicotine sulphate (50%) when mixed with the virus inoculum, caused loss in the infectivity of this virus (Singh and Mall 1979b). Singh *et al.* (1985) tested efficacy of 50 plant leaf extracts of which 42 were found inhibitory to mild as well as severe strains of the virus. The extract from *Capsicum annum* and *Datura stramonium* applied pre-inoculation, checked the infection in the pigeonpea variety Sharda.

5.14 Mild Mosaic

Some plants of pigeonpea at farm of Poona Agriculture College showed mild mosaic and slight puckering in the interveinal regions of leaves. These plants bore smaller leaves and fruits (Singh and Pandey 1979).

5.14.1 Causal Virus

Tobacco Mosaic Virus

The causal virus was transmitted easily by Sap but not by seed or aphids like *M. persicae, A.craccivora, A. gossypi, A. neri, Lipaphis pseudobrassicae* and *Rhopalosiphum maidis*.

The virus had the dilution end point and longevity *in vitro* as 10^{-7} to 10^{-8} and 30-31 days at 21-35°C respectively. The thermal death point was 80-85°C.

The virus produced mild mosaic symptoms on *Glycine max, Phaseolus vulgaris, P. lunatus, P. aureus, Desmodium gyrans, C. cajan;* local lesions on *Nicotiana glutinosa, Chenepodium amaranticolor, N. tabacum, N. rustica* and *N. glauca* while *Pisum sativum* and *Dolichos lablab* were symptomless carriers of the virus. Serologically it was related to tobacco mosaic virus (TMV).

On the basis of host range, symptoms produced on different hosts, transmission pattern, physical and serological properties, the virus was found different from all the viruses so far reported on pigeonpea specially cowpea mosaic virus, yellow and pale mosaic viruses, common bean mosaic virus, sterility mosaic, pigeonpea mosaic virus (Bisht and Banarjee 1965) and arhar mosaic virus (Singh and Mall 1976a). Thus, it is identified as a new strain of tobacco mosaic virus.

5.15 Mosaic

Mosaic in pigeonpea is reported to be caused by alfalfa mosaic virus and cowpea mosaic virus (Nene *et al.* 1996). The infection of pigeonpea seedlings by cowpea mosaic virus was reported under greenhouse conditions in Trinidad and Tobago (Dale 1943) and Puerto Rico (Adsur 1964). The symptoms of the virus on pigeonpea were described by Dale (1949) who found *Ceratoma ruficornis*, a beetle to be the efficient vector of the virus. Perez & Cortes-Monllor (1970) isolated a virus from naturally infected cowpea which was transmitted by *C. ruficornis* and could infect pigeonpea producing yellow mosaic symptoms in Puerto Rico. This isolate resembled the Arkansas cowpea mosaic virus and was considered as a potential threat to pigeonpea crop in Puerto Rico.

Another virus with spherical particles of 28-32 nm size, 5×10^{6} dilution end point and 60°C at 10 minutes as the thermal inactivation point was isolated from cowpea in Kenya Coast Province (Bock 1971). It was transmitted to pigeonpea mechanically and by another beetle *Ootheca mutabilis* and was identified as the yellow mosaic or Nigerian strain of cowpea mosaic virus on the basis of morphological and serological studies. The pigeonpea is considered as the reservoir for carry over of this virus in Kenya (Bock 1971).

5.16 Other Viruses

In addition to above described diseases caused by viruses and MLOs, several viruses have been found to infect pigeonpea and cause typical disease symptoms in the greenhouse test. Some of these have potential to become a problem for pigeonpea cultivation.

5.16.1 Foliar Vein Yellowing

A bullet shaped (Rhabdo) virus was found associated along with the mycoplasma like organism in the phloem of pigeonpea plants showing witches broom symptoms in Dominican Republic near Haiti (Maramorosch and Hichez 1973, Hirumi *et al.* 1973). The diseased plants were collected in Puerto Rico also which exhibited presence of MLO and in some cases particles of rhabdo virus were also seen (Maramorosch *et al.* 1974a and 1974b). Later, it was established that MLO was responsible for witches broom while rhabdo virus caused another disease which was named as "pale mosaic" by Licha-Baquero (1980). McKoy *et al.* (1983) also studied the disease and concluded that MLO was responsible for witches broom symptoms in pigeonpea while rhabdo virus particles were associated with plants showing "Foliar vein yellowing" only. The rhabdo virus particles were 45-55 nm in diameter and 240-260 nm in length (Maramorosch and Hichez 1973).

5.16.2 Clitoria Yellow Vein Virus

The pigeonpea was found very much susceptible to Clitoria yellow vein virus (CYVV), a tymovirus isolated from the wild legume *Clitoria ternatea* in greenhouse inoculation tests in Kenya (Bock *et al.* 1977). The symptoms on pigeonpea are stunting of plant and persistent systemic chlorotic vein net of the foliage. The disease seems to be potentially important to all food legumes grown in the costal areas of Kenya.

5.16.3 Tobacco Streak Virus

A new stain of tobacco streak virus from peas infected pigeonpea in greenhouse inoculation tests and produced yellow mottle symptoms (Patino and Zaumeyer 1959).

5.16.4 Tomato Black Ring Virus

An isolate of tomato black ring virus (TBRV) from potato infected pigeonpea variety T 21 systemically in sap inoculation test in Kenya (Kaiser, *et al.* 1978). The virus was transmitted in the seed from the infected pigeonpea plants.

5.16.5 Alfalfa Mosaic Virus

An east African isolate of alfalfa mosaic virus (AMV) from alfalfa and potato, when inoculated in greenhouse, produced necrotic local lesions and/or mosaic and leaf deformation symptoms in pigeonpea variety T 21 (Kaiser and Robertson 1976).

5.16.6 Cowpea Aphid Borne Mosaic Virus

Two of the east African strains of cowpea aphid borne mosaic virus infected pigeonpea in greenhouse (Bock 1973). The infection was systemic but no symptoms were produced in pigeonpea.

5.16.7 Bean Yellow Mosaic Virus

The pigeonpea was found a host of bean yellow mosaic virus in the inoculation tests in U.S.A. (Zaumeyer and Thomas 1957). Another strain of this virus obtained from diseased *Vicia faba* in Kenya was able to infect the pigeonpea. This strain was identified as pea mosaic virus (PMV) by Bock *et al.* (1973).

5.16.8 Urdbean (Blackgram) Leaf Crincle Virus

The pigeonpea has been reported as the additional host of blackgram leaf crinkle virus showing crinkling of leaf margins (Narayanaswamy and Jaganathan 1974).

5.16.9 Ring Spot Disease

Bright golden yellow pin head size ring spots were observed in several genotypes in Zambia which were suspected to be caused by a virus. Sometimes large chlorotic ring spots were also observed on pigeonpea (Kannaiyan and Haciwa 1990). The etiology is not worked out.

5.16.10 Gall Disease

A gall disease was observed on pigeonpea in addition to cacao and mango. In case of cacao, the disease was transmitted by washings of galls and by extracts of macerated gall tissues from mango or pigeonpea (Archibald 1961). It was suggested not to grow mango or pigeonpea in close proximity of cacao.

5.16.11 Spike Disease

In the regeneration plots, the sandal plants associated with pigeonpea plants as host which favour a rapid growth of the parasite, succumbed to spike disease (Sreenivasaya 1932).

5.16.12 Mosaic

Moderate to severe mosaic symptoms were recorded on pigeonpea varieties BDN 1, NP (WR) 15, ICPL 81, 362, 326, 32, GW 3 and C 11. In Zambia and Kenya of which causal organism is not identified (Kannaiyan and Haciwa 1990).

5.17 Mosaic Mottle

A mosaic mottle disease of pigeonpea was reported from New Delhi, India (Bhattiprolu 1993). The affected plants exhibited mosaic mottling, reduced leaf size, stunting and absence of flowering. The disease was caused by a low molecular weight RNA which could infect *Chenopodium amaranticolor, Nicotiana glutinose* and *N. Clevelandi* also. This viroid differred from the *N. glutinose* stunt viroid, the only viroid reported so far to infect legumes, with respect to size and symptoms produced on pigeonpea. It is transmitted mechanically. The name pigeonpea mosaic mottle viroid is proposed for it.

REFERENCES

Adsur, J. 1964. A mosaic disease of cowpea (*Vigna sinesis* Savi) in Puerto Rico. *Journal of Agriculture of the University of Puerto Rico* 48 : 264.

Alam, M. 1933. Rahar Sterility. Proceedings of 20th Annual Meeting, Indian Science Congress, Poona : Sect. Agriculture 43 : 15-16.

Amin, K.S., Reddy, M.V., Nene, Y.L., Raju, T.N., Shukla, P., Zote, K.K., Arjunan, G., Bendre, N.J., Rathi, Y.P.S., Sinha, B.K., Gupta, R.P., Anilkumar, T.B., Chauhan, V.B., Bidari, V.B., Singh, G., Jha, D.K. and Gangadharan, K. 1993.

Multilocation evaluation of pigeonpea (*Cajanus cajan*) for broad based resistance to sterility mosaic disease in India. *Indian Journal of Agricultural Sciences* 63 : 542-546.

Anonymous. 1990. Pigeonpea disease survey in Myanmar. *International Pigeonpea Newsletter* 12 : 4.

Anonymous. 1992. All India Coordinated Pulses Improvement Project, Kharif Pulses Workshop 1992, highlights. *International Pigeonpea Newsletter* 16 : 3-4.

Archibald, J.F. 1961. Transmission of gall disease of cacao, mango and pigeonpea. *Nature* (UK) 190 : 284.

Beniwal, S.P.S, Deena, E. and Nene, Y.L. 1983. Effect of yellow mosaic on yield and its component in post-rainy season pigeonpea. *International Pigeonpea Newsletter* 2 : 48.

Bhatnagar, P.S., Gangwar, L.C. and Kumar, V. 1966. Phyllody in pigeonpea (*Cajanus cajan* L. Millsp.). *Kanpur Agriculture College Magazine* 26 : 51-52.

Bhatnagar, V.S., Nene, Y.L. and Jadhav, D.R. 1984. Sterility mosaic disease of pigeonpea in a Sorghum based cropping system. *International Pigeonpea Newsletter* 3 : 37-38.

Bhatt, A. 1980. Biochemical changes in pigeonpea leaves in relation to resistance against SMD. M.Sc. Thesis, G.B. Pant University of Agriculture and Technology, Pantnagar, India. pp. 1-90.

Bhattiprolu, S. L. 1993.Occurrence of mosaic mottle, a viroid disease of pigeonpea (*Cajanus cajan*) in India. *Journal of Phytopathology* 137 : 55-60.

Bhite, B.R., Chavan, J.K. and Kachare, D.P. 1997. A biochemical marker for resistance to sterility mosaic disease in pigeonpea. *Journal of Maharashtra Agricultural Universities* 22 : 340-341.

Bird, J. 1962. A whitefly transmitted mosaic of *Rhynchosia minima* and its relation to tobacco leaf curl and other virus diseases of plants in Puerto Rico. *Phytopathology* 52 ; 286 (Abst.).

Bird, J. and Sanchez, J. 1971. Whitefly transmitted virus in Puerto Rico. *Journal of Agriculture of the University of Puerto Rico* 55 : 461-467.

Bird, J., Sanchez , J., Rodriguez, R.L. and Julia, F.J. 1975. Rugaceous (Whitefly transmitted) viruses in Puerto Rico. Pages 3-25 *in* Tropical diseases of legumes (Eds. J.Bird, and K. Maramorosch). Academic Press, New York, USA.

Bisht, N.S. and Banerjee, A.K. 1965. Occurrence of two new virus diseases in Uttar Pradesh. *Labdev Journal of Science and Technology* 3 : 271-272.

Bock, K. R. 1971. Notes on East African plant virus diseases. I. Cowpea mosaic virus. *East African Agricultural and Forestry Journal* 37 : 60-62.

Bock, K.R. 1973. East African stains of cowpea aphid borne mosaic virus. *Annals of Applied Biology* 74 : 75-83.

Bock, K.R., Guthrie, E.J. and Kulkarni, H.Y. 1973. Notes on East African Plant virus diseases. 2. pea mosaic virus. *East African Agricultural and Forestry Journal* 39 : 77-81.

Bock, K.R., Guthrie, E.J. and Meridith, G. 1977. Clitoria yellow vein virus, a tymovirus from Kenya. *Annals of Applied Biology* 85 : 97-103.

Brathwaite, C.W.D. 1981. Disease of pigeonpea in the Caribbean areas. Pages 129-136 *in* Proceedings of the International Workshop on Pigeonpea Vol. I, 15-19th December 1980, ICRISAT centre Patancheru, India.

Capoor, S.P. 1950. Report on pigeonpea sterility with symptoms and transmission. *Proceedings of the Indian Science Congress* 37 (Pt. 3) : 56-59.

Capoor, S.P. 1952. Observations on the sterility disease of pigeonpea in Bombay. *Indian Journal of Agricultural Sciences* 22: 271-274.

Chadha, K.C. and Raychaudhary, S.P. 1965. Interaction between sterility virus and *Fusarium udum* Butl. in pigeonpea. *Indian Journal of Agricultural Sciences* 36 : 133-139.

Chaube, H.S. 1968. Combating diseases of arhar and gram. *Indian Farmers Digest* 1 : 26-27.

Chaudhary, R.G., Vishwadhar and Naimuddin. 1995. Relationship between vexillum colour and sterility mosaic in pigeonpea. *Indian Journal of Mycology and Plant Pathology* 25 : 60 (Abst.).

Chauhan, V.B., Singh, U.P. and Nandan, R. 1991. Raction of some advanced breeding/germplasm lines of pigeonpea to sterility mosaic. *International Pigeonpea Newsletter* 13 : 19-20.

Chaurasia, P.C. 1993. Comparison of strains of sterility mosaic of pigeonpea in Nepal and India. *International Pigeonpea Newsletter* 17 : 24.

Chenulu, V.V., 1984. Plant Virology in India—Past, present and future. *Indian Phytopathology* 37 : 1-20.

Dabek, A.J. 1983. Leaf hopper transmission of Rhynchosia little leaf, a disease associated with mycoplasma like organism in Jamaica. Annals of Applied Biology 103 : 431-438.

Dahal, G. and Neupane, K.R. 1991. Incidence and effect of sterility mosaic disease of pigeonpea in Nepal. *International Pigeonpea Newsletter* 13 : 23-24.

Dale, W. T. 1943. Preliminary studies of the plant viruses of Trinidad. *Tropical Agriculture* 20 : 228-235.

Dale, W. T. 1949. Observations on a virus disease of cowpea in Trinidad. *Annals of Applied Biology* 36 : 327-333.

Das, N.D. and Gupta, S.K. 1992. Evaluation of some pigeonpea lines for resistance to wilt and sterility mosaic. *International Pigeonpea Newsletter* 15 : 23-24.

De, Rajib K., Vishwadhar and Rathore, Y.S. 1995. Bioefficacy of Neem based insecticides on sterility mosaic and yellow mosaic of pigeonpea. Proceedings National Symposium on Perspectives in Ecofriendly Approaches of Plant Protection, New Delhi 7-8 September 1995, pp. 49.

De, Rajib K., Vishwadhar and Rathore, Y.S. 1996. Control of sterility mosaic in pigeonpea with insecticides and acaricides. *Indian Journal of Pulses Research* 9: 87-89.

Desai, B.G., Vora, M.S. and Patel, J.C. 1981. A note on survey of pigeonpea diseases in Gujarat state. *Pulse Crop Newsletter* 1 (3) : 54.

Dwivedi, Kushum and Shukla, P. 1986. Screening of pigeonpea lines for resistance to sterility mosaic disease. *Indian Journal of Mycology and Plant Pathology* 16 : 75-76.

Gangadharan, Koushalya, Arjunan, G., Krishnamohan, G. and Kandaswamy, T.K. 1980. Screening of pigeonpea cultivars for sterility mosaic disease. Pages 66-67 in Proceedings of the National Seminar on Disease Resistance in Crop Plants, Tamil Nadu Agricultural University, Coimbatore, India.

Garg, Rahul, Bajpai, G.C., Gupta, A.K. and Garg, R. 1996. Genotype sensitivity to sterility mosaic and phytophthora blight in pigeonpea. *Agricultural Science Digest, Karnal* 16 : 97-100.

Ghanekar, A.M., Sheila, V.K., Beniwal, S.P.S., Reddy, M.V. and Nene, Y.L. 1992. Sterility mosaic of pigeonpea. pp. 415-428 *in* Plant Diseases of International Importance Vol. 1. Diseases of Cereals and Pulses (Eds. U.S. Singh, A.N. Mukhopadhyay, J. Kumar and H.S. Chaube), Prantice Hall Inc. Englewood, Cliffs, New Jersy, U.S.A.

Gupta, R.P., Singh, D.P. and Katiyar, R.P. 1988a. Response of pigeonpea lines/germplasm to sterility mosaic. *International Pigeonpea Newsletter* 7 : 32-34.

Gupta, R.P., Singh, B.B., Singh, D.P. and Singh, Vinod. 1988b. Screening for resistance to sterility mosaic disease of pigeonpea (*Cajanus cajan*). *Indian Journal of Agricultural Sciences* 58 : 893-894.

Gupta, S.C., Reddy, M.V. and Nene, Y.L. 1981. Sterility mosaic resistant lines of early maturing pigeonpea developed at ICRISAT. *International Pigeonpea Newsletter* 1 : 20.

Gurha, S.N., Singh, D.N. and Gangal, L.K. 1983. Effect of population density on the incidence of sterility and yellow mosaic diseases in pigeonpea. *International Pigeonpea Newsletter* 2 : 47-48.

Haque, S.Q. 1979. Status of virus diseases of grain legumes in the Commonwealth Caribbean. pp. 7-8 *in* Proceedings of Regional Workshop on Tropical Grain Legumes, University of West Indies St. Augustine, Trinidad, Trinidad and Tobago.

Hirumi, H., Maramorosch, K. and Hichez, E. 1973. Rhabdo virus and mycoplasma like organism : Natural dual infection of *Cajanus cajan*. *Phytopathology* 63 : 202 (Abstr.).

Janarthanan, R., Navaneethan, G., Subramanian, K.S. and Samuel, G.S. 1972a. Some observations on the transmission of sterility mosaic of pigeonpea. *Current Science* 41 : 646-647.

Janarthanan, R., Navaneethan, G., Subramanian, K.S. and Samuel, G.S. 1972b. A method of assessment of eriophyid mites on pigeonpea leaves. *Madras Agricultural Journal* 59 : 437.

Janarthanan, R., Samuel, G.S., Subramanian, K.S., Navaneethan, G. and Kandaswamy. T.K. 1973. A report on the survey of sterility mosaic disease incidence on red gram in Tamil Nadu. *Madras Agricultural Journal* 60 : 41-44.

Jayraj, S. and Seshadri, A.R. 1967. Preference of the leaf hopper *Empoasca kerri* Pruthi (Homoptera : Jassidae) for pigeonpea (*Cajanus cajan* (L.) Millsp.) plants infected with sterility mosaic virus. *Current Science*, 36 : 353-355.

Kaiser, W.J. 1979. Natural infection of cowpea and mung bean by alfalfa mosaic virus in Iran. *Plant Disease Reporter* 63 : 414-18.

Kaiser, W.J., Bock, K.R., Guthrie, E.J. and Meridith, G. 1978. Occurrence of tomato black ring virus in potato cultivar Anett in Kenya. *Plant Disease Reporter* 62 : 1088-1092.

Kaiser, W.J. and Robertson, D.G. 1976. Notes on east African plant virus diseases. II. Alfalfa mosaic virus. *East African Agricultural and Forestry Journal* 42 : 47-54.

Kandaswamy, T.K. and Ramakrishnan, K. 1960. An epiphytotic of pigeonpea sterility mosaic at Coimbatore. *Madras Agricultural Journal* 47 : 440-441.

Kannaiyan, J. and Haciwa, H.C. 1990. Diseases of pigeonpea in Zambia. *International Pigeonpea Newsletter* 12 : 22-23.

Kannaiyan, J., Nene, Y.L., Reddy, M.V. and Raju, T.N. 1981a. International survey of pigeonpea diseases. Pulse Pathology Progress Report No. 12, Patancheru, A.P. 502324, ICRISAT, 82 pp.

Kannaiyan, J., Nene, Y.L., Reddy, M.V., Ryan, J.G. and Raju, T.N. 1984. Prevalence of pigeonpea diseases and associated crop losses in Asia, Africa and Americas. *Tropical Pest Management* 30 : 62.

Kannaiyan, J., Reddy, M.V., Nene, Y.L. and Raju. T.N. 1981b. Prevalence of pigeonpea wilt and sterility mosaic in India (1975-80). *International Pigeonpea Newsletter* 1 : 25.

Keifer, H.H. 1952. The eriophyid mites of California. *Bulletin of the California Insect Survey* 2 (1) : 1-123.

Lakshmikantha, B. P., Prabhuswamy, H. P. and Jagadish, K. S. 1997. Effect of staggered sowing on the incidence of pigeonpea sterility mosaic. *Mysore Journal of Agricultural Sciences* 31 : 29-32.

Lal, S. and Rathore, Y. S. 1994. Control of sterility mosaic disease of pigeonpea. *Indian Farming* 43 (10) : 8.

Licha-Baquero, M. 1980. The witches broom disease of pigeonpea in Puerto Rico. *Journal of Agriculture of the University of Puerto Rico* 64 : 424-441.

Mahalinga, D. M., Suryanarayana, V., Gundappagol, R. C. and Jayalaxmi, S. K. 1998. Status of pigeonpea diseases in northern Karnataka. Abstracts National Symposium on Biotic and Abiotic stresses in Pulse Crops, 26-28th June 1998, IIPR, Kanpur, pp. 113.

Mali, V. R., Shirsat, A. M. and Godbole, G. M. 1977. Occurrence of pigeonpea sterility mosaic in Marathwada. *Research Bulletin of the Marathwara Agricultural University* 1: 148-149.

Mall, T. P. 1975. Studies on some virus diseases of pigeonpea, *Cajanus cajan* (L.) Millsp. Ph.D. thesis, University of Gorakhpur, Gorakhpur, Uttar Pradesh, India.

Maramorosch, K. and Hichez, E. 1973. Rhabdovirus and mycoplasma like organism: Natural dual infection of *Cajanus cajan*. *Phytopathology* 63: 202.

Maramorosch, K. Hirumi, H., Kimura, M., Bird, J. and Vakili, N.G. 1974a. Diseases of pigeonpea in the Caribbean area : an electron microscopy study. *FAO Plant Protection Bulletin* 22 : 32-36.

Maramorosch, K., Hirumi, H., Kimura, M., Bird, J. and Vakili, N.G. 1974b. Pigeonpea witches broom disease. *Phytopathology* 64 : 582-583 (Abstr.).

Maramorosch, K., Kimura, M. and Nene, Y.L. 1976. Mycoplasma like organisms associated with pigeonpea rosette disease in India. *FAO Plant Protection Bulletin* 24: 33-35.

Marekar, R.V. 1980. A case of phyllody in pigeonpea. *Indian Journal of Heredity* 12 : 63.

McCoy, R. E., Tsai, J. H., Norris, R. C. and Gwin, G. H. 1983. Pigeonpea witches broom in Florida. *Plant Disease* 67: 443-445.

McRae, W. 1932. Report of the Imperial Mycologist. Scientific reports of the Imperial Institute of Agricultural Research, Pusa, 1930-31, pp. 73-86.

Mishra, B. and Prasad, S. M. 1989. Screening of advanced pigeonpea germplasm lines for resistance to sterility mosaic. *Journal of Research Birsa Agricultural University* 1 (1): 27-29.

Mishra, D.P. and Gurha, S. N. 1980. Losses due to yellow mosaic in winter crop of pigeonpea in India. *Tropical Grain Legume Bulletin* 19 : 18-19.

Mitra, M. 1931. Report of the Imperial Mycologist. Scientific Report of the Agricultural Research Institute, Pusa, 1929-30, pp. 58-71.

Muniyappa, V. and Nangia, N. 1982. Pigeonpea cultivars and selections for resistance to sterility mosaic in relation to prevalence of eriophyid mites *Aceria cajani* Channabasavanna. *Tropical Grain Legume Bulletin* No. 25 : 28-30.

Muniyappa, V., Rajeshwari, R., Bharathan, N., Reddy, D. V. R. and Nolt, B. L. 1987. Isolation and characterization of a gemini virus causing yellow mosaic disease of horsegram (*Macrotyloma uniflorum* (Lam.) Verdc.) in India. *Journal of Phytopathology.*

Muniyappa, V. and Veeresh, G. K. 1984. Plant virus disease transmitted by white flies in Karnataka. *Proceedings of the Indian Academy of Sciences* (*Animal Science*) 93 : 397-406.

Murugesan, S., Murugan, E. and Natarajan, N. 1997. Inheritance of duration, leaf colour, sterility mosaic disease resistance and growth habit in pigeonpea. *Madras Agricultural Journal* 84 : 10-12.

Nambiar, K.K.N. and Ramakrishnan, K. 1968. Studies on pigeonpea sterility mosaic disease. VI. Effect of disease on carbohydrates. *Proceedings of the Indian Academy of Sciences*, Section B68 : 295-300.

Nambiar, K.K.N. and Ramakrishnan, K. 1969a. Studies on pigeonpea sterility mosaic disease. VII. Effect on mineral metabolism. *Proceedings of the Indian Academy of Science*. Section B70:37-41.

Nambiar, K.K.N. and Ramakrishnan, K. 1969b. Studies on pigeonpea sterility mosaic virus. VIII. Effect on photosynthesis and nucleic acids of pigeonpea leaves. *Phytopathologische Zeitschrift* 66 : 91-94.

Nambiar, K.K.N. and Ramakrishnan, K. 1969c. Studies on pigeonpea sterility mosaic disease. IX. Effect on nitrogen metabolism. *Proceedings of the Indian Academy of Sciences,* Sect. B 70:200-7.

Narayanaswamy, P. and Jaganathan, T. 1974. Characterization of leaf crinkle virus. *Madras Agricultural Journal* 61 : 979-982.

Narayanaswamy, P. and Ramakrishnan, K. 1965a. Studies on sterility mosaic disease of pigeonpea. I. Transmission of the disease. *Proceedings of the Indian Academy of Sciences*, Sect. B 62:73-86.

Narayanaswamy, P. and Ramakrishnan, K. 1965b. Studies on sterility mosaic disease of pigeonpea. II. Carbohydrate metabolism of infected plants. *Proceedings of the Indian Academy of Sciences*. Sect. B 62 : 130-139.

Narayanaswamy, P. and Ramakrishnan, K. 1966a. Studies on the Sterility mosaic disease of pigeonpea. III. Nitrogen metabolism of infected plants. *Proceedings of the Indian Academy of Sciences*, Sect.B 63:288-296.

Narayanaswamy, P. and Ramakrishnan, K. 1966b. Studies on sterility mosaic disease of pigeonpea. IV. Changes in activity of enzymes in diseased plants. *Proceedings of the Indian Academy of Sciences*, Section B 64 : 78-82.

Narayanaswamy, P. and Ramakrishnan, K. 1966c. Studies on sterility mosaic disease of pigeonpea. V. Organic acid metabolism and respiration of infected plants. *Proceedings of the Indian Academy of Sciences,* Section B 63 : 135-142.

Narayanaswamy, P., Seshadri, A.R. and Ramakrishnan, K. 1963. Preliminary note on suspected nematode transmission of red gram sterility mosaic virus. *Madras Agricultural Journal* 50 : 109-110.

Natarajan, K. and Dhahira Beevi, N. 1992. Control of *Aceria cajani* (Eriophidae : Acarina) on pigeonpea *Cajanus cajan* (L.) Millsp. *International Pigeonpea Newsletter* 16 : 22-24.

Naylor, A. G. 1974. Disease of plants in Jamaica. Kingston, Jamaica: Ministry of Agriculture, Agril. Information Services, 129 pp.

Nene, Y. L. 1972. A survey of viral diseases of pulse crops in Uttar Pradesh. Research Bulletin No. 4. Pantnagar, Uttar Pradesh, India: GBPU of Agriculture and Technology. 191 pp.

Nene, Y.L. 1973. Virus diseases of some warm weather pulse crops in India. *Plant Disease Reporter* 57 : 463-467.

Nene, Y. L. 1995. Sterility mosaic of pigeonpea, the challenge continues. *Indian Journal of Mycology and Plant Pathology* 25 : 1-11.

Nene, Y. L., Kannaiyan, J. and Reddy, M. V. 1981a. Pigeonpea diseases : Resistance screening technique.*Information Bulletin* No. 9. Patancheru, India: ICRISAT, pp 1-14.

Nene, Y. L., Kannaiyan, J., Reddy, M. V. and Ramanandan, P. 1981b. Sources of resistance to selected pigeonpea disease. Pulse Pathology Progress Report No. 16. Patancheru, A.P. 502324, India: International Crops Research Institute for the Semi-Arid Tropics. 34 pp.

Nene, Y. L. and Reddy, M.V. 1976a. Screening for Resistance to sterility mosaic of pigeonpea. *Plant Disease Reporter* 60 : 1034-36.

Nene, Y. L. and Reddy, M. V. 1976b. A new technique to screen pigeonpea for resistance to sterility mosaic. *Tropical Grain Legume Bulletin* 5 : 23.

Nene, Y. L. and Reddy, M. V. 1977. Leaf stappling technique to screen pigeonpea for resistance to sterility mosaic. *Indian Phytopathology* 30 : 153.

Nene, Y. L., Reddy, M. V. and Deena, E. 1981c. Modified infector row technique to screen pigeonpea for sterility mosaic resistance. *International Pigeonpea Newsletter* 1:27.

Nene, Y.L., Reddy, M.V., Beniwal, S. P. S., Mahmood, S., Zote, K. K., Singh, R. N. and Sivaprakasham, K. 1989. Multilocational testing of pigeonpea for broad based resistance to sterility mosaic in India. *Indian Phytopathology* 42 : 444-448.

Nene, Y. L. and Sheila, V.K. 1992. Callus induction from sterility mosaic infected pigeonpea leaves. *International Pigeonpea Newsletter* 15 : 20-21.

Nene, Y. L., Sheila, V. K. and Sharma, S. B. 1996. A world list of chickpea and pigeonpea pathogens. 5th edn. Patancheru, A. P., India : ICRISAT, pp. 1-27.

Newton, W. and Peiris, J. W. L. 1953. Virus diseases of plants in Ceylon. *FAO Plant Protection Bulletin* 2 : 17-21.

Oldfield, G. N. 1970. Mite transmission of plant viruses. *Annual Review of Entomology* 15 : 343-380.

Oldfield, G.N., Reddy, M. V., Nene, Y. L. and Reed, W. 1981. Preliminary studies of the eriophyid vector of sterility mosaic. *International Pigeonpea Newsletter* 1 : 25-27.

Padule, D. N., Newase, A. G. and Patil, B.P. 1982. Survey for incidence of fusarium wilt and other diseases of pigeonpea in central parts of western Maharashtra. *Journal of Maharashtra Agricultural Universities* 7 (2) : 159-161.

Pal, B. P., Shukla, A. and Rathi, Y.P. S. 1989. Reaction of pigeonpea lines to sterility mosaic and Phytophtora blight. *International Pigeonpea Newsletter* 10 : 25-26.

Patino, G. and Zaumeyer, W. J. 1959. A new strain of tobacco streak virus from peas. *Phytopathology* 49 : 43-48.

Pawar, K. B., Bhor, S. B., Bendre, N.J. and Deshmukh, R.B. 1993. Pigeonpea lines resistant to sterility mosaic. *Indian Journal of Pulses Research* 6 (1) : 110-111.

Perez, J. E. and Cortes-Monllor, A. 1970. A mosaic virus of cowpea from Puerto Rico. *Plant Disease Reporter* 54 : 212-216.

Prameela, H.A., Joshi, S. S., Vishwanath, S. and Anilkumar, T. B. 1990a. Histopathological and histochemical changes in pigeonpea due to single and dual infections by powdery mildew and sterility mosaic virus. *Biochem. Physiol. Pflanzen* 186 : 55-61.

Prameela, H. A., Vishwanath, S. and Anilkumar, T. B. 1989 a. Physiological and biochemical changes in pigeonpea (*Cajanus cajan* (L) Millsp.) due to single and dual infection with powdery mildew and sterility mosaic. *Biochem. Physiol. Pflanzen* 184 : 439-445.

Prameela, H. A., Vishwanath, S. and Anilkumar, T. B. 1989b. The predisposing effect of sterility mosaic to powdery mildew infections in pigeonpea. *Zentralblatt fur Mikrobiolgie* 144 : 110-114.

Prameela, H. A., Vishwanath, S. and Anilkumar, T.B. 1990b. Effect of single and combined infections of powdery mildew and sterility mosaic on nodulation and biomass of pigeonpea. *Zentralblatt Mikrobiologie* 145 : 37-39.

Prasad, S. N. 1965. Studies on sterility mosaic of 'Rahar' (*Cajanus cajan*). *Allahabad Farmer* 39 : 235-237.

Raguchander, T., Arjunan, G. and Samiappan, R. 1995. Field performance of pigeonpea genotypes to sterility mosaic. *Madras Agricultural Journal* 82 ; 319-320.

Ramakrishnan, K. and Kandaswamy, T. K. 1972. Investigations on virus diseases of pulse crops in Tamil Nadu : final technical report. Coimbatore, Tamil Nadu, India : Tamil Nadu Agricultural University, 53 pp.

Rangaswamy, K.T., Anilkumar, T. B., Vishwanath, K. P. and Shambulingappa, K. G.

1993. Severe recurrence of pigeonpea phyllody at GKVK, Bangalore. *Plant Protection Bulletin* (Faridabad) 45 : 53.

Rangaswamy, K. T., Veeresh, L.C., Anilkumar, T. B. and Shambulingappa, K. G. 1990. A severe outbreak of pigeonpea phyllody at Bangalore. *International Pigeonpea Newsletter* 12 : 18-19.

Rao, B.L.S., Nene, Y.L. and Jambunathan, R. 1985. Sterility mosaic infection in different pigeonpea genotypes. I. Studies on different N compounds of the host. *Indian Journal of Plant Pathology* 3 (1) : 108-118.

Rathi, Y.P.S. 1979. Temik treatment of pigeonpea seeds for prevention of sterility mosaic. *Acta Botanica Indica* 7 : 90-91.

Rathi, Y.P.S. 1983. Studies on sterility mosaic disease of pigeonpea (*Cajanus cajan* (L) Millsp.). *Final Technical Report,* GBPU of Agriculture and Technology, Pantnagar, India, 1-31 pp.

Rathi, Y. P. S. and Nene, Y. L. 1976. Influence of different host combinations on virus-vector relations of mung bean yellow mosaic virus. *Pantnagar Journal of Research* 1 : 107-111.

Rathi, Y. P. S. and Tripathi, H. S. 1989. Management of mung been yellow mosaic and pigeonpea sterility mosaic. *Indian Phytopathology* 42 : 314-315 (Abstr.).

Rathi, Y.P.S. and Tripathi, H. S. 1993. Identification of sources of resistance to pigeonpea sterility mosaic virus (?) and mung bean yellow mosaic virus. *Indian Phytopathology* 44 & 45 (Suppl.) LXX (Abst.).

Ravi, K. S. and Reddy, H. R. 1987. Association of mycoplasma like organism with pigeonpea Phyllody. *Current Science* 56 : 29-30.

Reddy, H.R. and Ravi, K.S. 1984. Phyllody disease in pigeonpea. *International Pigeonpea Newsletter* 3 : 39-40.

Reddy, H. R., Siddappaji, C., Channabasavanna, G. P., Janardhana, A. and Ravi, K. S. 1983. Occurrence of pigeonpea phyllody in Karnataka State of India. *Legume Research* 6 (1) : 41-42.

Reddy, M. V., Arjunan, G. and Munyappa, V. 1990a. Survival of pigeonpea sterility mosaic pathogen and its vector during summer in southern India. *International Pigeonpea Newsletter* 11: 16-17.

Reddy, M. V., Beniwal, S. P. S., Sheila, V. K., Sithanantham, S. and Nene, Y. L. 1989a. Role of an eriophyid mite *Aceria cajani* (Acari : Eriophyidae) in transmission and spread of sterility mosaic of pigeonpea. Pages 121-127 *In* Progress in acarology (Eds. G.P. Channabasavanna and C.A. Viraktamath). New Delhi, India : Oxford & IBH Publishing Co.

Reddy, M.V., Jain, K.C., Chauhan, Y.S. and Singh, Laxman, 1995. Wilt and sterility mosaic resistant pigeonpea genotype ICPL 87119 benefits farmers in Medak district of Andhra Pradesh, India, *International Pigeonpea Newsletter* 2 : 71-72.

Reddy, M.V., Kannaiyan, J. and Nene, Y.L. 1984. Increased susceptibility of sterility mosaic infected pigeonpea to powdery mildew. *International Journal of Tropical Plant Disease* 2: 35-40.

Reddy, M. V. and Nene, Y. L. 1979. Ringspot symptom : a genotypic expression of pigeonpea sterility mosaic. *Tropical Grain Legume Bulletin* 15 : 27-29.

Reddy, M.V. and Nene, Y.L. 1980. Influence of sterility mosaic resistant pigeonpeas on multiplication of mite vector. *Indian Phytopathology* 33 : 61-63.

Reddy, M.V. and Nene, Y.L. 1981a. Estimation of yield losses in pigeonpea due to sterility mosaic. Pages 305-312 *in* Proceedings of the International Workshop on Pigeonpeas, 15-19 December 1980, ICRISAT Centre, India. Vol. 2. Patancheru, A.P., India.

Reddy, M. V. and Nene, Y.L. 1981b. Some aspects of field screening of pigeonpea for resistance to sterility mosaic disease, pages 285-289 *in* Proceedings of the International Workshop on Pigeonpeas, 15-19 December 1980, ICRISAT Centre, India.Vol. 2. Patancheru, A.P., India.

Reddy, M. V., Nene, Y. L., Raju, T. N., Sheila, V. K., Kannaiyan, J. and Beniwal, S.P.S. 1989b. Evaluation of pigeonpea lines for resistance to wilt, sterility mosaic and phytophthora blight. *International Pigeonpea Newsletter* 10 : 22-24.

Reddy, M. V. and Raju, T. N. 1993. Some clues to increased incidence and seasonal variation of pigeonpea sterility mosaic in the peninsular India. *International Pigeonpea Newsletter* 18: 22-24.

Reddy, M. V., Raju, T. N. and Nene, Y.L. 1991. Appearance of a new strain of pigeonpea sterility mosaic pathogen. *International Pigeonpea Newsletter* 14 : 22-23.

Reddy, M.V., Raju, T. N., Nene, Y. L., Ghanekar, A. M., Amin, K. S., Arjunan, G., Astaputre, J. V., Sinha, B. K., Muniyappa, V., Reddy, S.V., Gupta, R.P. and Gangadharan, Kaushalya. 1993a. Variability in sterility mosaic pathogen of pigeonpea in India. *Indian Phytopathology* 46 : 206-212.

Reddy, M. V., Raju, T. N., Sharma, S. B., Nene, Y.L. and McDonald, D. 1993b. Handbook of pigeonpea diseases. Patancheru, India ; ICRISAT. Information Bulletin No. 42, pp. 61.

Reddy, M. V., Reddy, D. V. R. and Sacks, W. R. 1994. Epidemiology and management of sterility mosaic disease of pigeonpea. Pages International Symposium on Rose rosette and other eriophyid mite transmitted plant diseases agents of uncertain etiology, 19-21 May 1994, Iowa State University, Ames, Iowa, USA.

Reddy, M. V., Saxena, K. B., Jayasekara, S. J. B. A. and Faris, D. G. 1992a. Assessment of diseases on short duration pigeonpea in Sri Lanka. *International Pigeonpea Newsletter* 15 : 15-17.

Reddy, M. V., Sharma, S. B. and Nene, Y.L. 1990b. Pigeonpea: Disease management. Pages 303-347 *in* the Pigeonpea (Eds. Y.L. Nene, Hall, S. D. and Sheila V. K.), Wallingford, Oxon, UK. CAB International.

Reddy, M. V., Sheila, V. K. and Nene, Y.L. 1993b. *Cajanus scarabaeoides* and alternative host of pigeonpea sterility mosaic pathogen and its vector *Aceria cajani*. *International Pigeonpea Newsletter* 18 : 24-27.

Reddy, M. V., Sheila, V. K., Murthy, A. K. and Padma, N. 1995. Mechanism of resistance to *Aceria cajani* in pigeonpea. *International Journal of Tropical Plant Diseases* 13 : 51-57.

Reddy, M. V., Vishwa Dhar, Lenne, J. M. and Raju, T.N. (Editors). 1996 Proceedings of the Asian Pigeonpea Pathologists Group Meeting and Monitoring Tour, ICRISAT Asia Centre, India : 20-25 Nov. 1995. Patancheru, India : ICRISAT, pp. 28.

Reddy, S. V., Reddy, M. V., Ghanekar, A. M., Nene, Y. L. and Amin, K. S. 1988. Annual recurrence of pigeonpea sterility mosaic in eastern Uttar Pradesh, India. *International Pigeonpea Newsletter* 7: 30-31.

Rishi, Narayani and Sharma, Pradip. 1999. Economically important viral diseases of pulse crops and their management. *Indian Journal of Pulses Research* 12 : 143-172.

Samiyappan, R. and Arjunan, G. 1986. Resistance of pigeonpea to sterility mosaic diseases in southern India. *International Pigeonpea Newsletter* 5 : 37-38.

Samiyappan, R. and Sivaprakasham, K. 1985. Reaction of some pigeonpea lines to sterility mosaic disease. *Tropical Pest Management* 31 (3) : 235-236.

Saxena, K. B., Gupta,M. D., Kumar, R. V., Latif, S. S. and Reddy, M.V. 1992. ICPL 371, a promising long duration pigeonpea line tolerant to pod fly and sterility mosaic. *International Pigeonpea Newsletter* 15 : 9-10.

Seth, M. L. 1962. Transmission of pigeonpea sterility by an eriophid mite. *Indian Phytopathology* 15 : 225-227.

Seth, M. L. 1965. Further observations and studies on pigeonpea sterility. *Indian Phytopathology* 18 : 317-319.

Sharma, D., Gupta, S.C., Rai, G. S. and Reddy, M. V. 1983. Inheritence of resistance to sterility mosaic disease in pigeonpea. *International Pigeonpea Newsletter* 2 : 45-47.

Sharma, D., Gupta, S. C., Rai, G. S. and Reddy, M. V. 1984. Inheritence of resistance to sterility mosaic disease in pigeonpea. *Indian Journal of Genetics and Plant Breeding* 44 : 84-90.

Sheila, V. K., Manohar, S. K. and Nene, Y.L. 1988. Biology and Morphology of *Aceria cajani*. *International Pigeonpea Newsletter* 7: 28-29.

Shirshikar, S. P., Astaputre, J. V., Shinde, V. K. and Deshmukh, R. B. 1990. Screening of pigeonpea entries against wilt and sterility mosaic disease. *Indian Phytopathology* 43 : 307.

Singh, A. B. and Pandey, P.K. 1979. A new strain of tobacco mosaic virus causing mosaic disease of pigeonpea. *Current Science* 48 : 261.

Singh, A. K. and Rathi, Y.P.S. 1994. Nature of losses caused by sterility mosaic in pigeonpea. *Journal of Applied Biology* 4: 35-37.

Singh, A. K. and Rathi, Y.P.S. 1996a. Histopathological studies in sterility mosaic affected pigeonpea using fluorescent and light microscopy. *Indian Journal of Virology* 12 : 151-153.

Singh, A. K. and Rathi, Y.P.S. 1996b. Nuclear inclusion produced in phloem cells of pigeonpea diseased mid-vein infected with pigeonpea sterility mosaic virus (PSMV). *Indian Journal of Virology* 12 (2) : 147-149.

Singh, A. K. and Rathi, Y.P.S. 1996c. Effect of different dates of sowing on the first symptoms appearance and disease incidence of sterility mosaic of pigeonpea (*Cajanus cajan* (L) Millspaugh). *Advances in Plant Sciences* 9 : 61-64.

Singh, A. K. and Rathi, Y.P.S. 1997. Epidemiology of vector of pigeonpea sterility mosaic virus. *Indian Journal of Virology* 13 : 143-145.

Singh, A.K., Agrawal, K.C. and Rathi, Y.P.S. 1999a. Occurrence and sources of resistance of sterility mosaic of pigeonpea. *Indian Phytopathology* 52 : 156.

Singh, A.K., Rathi, Y.P.S. and Agrawal, K.C. 1999b. Sterility mosaic of pigeonpea : a challenge of 20th Century. *Indian Journal of Virology* 15 : 85-92.

Singh, B.B., Singh, D.P., Singh, N.P. and Kumar, R. 1995. Evaluation of pigeonpea germplasm for resistance to sterility mosaic. *International Chickpea and Pigeonpea Newsletter* 2 : 69-70.

Singh, Brij Vir, Pandya, B.P., Gautam, P.L., Beniwal, S.P.S. and Pandey, M.P. 1983. Inheritence of resistance to sterility mosaic virus in pigeonpea. *Indian Journal of Genetics and Plant Breeding* 43 : 487-493.

Singh, O., Sah, R.P., Joshi, Sharada, Shrestha, D., Karna, R. S. L. and Bharati, M.P. 1989. Pigeonpea germplasm resistant to sterility mosaic identified in Nepal. *International Pigeonpea Newsletter* 9 : 21-22.

Singh, K., Dahiya, B. S. and Chohan, J. S. 1975. Evaluation of arhar (*Cajanus cajan*) germplasm lines against the sterility disease in Punjab. *Journal of Research, Punjab Agricultural University* 12 : 327-328.

Singh, N. B., Reddy, M.V., Nageswara Rao A., Raju, T. N., Singh, L. and Gupta, S.C. 1996. Newly developed extra short duration pigeonpea lines with combined resistance to wilt and sterility mosaic, ICRISAT Asia Centre. *International Chickpea and Pigeonpea Newsletter* 3 : 87-88.

Singh, R. and Mall, T.P. 1974a. Effect of arhar mosaic virus on yield and chemical constitution of seeds of some legumes. *Labdev Journal of Science and Technology* 12 : 145-149.

Singh, R. and Mall, T.P. 1974b. Studies on the nodulation and nitrogen fixation by infected leguminous plants. I. Effect of arhar mosaic virus infection on nitrogen value, nodulation and nitrogen fixation by some pulse crops. *Plant and Soil* 41 : 279-86.

Singh, R. and Mall, T.P. 1975. Effect of arhar mosaic virus infection on nodulation of pigeonpea. *Indian Journal of Experimental Biology* 13 : 322-323.

Singh, R. and Mall, T.P. 1976a. A new virus disease of arhar (*Cajanus cajan* (L) Millsp.). *Current Science* 45 : 635-636.

Singh, R. and Mall, T.P. 1976b. Effect of infection by arhar mosaic virus on the Hill reaction and primary productivity of pigeonpea (arhar) leaves. *Indian Journal of Experimental Biology* 14 : 376-377.

Singh, R. and Mall, T.P. 1978a. Effect of arhar (pigeonpea) mosaic virus on the yield and reproductive capacity of pigeonpea cultivars. *Indian Journal of Mycology and Plant Pathology* 8 : 171-181.

Singh, R. and Mall, T.P. 1978b. Changes in chemical composition of pigeonpea fruits due to arhar (pigeonpea) mosaic virus infection. *Acta Phytopathologica Academiae Scientiarum Hungaricae* 13 : 41-44.

Singh, R. and Mall, T.P. 1979a. Chlorophyll and carbohydrate contents of a virus diseased pigeonpea plant. *Indian Journal of Mycology and Plant Pathology* 9: 269-271.

Singh, R. and Mall, T.P. 1979b. Screening of some chemicals for antiviral properties. *Science and Culture* 45 : 66-68.

Singh, R., Mall., T.P. and Singh, R.R. 1985. Inhibitory activity of leaf extracts on the infectivity of arhar (pigeonpea) mosaic viruses. *International Pigeonpea Newsletter* 4 : 38-40.

Sivaprakasam, K. and Anbalagam, R. 1983. A new sterility mosaic resistant pigeonpea line. *International Pigeonpea Newsletter* 2 : 45.

Slykhuis, J. T. 1980. Mites. Pages 325-356 *in* Vectors of plant pathogens (Eds.K. F. Harris and K. Maramorosch). New York USA: Academic Press.

Sreenivasaya, M. 1932. Present position of the problem of spike disease. *Cajanus indicus. Current Science* 1 : 126.

Srinivas, T., Jain, K. C. and Reddy, M.S.S. 1998. Combining ability studies of sterility mosaic resistant pigeonpea (*Cajanus cajan* (L.) Millsp.). *Crop Research* (*Hisar*) 15 (1) : 99-103.

Srinivas, T. and Reddy, M.V. 1995. Pigeonpea lines resistant to old and new strains of sterility mosaic disease. *International Chickpea and Pigeonpea Newsletter* 2 : 67-69.

Srinivas, T., Reddy, M.V., Jain, K. C. and Reddy, M.S.S. 1997a. Screening for resistance to two isoiates of sterility mosaic pathogen in pigeonpea (*Cajanus cajan* (L.) Millsp.). *Crop Research Hisar* 13: 169-175.

Srinivas, T., Reddy, M.V., Jain, K.C. and Reddy, M.S.S. 1997b. Studies on inheritence of resistance and allelic relationships for strain 2 of pigeonpea sterility mosaic pathogen. *Annals of Applied Biology* 130 : 105-110.

Srinivas, T., Reddy, M. V., Jain, K. C. and Reddy, M. S. S. 1997c. Inheritence of resistance to two isolates of sterility mosaic pathogen in pigeonpea (*Cajanus cajan* (L.) Millsp.). Inheritence to isolates of sterility mosaic. *Euphytica* 97 : 45-52.

Srivastava, A.K. and Singh, R. B. 1978. Effect of pigeonpea mosaic virus on rhizosphere fungal flora of pea. *Legume Research* 1 : 92-96.

Su, U. 1931. Plant Disease in Burma. *International Bulletin of Plant Protection* 5 : 141-142.

Subramanian, K. S., Samuel, G. S., Janarthanan, R. and Kandaswamy, T. K. 1973. Studies on the varietal resistance of pigeonpea (*Cajanus cajan* L.) to sterility mosaic disease. *Madras Agricultural Journal* 60 : 38-40.

Suryanarayana,V., Muniyappa, V., Singh, S. J., Viraktamath, C.A. and Reddy, H. R. 1997a. Phytoplasma-vector relationship of pigeonpea phyllody disease. *Pest Management in Horticultural Ecosystem* 3 (1) : 1-6.

Suryanarayana, V. and Ravi, K. S. 1994. Seasonal occurrence of pigeonpea phyllody, a plant mycoplasma disease. *Indian Phytopathology* 47 : 333 (Abstract).

Suryanarayana, V., Viraktamath, C.A., Muniyappa, V. and Reddy, H. R. 1997b. Vector transmission studies of pigeonpea phyllody. *Journal of Mycology and Plant Pathology* 27 : 108-109.

Thiyagarajan, K., Natarajan, C., Arjunan, G., Vijayakumar, G., Jehangir, K. S. and Rathnaswamy, R. 1987. Reaction of arhar (pigeonpea) coordinated trial lines to sterility mosaic in Tamil Nadu, India. *International Pigeonpea Newsletter* 6 : 53-54.

Vakili, N. G. and Maramorosch, K. 1974. "Witches broom" disease caused by mycoplasma like organism on pigeonpea (*Cajanus cajan*) in Puerto Rico. *Plant Disease Reporter* 58 : 96.

Van Velson, R. J. 1961. Witches broom on pigeonpea induced by mealy bug (*Planococcus*); i.e. *Pseudococcus citri* infestation. *Journal of Papua New Guinea Agriculture* 14 : 129.

Vishwa Dhar and Rathore, Y. S. 1994. Pattern of population distribution of *Aceria cajani* on pigeonpea plant. *Indian Journal of Pulses Reaserch* 7: 137-143.

Vishwa Dhar, Rathore, Y. S. and De, R. K. 1994. Identification of stable resistance against pigeonpea sterility mosaic. *Indian Phytopathology* 47 : 313 (Abstract).

Vishwa Dhar, Rathore, Y. S. and De, R. K. 1995. Studies on the population dynamics of *Aceria cajani*, the vector of pigeonpea sterility mosaic disease. *Indian Journal of Mycology and Plant Pathology* 25 : 72-73.

Vishwa Dhar, Rathore, Y. S., De, R. K. and Lal, S. 1997. The sterility mosaic of pigeonpea. Indian institute of Pulses Research, Kanpur, India., pp. 1-19.

Wellman, F. L. 1972. Tropical American Plant Diseases. Metuchen, New Jersey, USA : Scarecrow Press.

Williams, F. J., Grewal, J. S. and Amin, K. S. 1968. Serious and new diseases of pulse crops in India in 1966. *Plant Disease Reporter* 52 : 300-304.

Zaumeyer, W. and Thomas, H. R. 1957. A monographics study of bean diseases and methods for their control. Technical Bulletin No. 868. Washington, D. C., USA. : United States Department of Agriculture 255 pp.

Zote, K.K., Astaputre, J.U. and Shirshikar, S.S. 1993. Management of sterility mosaic disease through resistant breeding. *Indian Phytopathology* 44 & 45 (Suppl.) : XXII (Abstract).

Zote, K.K. and Dandnaik, B.P. 1986. Comparative performance of pigeonpea cultivars to sterility mosaic. *Indian Phytopathology* 39: 304-306.

Zote, K.K. and Dandnaik, B.P. 1987. Screening of pigeonpea for multiple disease resistance. *Indian Phytopathology* 40: 59-62.

Zote, K.K. and Dandnaik, B.P. 1989. Multilocation testing of some pigeonpea lines to sterility mosaic disease. *Indian Phytopathology* 42 : 338 (Abstract).

Zote, K. K., Dandnaik, B.P. and Khalikar, P.V. 1983a. Reaction of Maharashtra cultivars of pigeonpea to wilt and sterility mosaic. *International Pigeonpea Newsletter* 2 : 44-45.

Zote, K. K., Dandnaik, B.P., Khalikar, P.V. and Raut, K. G. 1988. Effect of intercropping with sorghum and pearl millet on the incidence of pigeonpea sterility mosaic. *International Pigeonpea Newsletter* 7: 26-27.

Zote, K. K., Mali, V. R., Mayee, C.D., Kulkarni, S.V. and Mote, T. S. 1991. Outbreak of sterility mosaic disease of pigeonpea in Marathwada region, Maharashtra, India. *International Pigeonpea Newsletter* 14 : 19-21.

Zote, K.K., Mali, V. R., Mayee, C.D., Saikh, M.H., Katare, R. A., Kulkarni, S. V. and Mote, T. S. 1997. Outbreak of sterility mosaic disease of pigeonpea in Marathwada region. *Indian Phytopathology* 50 : 141-143.

Zote, K.K., Thombre, P. G., Khalikar, P. V., Dandnaik, B. P., Chavan, G. V. and Olekar, S. S. 1983b. Breeding pigeonpea for resistance to wilt and sterility mosaic. *International Pigeonpea Newsletter* 2: 43-44.

6

Diseases Caused by Nematodes

Large number of nematodes have been found associated with pigeonpea. In general, the plant parastitic nematodes are minute and vermiform animals ranging from 0.3 mm (*Paratylenchus* spp.) to 10 mm (*Longidorus* spp.) in size. The sexual dimorphism is not very common except that in species of *Meloidogyne, Heterodera, Globodera, Punctodera* and *Nacobus* in which females are markedly different than males morphologically. All the plant parasitic nematodes possess the stylet or mouth spear which is used to pierce plant cells and feeding. They are dependent on water film for motility and become inactive or die in its absence. In addition to direct losses caused to plant, nematodes may help in increasing severity of some soil borne diseases caused by fungi. They may also act as vector of some pathogens. In soil, many saprophytic nematodes are present which do not possess stylet and are beneficial as they break down organic material and aid the distribution of helpful microorganisms.

All the members of a particular genus of nematodes are not necessarily the plant pathogens. Great variability occurs within a genus and even within a species with regard to their habit and degree of penetration of host tissues, host preference etc.

The namtodes may be classified on the basis of their habitat as follows:

(i) *Above ground* : Species of *Anguina, Aphelenchoides, Ditylenchus, Neotylenchus, Pratylenchus coffeae, Scutelonema brachyurum,* etc. Normally root parasites may occur in crown or bark tissues of host.

(ii) *Root Parasites* : They may be :

a. *Ectoparasites* : They normally do not penetrate root and usually have long mouth spears. They may be sedentary like *Criconema, Criconemoides, Hemicriconemoides, Macroposthonia* and *Pratylenchus* etc. or may be migratory like *Belonolaimus, Dolichodorus, Longidorus, Trichodorus, Xiphinema* etc.

b. *Semiendparasites* : They usually feed with front end of their body in the root. Some of the species tend towards full endoparasites. They may be sedentary like *Rotylenchulus, Sphaeronema, Tylenchulus semipenetrans* etc. or migratary like *Helicotylenchus, Hoplolaimus, Rotylenchus, Scutelonema, Tylenchorhynchus* etc.

c. *Endoparasites* : They penetrate in the host tissues and may be sedentary in which females are saccate or much swellen such as *Heterodera, Meloidogyne, Meloidodera, Nacobus, Punctodera* etc. or active migratory in which females are vermiform like *Ditylenchus,* some species of *Helicotylenchus, Pratylenchoides, Pratylenchus, Radopholus, Rotylenchoides* spp.

The above ground symptoms are the adverse effect on plant growth due to injury of roots. These symptoms are often similar to those produced when a plant is deprived of an adequate root system or specific nutrients. In general, symptoms are more pronounced if the plants are already affected by adverse conditions or attack of other root pathogens. The plants growing under favourable conditions may not show any symptoms even if they are attacked by the nematodes. They can be most destructive in association with other pathogens. Frequently, the symptoms on a plant result from the combined action of several species of nematodes.

The mechanical injury to plant tissues is caused due to movement of nematodes through or between the cells. Some may secrete pectinase which dissolves the middle lamella. The necrosis or other changes in the cell contents may be caused by salivary secretion resulting in deformities in host tissues in the form of galls/knots, proliferations, hypoplasia, necrosis etc.

The earliest report of nematode on pigeonpea is that of root knot nematodes by Bessy (1911). Since then large number of species have been found associated and the available information has been reviewed from time to time (Kaiser 1981, Swarup 1983, Rajak *et al.* 1986, Sharma 1985a, Sharma 1988, Gill and Singh 1990, Sharma and McDonald 1990, Nene *et al.* 1996). There are some reports on systematic survey on nematode fauna associated with pulse crops including pigeonpea (Starr

1979, Sharma *et al.* 1985, Ali 1987, Anonymous 1987, Sharma *et al.* 1992b, 1993a & 1993c, Ali 1993, Sharma *et al.* 1996). Information has also been compiled on aspect of diseases caused by nematodes in pigeonpea (Yadava 1986, Sasser 1989, Reddy *et al.* 1990, Sharma *et al.* 1992c and Ali and Sharma 1997).

Nematodes are responsible to cause considerable yield losses in pigeonpea. On global basis plant parasitic nematodes cause about 13.2% losses to pigeonpea annually (Sasser and Frekman 1987) which comes to about 177 million dollars. The status of nematology with special reference to pigeonpea/pulse crops has been reviewed by Sharma (1988), Sharma and McDonald (1990) and Tiwari and Sharma (1997).

Control of nematodes in the field has been a great problem. Efforts have been made to regulate their population through the biological agents (Stirling 1991), soil solarization (Sharma and Nene 1990b), crop rotation etc. (Gonzga and Lordello 1960, Sharma *et al.* 1996b), Important nematode diseases of pigeonpea are :

6.1 Pearly Root Disease

The pearly root disease of pigeonpea is caused by pigeonpea cyst nematode, *Heterodera cajani*. The literature on cyst forming nematodes has been reviewed in detail (Sharma and Swarup 1984, Swarup and Gokte 1986 and 1987). The disease has been reported from India and Egypt (Nene *et al.* 1996) only. In India, the nematode occurs on pigeonpea in the states of Delhi (Swarup *et al.* 1964), Tamil Nadu (Janarthanan 1972), Rajasthan (Verma and Yadava 1975), Andhra Pradesh (Starr 1979), Maharashtra (Darekar *et al.* 1985), Haryana (Walia *et al.* 1985), Bihar (Nath 1986). Karnataka (Saxena and Reddy 1987), Gujarat (Ali 1992) and Uttar Pradesh (Koshy and Swarup 1971). The nematode is very widespread and has been detected from most of the locations surveyed in U.P. (Hussain *et al.* 1989 and Sharma *et al.* 1996a) and Gujarat (Sharma *et al.* 1993a). However, in some of the areas of eastern Uttar Pradesh, many of the cysts of *H. cajani* looked quite old and empty (Singh and Rao 1974, Ganguli and Khan 1989). The pest is economically important in states of U.P., Bihar, Haryana and Karnataka (Anonymous 1988).

The cyst nematode may cause heavy losses to pigeonpea crop. In a heavily infested field with nematode, an yield loss of 30% was recorded (Saxena and Reddy 1987). The losses in yield is through adverse effect of nematodes on growth of plants. It causes significant reduction in shoot length and weight, root weight, leaflet area and number and nodule numbers etc. (Sharma 1985b, Sharma and Nene 1988, Sharma *et al.* 1992, 1993b). However, low inoculum levels are not able to exhibit such effects. These effects were significant at 40-45 days of incubation and 1000 larvae/kg. of soil (Singh and Singh 1988b). On the other hand, highly significant reduction in growth parameters of plants could be recorded even at 100 larvae per kg of soil also (Zaki and Bhat 1986b). Sharma and McDonald (1990) have also reported the threshold level of *H. cajani* as 0.1 to 1.0 nematodes/g of soil (100-1000 larvae/kg. of soil). According to Nath (1986), the economic threshold population of cyst nematode is 100/kg of soil at which plant growth is reduced significantly. An initial population of less than 1/cm^3 of soil is sufficient to reduce the plant growth by the cyst nematode (Sharma 1988).

6.1.1 Symptoms

The symptoms produced by *H. cajani* on pigeonpea are distinct at 30-45 days after inoculation only (Koshy and Swarup 1979, Sharma 1985b, Sharma *et al.* 1992c). The infected plants look stunted with smaller internodes and leaves. Expression of symptoms may vary with the genotypes. The yellowing of foliage in general is not very apparent but it is observed in genotypes ICPL 366 (Sharma 1985b) T 15-15 and BDN 2 (Sharma *et al.* 1992a). The affected plants are observed in patches. The nodulation is reduced with smaller root biomass. The nematode damage epidermis and cortex of roots. Many pearly white females with their necks embedded in root tissues are seen attached to root system and even on the root nodules. These females gradually mature, turn brown and mostly dislodge from the root when the plants are lifted for examination. The nematode infestation delays flowering and pod formation by more than a week (Sharma and McDonald 1990).

Manifestation of symptoms depends on level of the inoculum as well as time of inoculation. The plants inoculated at higher levels of inoculum (2500 larvae/pot) show yellowing and stunting after one month and higher reduction in height and weight of plants, weight of root, number and area of leaves and their chlorophyll contents. The degree of symptom manifestation decreases with the lower inoculum level and the much lower inoculum (10 larvae/pot) may even stimulate the plant growth slightly (Singh and Singh 1988a). Similarly inoculation by 1000 larvae/ pot at sowing time has been observed to be more inhibitory with poorly developed root system. The degree of symptom manifestation decreased with increase in the age of plant at inoculation (Singh and Singh 1988b).

6.1.2 Causal Nematode

Heterodera cajani Koshy

The pigeonpea cyst nematode was first reported from Delhi by the name *Heterodera trifolii* by Swarup *et al.* (1964) and simultaneously by Prasad *et al.* (1964). Later, Koshy (1967) studied it in detail and named *Heterodera cajani* as a new species. On cowpea, *Heterodera vigni* was described (Edward and Mishra 1968 and Gupta and Edward 1974) which was later synonymized with *Heterodera cajani* (Kalha and Edward 1979). Other species of cyst nematodes reported on pigeonpea are *H. avenae* (Prasad *et al.* 1959) and *H. mothi* (Ali 1993). However *H. cajani* is the common and widely spread species described in details.

Morphology : The morphology of *H. cajani* has been studied in detail by Koshy (1967), Koshy (1968) and Sharma and Swarup (1984).

Second Stage Larvae: Body cylindrical, tapering at both the ends; slightly set off with 4-5 annules in lip region; lateral field with 4 inscisures, approximately covering 1/5 of the body width. Head well scelerotized, 4-5 μ long and 7-10 μ wide. Stylet well developed with anteriorly directed knobs. Spear knob length 2-3 μ and width 4-5 μ. Dorsal oesophageal gland opening 3.3-4 μ from the base of the stylet. Metacorpus ovalish round in shape witn well developed valvular apparatus. Tail tapering to bluntly rounded, narrow terminus. Measurements are : length 275-456 μ (392 μ), a 22.23; b 2.6-3.1; c 7-10; spear 20-25 μ (23 μ); tail 39-54 μ (42 μ); tail terminal 14-34 μ (24 μ).

Females : Body is white, lemon shaped with protruding neck and vulva. Neck longer than the posterior protuberance and cuticle with zigzag pattern. Stylet with round to posteriorly sloping and anteriorly pointed knobs of 3-4 μ length and 4-5 μ width. Opening of dorsal oesophageal gland located at 4-7 μ from base of the stylet. Median bulb well developed with prominent valve plates. Egg sac present and is half to sometimes double the size of female. Sub-crystalline layer present. The measurements are : length 681-943 μ, width 363-488 μ, length width ratio 1.4 -2.1 and spear 20-30 μ.

Males: Body cylindrical with annulated cuticle, very prominent cephalic sclerotization bearing 4-6 annules, lateral field with 4 inscisures.

Head offset with body contour, 5-6 μ long and 8-10 μ wide. Stylet knobs dorsoventrally flat to anteriorly directed 2-4 μ long and 4-6 μ wide. Tail very short and bluntly rounded. Measurements are : length 844-1666 μ (1040 μ), spear 23-29 μ (26 μ), spicules 32-43 μ (36 μ).

Cyst: They are light to dark brown, lemon shaped with cuticular pattern zigzag. Egg sac is present as also a white subcrystelline layer evident on some cysts. They measure as length 325- 850 μ (625μ), width 206-565 μ (373 μ) and length width ratio 1.65. The cone top structures ambifenestrate bounded by a basin. Fenestra 22-42 μ (32 μ) wide and 25-42 μ (36 μ) long with individual semifenestrae 11-19 μ (15μ) across. The semifenestrae are separated by well formed vulva bridge. Vulval slit is long 36-48 μ (44 μ). The under bridge is well developed with a thin, transparent circular mass attached in the centre of under bridge at the base. Bullae are present and are prominent, peripheral and many with variable size and shape. Some are forked at the base and present at 2 or 3 levels (i) above the level of under bridge, (ii) at the level of under bridge and (iii) below the level of under bridge. Some bullae seem to meet the under bridge probably forming a supporting frame for the reproductive structures. Vulval denticles pattern of the cyst wall is distinct with thick striae.

Eggs. Eggs are more than double in length (78-125 μ) than width (35-50 μ). Egg shell hyaline having second stage larva four folds inside.

The single cyst progeny population have slightly less values of almost all the characters than the field populations indicating that exposure to the natural conditions and continued culturing results in development of more variable forms (Sharma and Swarup 1984). The nematode *H. cajani* appears to have affinities with *H. glycines* and *H. trifolii*. From the later, it differs in length and other body measurements of second stage larvae and from the former by the length of second stage larvae and the cyst cone measurements, i.e. length and width of fenestrae and length of vulval slit.

Biology: The juveniles emerge from the cyst and egg sac at the temperature of 15-37°C with an optimum of 29°C (Koshy and Swarup 1971). Even a slight variation from the optimum may affect emergence significantly from cyst but not from egg sacs (Sharma and Swarup 1984). The emergence is increased by pre-conditioning cyst at 40°C. The pattern of emergence differs in white and brown cysts (Singh and Sharma 1996). In case of white cysts, 50-80% juveniles emerge at 25-30°C within one month and the remaining juveniles emerge gradually without any dependency on temperature. In case of brown cysts, 53, 52 and 5%

juveniles emerge at temperature of 25°C, 20°C and 15°C respectively and the remaining juveniles do not emerge even after incubation for 525 days at 25°C. At the optimum temperature of 28°C, the left out juveniles in the cyst are observed in the form of unhatched second stage larvae (5.7 %) and hatched larvae (7.2-8.6%). The hatching is favoured by *p*H 10.5 and constant light but it is unaffected by aeration (Koshy and Swarup 1971). Desiccation of cysts reduces the hatch (Gaur *et al.* 1996). The cysts stored in moist soil gave higher hatch percentage than those stored in dry soil. In dry soil they survived for 2 years (Koshy and Swarup 1971). Thus, emergence is immediate and high during July to September and declines during November-May (Koshy and Swarup 1971). The root leachates from host plants specially pigeonpea (Koshy and Swarup 1971), hyacinth bean, cowpea, moth bean and sesame (Yadava and Walia 1988) have been reported to stimulate the larval hatches from the cysts and that the stimulatory effect of leachates is higher at plant age of 30 days or less as compared to older plants (Singh and Sharma, 1996). The emergence is greater and rapid from egg sac than from cysts. It is 14 times more in case of free eggs as compared to encysted eggs. The cyst wall fragments and other cyst contents repressed the emergence of juveniles from egg.

The infective second stage larvae randomly penetrate the tap roots and lateral roots and the penetration is more and faster in roots of susceptible plants (Yadava and Walia 1988, Singh and Singh 1995). After penetration, the larvae reach the vascular tissues, place their heads adjacent to stele and start feeding forming syncytia. The larvae gradually pass through their third and fourth stages, swell and become adult females. The juveniles which establish in the cortex develop into males and those which feed in the stele region develop into females. The juveniles when transferred to cotyledons and shoot developed in males only probably due to lack of nutrition (Koshy and Swarup 1971c). The adult male matures in 10 days while swollen, lemon shaped female is formed in 12 days. The males are produced in large number but females can reproduce parthenogenitically (Koshy and Swarup 1971a, Sharma and Swarup 1984). The infective juveniles can be seen in soil 15 days after penetration of roots. The time required to complete the life cycle depends on the soil temperature being 16 days at 84°C and 45-80 days at 10-25°C (Koshy and Swarup 1971a). They are able to complete nine generations on pigeonpea in laboratory (Koshy and Swarup 1971b). The time taken for completion of the life cycle varied considerably on different hosts (Yadava and Walia 1988) species. On cluster bean, it did not develop beyond the third stage larvae. The most active period for multiplication of the nematode is from June to September and April to June. The males are necessary for rapid multiplication although, nematode can reproduce parthenogenitically. A female produces 10-300 eggs depending on the health of the host plant. The egg sac contains about 1/3 of the total number of eggs. The second stage larvae emerge from eggs and are ready to penetrate new host plant.

Population Dyanomics : The population analysis of *H.cajani* revealed higher population in Vertisols as compared to Alfisol (Anonymous 1985a, Sharma *et al.* 1992b). This pattern was observed even in field where pigeonpea was not grown for last five years (Sharma *et al.* 1985). It has been reported that soil types do not influence the pathogenicity of nematodes but they multiply best in sandy and sandy loam soils than loam and clay loam soils due to better root development in these soils (Walia 1987). In vertisol, the nematodes were recorded at 0-45 cm depth but cysts were present even at 75-90 cm (Sharma *et al.* 1992b). The summer fallow caused reduction in juveniles by 45% at depth up to 15 cm but not beyond that, although, number of eggs and juveniles were reduced in cysts up to 30 cm. The highest population densities were recorded at crop maturity, i.e. in January to February while maximum cyst population was in April and minimum in January.

The host species and the cropping system influence the population of *H. cajani* greatly. Number of cysts recorded were 28 on *Solanum indicum,* 15 on *Phaseolus aureus,* 9 on *C. cajan*, 8 on *P. mungo* and none on *Zea mays* (Verma and Yadava 1975). The nematode could survive up to 305 days in the soil in absence of host plant. Amongst various cropping systems tested, inter-copping of sorghum + pigeonpea, soybean + pigeonpea and green gram were found conducive for build up of H. *cajani* (Singh *et al.* 1994). Cowpea, mung bean and pigeonpea increase the population greatly. The population was 8 times lower in single crop system than double cropping with pigeonpea as compared to intercrops (Sharma *et al.* 1996b). Continuous crops of sorghum-safflower reduced the nematode population.

The densities of plant parasitic nematodes were lower in low input cropping systems than in the higher input cropping systems. The inorganic fertilizers increase the population of *H. cajani* while FYM reduces it considerably (Singh *et al.* 1994). The multiplication of *H. cajani* is decreased with increase in the initial inoculum (Devi and Gupta 1988).

Race Variation : The population of *H.cajani* from pigeonpea and

C. tetragonoloba differed with regard to their pathogenicity on 7 plant species. The population from *C.tetragonoloba* penetrated, developed and completed the life cycle in 3 weeks on all the host species. On the other hand, larvae from *C. cajani* penetrated the roots of *C. tetragonoloba* but their development was arrested (Walia and Bajaj 1986). The juveniles remaind in the second stage and degenerated within 8 weeks. The differences were also observed in the population of *H. cajani* collected from different locations (Walia and Bajaj 1988). The population from Bhiwani, multiplied on all the four differentials used, namely cluster bean, sunnhemp, sesame and pigeonpea. On the other hand, the population from other six locations, i.e. Ambala, Faridabad, Ludhiana, Delhi, Coimbatore and Hyderabad did not multiply on cluster bean and sunnhemp. Hence these two groups of population were designated as race B and A respectively. Exhistance of several races of *H. cajani* is possible.

6.1.3 Host Range

The nematode *H.cajani* was recorded on *C. cajani* and *Vigna sinensis* in the field while *Glycine max, Pisum sativum, Vicia sativa, Phaseolus mungo, P. aureus, P. aconitifolius* and *P. calcaratus* were infected in the laboratory (Koshy 1967). Later reports (Koshy and Swarup 1972, Bhatti and Gupta 1973, Sharma 1985 b, Sharma and Nene 1985b and Walia *et al.* 1985) indicated that the nematode is mainly confined to plant species belonging to family Leguminosae, namely *Cajanus cajan, C. platycarpus, C. crassus var. crassus, Cicer arietinum, Crotalaria juncea, Cymopsis tetragonoloba, Dolichos biflorus, D. lablab, Dunbaria ferruginea, Fleminga strobilifera, Glycine max, Phaseolus aconitifolius, P.acutifolius, P. atropurpurious, P.aureus, P.calcaratus, P.lathyroides, P.lunatus, P. mungo, P. vulgaris, Pisum sativum, Rhynchosia bracteata, R. cana, R. densiflora, Vicia narbonensis* and *V. sativa.* Amongst many of the non-legumes tested, *Sesamum indicum* and *Phyllanthus mediraspatensis* belonging to families Pedaliaceae and Euphorbiaceae respectively are the hosts (Koshy and Swarup 1972 and Sharma and Swarup 1984). The comparative susceptibility of host differs greatly. *C. cajan, Dolichos lablab, P. aureus, Vigna catjang* (Cowpea) and *Sesamum indicum* are the most favoured hosts of this nematode. The incidence as well as multiplication of *H.cajani* has been reported to be much more on *S.indicum* (Verma and Yadava 1975), *Cymopsis tetragonoloba* (Walia *et al.* 1985) as compared to pigeonpea. *Rhynchosia cana* has been found to be more susceptible than other wild relatives of pigeonpea (Sharma 1985b). The temperature levels may change the susceptibility of some hosts. The hosts *C. arietinum, Crotalaria juncea, G. max* and *P.sativum* were not infected by the nematode at minimum temperature of 6-15.2°C and maximum of 12.7-22.7°C (Jain *et al.* 1994). They reported *Sesbania aculeata, Sesmodium triflorum* and *Vigna trilobata* to support the population of nematode in winter.

6.1.4 Host Parasite Interaction

After entry, *H. cajani* interacts with the host in various ways disturbing its physiology, the phenology, internal morphology and its chemical composition. The histopathology has been described by Koshy and Swarup (1979) as follows :

The juveniles of *H. cajani* reach in the cortex in 48 h after inoculation of pigeonpea. They move intracellularly and reach vascular tissues within 72 h where they form syncytia in the stelar region. The cells near the feeding site become angular with thickened cell walls and the giant cells are formed containing granular cytoplasm with 4-5 nuclei. The females enlarge damaging cortex and epidermis by erupting through it. The xylem vessels are disrupted extensively causing their discontinuity. The juveniles which are established in the cortex develop into males while those in the stelar region, become females.

The inoculation of pigeonpea by *H. cajani* increases N and P in roots but decreases the same in top. The Na concentration on other hand decreases in roots and increases in top while K accumulation is decreased in root as well as in shoot. The microlements seem to be less prone to change due to infection. The decrease in Na, Zn, Cu, Mn and Fe in the infected roots may be attributed to increased leaching of these elements from roots to soil (Zaki and Bhatti 1986b). The interference of *H.cajani* in the translocation of N, P, K, Na, S, Cu, Zn, Mn and Fe in the pigeonpea plant has also been reported by other workers (Walia and Gupta 1986, Bhatti and Walia 1990). The infection by nematode altered the amino acid composition of pigeonpea seedlings also (Zaki and Bhatti 1987). Most of the 10 amino acids analyzed, were altered due to infection which may be due to highly specialized host-parasite relationship. Specific metabolism requirements to meet the high multiplication rate and formation of syncytia, the metabolic sinks in the conducting vessels leading to an imbalance in the normal amino acid composition may be important factors.

6.1.5 Inter-Relationship With Other Microbes

Heterodera cajani and *Fusarium udum* cause more damage to pigeonpea when used in combination as compared to alone (Edward and Singh 1979). The nematode increase wilt incidence and the increase is much more when plants are inoculated with nematodes six weeks prior to *F.udum* (Hasan 1984). High population of *H.cajani* has been observed in plots with higher wilt incidence (Singh and Jayawant 1985). The increase in wilt due to nematode has been recorded in susceptible variety but the reaction of wilt resistant variety is not affected (Sharma 1985b, Anonymous 1987b, Sharma and Nene 1989). It has been demonstrated by dual inoculations that *F. udum* enters pigeonpea through the injury created by protruding females of *H. cajani* (Rai and Singh 1996). However, the increase in wilt is not mearly due to injury created by nematodes because such effect has not been observed in cases of *Helicotylenchus indicus, Hoplolaimus indicus, Tylenchorthynchus vulgaris* (Hasan 1984). The pathogenicity of *F.udum* is enhanced by *H. cajani* but *F. udum* was antagonistic to nematode multiplication (Sharma and Nene 1989).

The infection of pigeonpea by cyst nematode reduces the root nodulation by *Rhizobium* (Sharma 1985b). In cowpea, *H. cajani* is reported to interfere with the leghaemoglobin contents of nodules (Sharma and Sethi 1975).

6.1.6 Host Resistance

There are only few reports, and that too from India, available on screening of pigeonpea against *H. cajani.* Most of the germplasms screened at ICRISAT centre did not show any resistance but some accessions of *Cajanus scarabaeoides* and others were found resistant (Anonymous 1989b, Saxena *et al.* 1990) and could be crossed easily with pigeonpea. The resistant sources identified, have been compiled in Table 6.1.

For screening and scoring against *H. cajani* a standarized green-house technique has been developed at ICRISAT (Anonymous 1989a, Sharma *et al.* 1991). It involves growing pigeonpea in nematode infested soil and counting the number of white cysts (females) in the root system 30 days after emergence of seedlings. The cysts are clearly visible on air dried soil. The scoring is done as per 9 point scale based on number of cysts per root system (1 being resistant with no cyst while 9 highly

Table 6.1: Sources of resistance in pigeonpea against *H. cajani*

Entries evaluated	*Entries found resistant*	*Reference*
—	Five cultivars	Anonymous (1981)
—	P 1148, P 1162/1	Anonymous (1982)
34	Co 3, Co 5	Velayutham (1988a)
173	Accessions of *Atylosia grandiflora* (ICPW 9), *A. scarabaeoides* (ICPW 94, ICPW 11), *Flemingia macrophyla* (ICPW 194), *F. striata* (ICPW 202), *F. strobilifera* (ICPW 203) and *Rhynchosia rothi* (ICPW 257)	Anonymous (1989b)
—	Accessions of *A. scarabaeoides*	Saxena *et al.* (1990)
—	10 accessions of *Atylosia* spp. and *Rhynchosia* spp.	Sharma *et al.* (1991)
24	Basant, T 15-15, PDM 1, KWR 1, Pusa 74	Devi and Gupta (1992)
21	Pant A 8, 8507, AF 276, 286, AL 13-31, 601, KPH 1160, MRG 66, P 605, 852, 856, PPH 19, T 92	Ali (1994)
61	GAUP 9003, 9004, H 86-14, KM 34, MA 5, PBNA 47-1, 47-2, Pusa 14, 22, 25, 30	Ali (1995a)
19	ICPW 62 and 69 of *C. platycarpa*	Saxená *et al.* (1996)
104	GAUP 9004, H 86-14, KM 34, Pusa 14, 22, 30 Pusa (B) 21, PBNA 47-1, 47-2	Siddiqui *et al.* (1998)

susceptible with more than 30 cysts. Siddiqui *et al.* (1998) used following scale for grading :

No cyst	= Highly resistant (HR)
1-5 cysts	= Resistant (R)
6-25 cysts	= Moderately resistant (MR)
26-50 cysts	= Susceptible (S)
51 or more cysts	= Highly susceptible (HS)

The number of cysts for above mentioned categories have been considered as 0, 1-25, 26-50, 51-100 and more than 100 respectively by Ali (1995a).

For proper counting, the cysts of *H.cajani* can be extracted by seiving the soil suspension through 20 and 60 mesh sieves followed by scanning the debris for cysts collected over a 80 mesh sieve (Sharma and Nene 1986). The eggs of *H. cajani* are produced in cysts and egg sac. About 1/3 or more eggs are produced in gelatinous egg sac which are difficult to count and they remain unaccounted. Sharma and Nene (1987) described a method to count them. It involves collection of infested roots, washing them gently, cutting in pieces and immersion of 1 g of pieces in 0.2% solution of sodium hypochloride (NaOCl) in 250ml beaker for 2-3 minutes. The root pieces are then homogenized and vigorously stirred with glass rod. The released eggs are collected using USA standard testing sieves Nos. 400 and 200 repeatedly.

6.1.7 Control

Chemical : Seed treatment of pigeonpea with aqueous solution of triazophos (0.01 and 0.001 %) has been reported to prevent penetration by *H. cajani* and slowering the development of the penetrated larvae (Prasad 1985). The nematode population was reduced significantly by seed soaking in 0.5 to 2 % concentrations of aldicarb, carbofuran, phorate or fensulphothion for 30 and 60 minutes (Zaki and Bhatti 1986c). Out of these, aldicarb was best and higher concentrations as well as soaking periods increased efficacy but adversely affected plant growth. Fensulphothion (2%) however, resulted in good growth of plants (Bhatti and Walia 1990). Contrarily, seed treatment with methy1 dimethoate, acephate, monocrotophos, phosphamidan, endosulfan, quinalphos and carbosulfan in water did not control cyst nematode on pigeonpea (Velayutham 1988b).

Effective control of the nematodes was achieved by soil application of carbofuran @ 4.5 kg a.i./ha and fensulphothion @ 1-2 kg a.i./ha (Gunasekaran *et al.* 1976); aldicarb 10 G, phorate 10 G or carbofuran 3 G each @ 5 kg/ha (Hasan 1989, Singh and Singh 1992c). These nematicides checked the nematode mediated wilt also. Carbofuran @ 2 and 4 kg a.i./ha checked the disease and increased the yield significantly (Ali 1991). Application of phenomiphos, oxamy1, phosalone and danusban as soil application or as foliar spray controlled cyst nematodes on pigeonpea. As spray, oxamy1 and phenomiphos were more effective (Mishra and Prasad 1990). These chemicals were not deleterious to plant as well as root nodulation.

Plant Products : The water extract of leaves of *Terminelia arjuna* has been reported to be toxic to second stage juveniles of *H.cajani*. Incorporation of 1-3 % powdered leaves in the soil reduced the nematode population greatly (Singh and Singh 1992a) and increased growth parameters of pigeonpea plants. Similarly soil amendment with 1% powder of Neem, Madar, Behaya, Saijan and Arjuna adversely affect entry of nematode in root, delay egg laying and development of nematode and finally, their population in soil (Singh and Singh 1992b). The water extract of these plants reduce egg hatching and emergence of juveniles from cysts. Maximum lethal effect is reported that of Madar followed by Behaya.

Soil amendments with oil cakes of Neem, Mustard and Mahua adversely affect the multiplication of *H.cajani* in soil and control the nematode mediated Fusarium wilt also (Rai and Singh 1995). This control is achieved due to certain antagonistic fungi which colonize the oil cakes. The culture filtrates of atleast 13 fungi including *Penicillium citrinum, Aspergillus niger, Cephalosporium roseogriseum* etc. isolated from Neem cake amended soil were found toxic to *H. cajani.* These extracts inhibited emergence of larvae from cysts/eggs and caused their death (Singh *et al.* 1989 and 1991).

Green manuring with sunnhemp, cowpea, Dhaincha and mung bean is also effective in reducing the population of cyst nematode (Devi and Gupta 1995).

Solarization : Solarization of soil by irrigation and then covering it with polythene sheets during the summer, drastically reduces the population of nematodes including *H.cajani* (Chauhan *et al.* 1988, Sharma and Nene 1985a and Nene 1990b). The population may be reduced by 93% and remains lower during the crop season. The solarization involves covering of soil with transparent 100 μ thick polythene sheets for 6-8 weeks during April/May after irrigation. It increases the soil temperature by 6-10°C in the 0-20 cm profile and is most useful where control of multiple pest and diseases is needed (Chauhan *et al.* 1988). Summer ploughing is also effective in controlling cyst nematode in pigeonpea (Sharma 1991).

Cultural : Rotation with cereals like Sorghum, maize, pearl millet etc. may help in reducing the population of nematodes. Some of the non-host species of plants are *Chionachne* sp., *Echinocloa colona, Paspalum scorbiculatum, Setaria italica, Zea mays* and *Z. maxicana* which may reduce population of *H. cajani* (Koshy and Swarup 1972, Sharma and Swarup 1984).

Biological Control : A bacterium *Pasteuria penetrans* was found to be most destructive to eggs and larvae of *H. cajani* reducing their infectivity and rate of development inside the pigeonpea root (Sharma and Swarup 1988). The bacterium was described to cause 'Sticky swarm disease' of *H. cajani* and *Meloidogyne javanica* (Sharma and Sharma 1989). The infected females are devoid of eggs and larvae and are filled with the spores of bacteria. The second stage larvae become sluggish with jerky movement. They tend to stick with other larvae when placed in water. The larvae and females of *M. javanica* are also infected and form loosely wooven masses when placed in water. It is due to endospores of bacterium attached to the cuticle of one larva which stick to the cuticle of other larvae. Initially 2-3 larvae clinge to each other but gradually more and more larvae join them to form a loosely wooven sticky swarm which increase in size as more and more larvae entangle. These larvae struggle to dislodge from the sticky swarm but in the process they are completely entangled and immobilized. The bacterium could infect the larvae of *Rotylenchulus reniformis* also. The pathogen *Pasteuria penetrans,* produces elliptical, saucer shaped endospores of 4-5 μ in diameter and randomly distributed on the body of the larva. The organism holds promise as a potential bio control agent for control of nematodes of pigeonpea. Walia *et al* (1990) isolated a *Pasteuria* sp. from *Heterodera cajani* which is distinct from *P. penetrans* in not parasitizing *M. incognita.*

In addition to *P. penetrans* several fungi like *Allomyces anomalus, Catenaria auxiliaris, C. vermicola, Nematophthora* sp. *Oidium* sp., *Pythium* sp and seven other unidentified species have been recovered from the females and cysts, eggs and larvae of *H. cajani* (Sharma and Swarup 1988). Of these *C. vermicola* was encountered most frequently followed by *C. auxiliaris* which adversely affected the infectivity and development of the larvae inside the root of pigeonpea. According to Siddiqui and Mahmood (1996b) application of *Glomus mosseae, Trichoderma harzianum* and *Verticillium chlamydosporum* reduced population of *H. cajani* and wilting index of pigeonpea and the reduction was more when all three were used together.

6.2 Root Knot

Root Knot disease of crops is caused by *Meloidogyne* spp. which produces typical galling of roots. First report of root knot of pigeonpea seems to be from U.S.A. (Bessey 1911) and then from Hawaii (Godfrey 1928) where the causal nematode was named as *Heterodera radicicola* causing only little injury to pigeonpea. The causal nematode was later reported by the name *Heterodera marioni* from Rhodesia (Collins 1938) and Malaya (Beeley 1939). However, now it is established that root knot disease is caused mainly by species of *Meloidogyne*. Atleast five species have been reported to be associated with pigeonpea from Australia, Bangladesh, Brazil, Ethiopia, Egypt, Fiji, India, Kenya, Malawi, Nepal, Nigeria, Philippines, Puerto Rico, Trinidad and Tobago, Tonga, Uganda,

USA, Zambia and Zimbabwe (Nene *et al.* 1996). However, the disease is more important in Brazil, Egypt, Ethiopia, Fiji, India, Malawi, Nepal, USA, Zambia and Zimbabwe (Sharma and McDonald 1990). Out of five species, *M. incognita* and *M. Javanica* occur widely in most of the pigeonpea growing areas of the world. Pigeonpea is not a good host for *M. arenaria* and *M. javanica* in some parts (Sasser and Hartman 1985). Similarly it has been stated to be the poor host for *M. incognita* by some workers (Roy 1972, Reddy *et al.* 1983).

The root knot nematodes are the hot weather organisms and are important in regions where summers are long with short winters. They cause about 15% loss in pigeonpea yield in tropical countries of the world (Sasser 1979). According to Bridge (1981) the nematode may cause 8-35% losses in yield of pigeonpea. In India, root knot of pigeonpea is distributed in most of the pigeonpea growing states but they are more important in states of Gujarat, U.P., Maharashtra (Anonymous 1988) and Bihar (Nath 1986) where avoidable yield losses in pigeonpea have been estimated as 14.2% (Patel and Patel 1993), 29.7% (Ali 1995a) and 83.7% (Anonymous 1987a). As per estimates by the Scientists of ICAR (Anonymous 1989c) nematode causes 25-30% losses while Sharma (1991) reported 15-20% losses in yield of pigeonpea. The loss in yield is due to the effect of nematodes on root nodulation and growth of the plant. The nematode hampers the development of root, shoot, floral branches, pods and root nodulation significantly (Mishra and Gaur 1987, Pathak *et al.* 1985). The infection by nematodes also causes reduction in the water absorption capacity of roots (Alam *et al.* 1991) and the pollen fertility (Tiyagi *et al.* 1989). These effects are responsible for reduction in the yield of pigeonpea (Anver *et al.* 1997).

6.2.1 Symptoms

The above ground symptoms of the disease are stunting, suppressed growth, i.e. reduced length of shoot and roots, reduction in leaf size, chlorosis etc. ultimately arresting the plant vigour and initiating early senescence. The number of floral branches are reduced and flowers drop in severe cases resulting in reduced pod setting (Ali 1993). The most characteristic symptoms are formation of root galls on secondary as well as tap roots (Raveendhran and Nadaka 1975, Ali 1993). The mild infection causes discrete galls specially on lateral roots but severe infection produces large galls on main as well as lateral roots. The symptoms oftenly appear in clearly defined patches in the field and are more obvious under adverse growing conditions specially drought and sandy soils.

Some populations of *M. incognita* and *M. javanica* in India, Nepal and Malawi have been found not to produce galls on pigeonpea roots but they produce many egg sacs (Sharma *et al.* 1992c). Due to this behaviour of nematode, stunting and other foliar symptoms on some genotypes of pigeonpea may not be apparent even after nematode infection.

6.2.2 Causal Nematodes

Meloidogyne incognita (Kofoid & White) Chitwood
Meloidogyne javanica (Treub) Chitwood
Meloidogyne arenaria (Neal) Chitwood
Meloidogyne incognita var. *acrita* Chitwood
Meloidogyne hapla Chitwood
Meloidogyne acronea Coetzee

The *Meloidogyne* spp. in general possess the following characters (Ali 1995b):

Females : They are round to pear shaped with short projecting neck, white, sedentary with vulva and anus closely situated. Phasmids are dot like, slightly above and on either side of anus. Cuticle striated; stylet slender, 12-15 μ with small knobs. Excretory pore anterior to median bulb; ovaries paired, prodelphic convulated; rectal glands six, large and secrete geletinous material in which eggs are deposited. The eggs are not retained in the body.

Males : They are vermiform up to 2 mm long, tail end twisted. Cuticle strongly annulated, lateral field with four incisures, cephalic regions not offset with distinct labial disc and few annules; lateral sectors wider than sub-medians appearing as cheeks. Stylet robust, 18-25 μ long with large knobs; oesphageal glands mostly ventral to intestine. Spicules slender, generally 25-33 μ long; gubernaculum 7-11 μ long; testis single or paired when sex reversal occurs. Tail rounded and bursa absent.

Juveniles : First stage with blunt tail tip, moult within the egg. Second stage larvae infective, vermiform migratory, straight to acute on death; cephalic regions with coarse, 1-4 annules, distinct labial disc, framework lightly sclerotized, lateral sector wider than sub-medians.

Stylet slender, under 20 μ, excretory pore posterior to hemizonid. Median bulb with large oval valve plates. Tail with conspicuous hyaline region, tip narrow and irregular in outline. Third stage larvae sedentary, swollen sausage-shaped with a short blunt tail; stylet absent. Fourth stage sedentary, swollen with terminal anus, stylet absent.

Six species of *Meloidogyne* have been found associated with pigeonpea and may be identified on the basis of the following characters (Ali 1995b).

(i) *M. incognita* : This nematode was reported on pigeonpea in India by Prasad (1960) and later from Uganda (Mukiibi 1976), USA (Ingram and Rodriguez Kabana 1977) and several other countries including Australia, Bangladesh, Egypt, Malawi, Nepal, Ethiopia, Philippine, Trinidad and Tobago etc. (Nene *et al.* 1996). It is reported to cause the root knot disease of pigeonpea in field situations. The nematode has following important characteristic features :

Females : The perineal patterns with distinct high dorsal arch composed of small to heavy striae some of which fork near the lateral lines without distinct lateral incisures. Often there are striae bending towards vulva. The stylet cone is distinctly curved dorsally with anterior portion cylindrical and posterior half conical. The shaft is slightly wider posteriorly, stylet knobs are broadly elongate, set off from the shaft and anteriorly indented.

Males : Head region is marked by 2-3 incomplete annulation with labial disc large, round, centrally concave and raised above the medial lips. The stylet is blunt and wider than the medial portion of the cone with knobs set off from the shaft, anteriorly indented and broadly elongate to round.

Four host races of *M. incognita* have been identified. Race 1 do not reproduce on tobacco or cotton, race 2 reproduce on tobacco but not cotton, race 3 do not reproduce on tobacco but on cotton while race 4 reproduce on both.

(ii) *M. Javanica* : This is also a wide spread species causing root knot disease of pigeonpea. *M. javanica* infecting pigeonpea was reported from Zambia (Angus 1962), although, *M. javanica bauruensis* was reported from Brazil as early as 1956 by Lordello and Vaz De Arruda. This species of nematode also occur in Australia, Bangladesh, India, Kenya, Malawi, Nepal, Philippines, Puerto Rico and Zimbabwe infecting pigeonpea (Nene *et al.* 1996). The characteristic features of the nematode are as follows :

Females : Perineal patterns have a rounded to flattened dorsal arch, distinct lateral incisures separating the pattern into dorsal and ventral regions, no or only few striae crossing the lateral incisures and some striae bending towards vulva. Stylet with cone not having any curve dorsally and has increasing width posteriorly. Shaft widens slightly posteriorly. Knobs are short, wide and often anteriorly indented.

Males : They have high head which is as wide as the head region. Stylet cone narrow anteriorly and very wide posteriorly with shaft cylindrical and often narrow near joint with knobs. The stylet knobs are low and wide set off from the shaft.

M. javanica reproduces on root knot resistant tobacco, water melon and tomato. Most population do not reproduce on cotton, pepper and only few can reproduce on peanut.

(iii) *M. arenaria* : This species has been reported to occur on pigeonpea only from U.S.A. (Killinger 1968b), although, it has proved to be highly pathogenic (Sasser and Hartman 1985). It is characterized as follows :

Females : The dorsal arch flattened to rounded with striae slightly indented at lateral lines generally from shoulder on the arch. Often the dorsal and ventral striae meet an angel at the lateral lines. Some striae fork, short and irregular near lateral lines. Striae are smooth to wavy and some bend towards vulva. There are striae that extend laterally to form one or two wings. Stylet very robust with broad cone and shaft. The shaft widens posteriorly and gradually merges with the stylet knobs. The knobs are wider and rounded posteriorly.

Males : Head cap low and slopes posteriorly with 2-3 incomplete annulations on the head region. Stylet with pointed cone having posterior portion much wider than the anterior portion of shaft. Knobs are anteriorly indented, very large and gradually merging with the shaft.

The population differentiated into race 1 reproducing on peanuts while race 2 do not.

(iv) *M. incognita* var *acrita* : It was recorded on pigeonpea in India by Rajak *et al.* (1986). It is synonymous to *M. acrita* and does not occur widely on pigeonpea.

(v) *M. hapla* : It was found associated with pigeonpea in Australia, India and U.S.A. (Nene *et al.* 1996). Pigeonpea has been found to be a very poor host of *M. hapla* (Sasser and Hartman 1985).

(vi) *M. acronea* : This nematode has been reported to be associated with pigeonpea in Malawi (Nene *et al.* 1996).

Biology and Disease Cycle : One-celled egg passes through embryogenesis resulting in first stage juveniles within the egg. The first moulting is inside the egg producing the second stage infective juveniles. They move towards the root tips, penetrate the root, migrate through the root cells and reach the vascular system. They become sedentary, induce formation of giant cells and start feeding. The juveniles moult three times and develop to sacciform females or worm like and free living males. The third and fourth stage juveniles do not possess stylet but it reappears when final moult occurs. Galls are initiated after infection but not necessary for the growth of nematode. The nematodes remain sedentary during the feeding. The male is sedentary parasite during its juvenile development and emerges as a slender worm possessing stylet, oesophagus with median bulb, spicules and sperms in the testis. The male in general, is not involved in the reproduction. The fertilized females extrude a geletinous matrix in which 500 to 1500 eggs are laid down during the life span forming an egg mass. The eggs of *M. incognita* and *M. javanica* hatch soon and initiate another generation. The total duration for completing the life cycle at optimum temperature (25-30°C) is 3-4 weeks. Many generations are completed in a crop season.

6.2.3 Host Parasite Interaction

The juveniles invade young roots and initiate hyperplasia and hypertrophy of root tissues surrounding the feeding site causing swelling or root galls. While in tissues, the nematode interrupts the function of xylem and phloem ultimately reducing the water absorption capacity of plant (Alam *et al.* 1991). In addition to reduction in growth of plant, parasite reduces the chlorophyl l content of leaves and bulk density of stem parts (Anver and Alam 1989). The roots of pigeonpea inoculated by *M. javanica* showed higher peroxidase, polyphenol oxidase and total phenol contents than the uninoculated roots (Patel *et al.* 1992).

6.2.4 Damage Threshold

The damage threshold of *Meloidogyne* spp. on pigeonpea has been calculated as 4.0 nematodes/g of soil in Fiji while in India it is mentioned as 1-2 and 1 for *M. incognita* and *M. javanica* respectively (Sharma 1988, Sharma and McDonald 1990). According to Nath (1986) the economic threshold population of root knot nematode is 100/kg of soil.

6.2.5 Interaction With Other Microorganisms

The nematode *M. javanica* has been reported to interact with *F. udum* showing synergistic effect. The pigeonpea plants wilt sooner in presence of both the organisms (Salam and Khan 1986). This effect has been observed even in wilt resistant variety ICP 8863 (Sharma and Nene 1990a). It is to the extent that the resistant varieties like ICP 9145 may show susceptible reaction to *F. udum* in presence of root knot nematodes (Marley and Hillocks 1996). It could happen even when nematodes are present in soils and the wilt fungus is inoculated on stem of the same plant. It is the evidence of translocable factor or systemic effect produced by nematodes. However, such effect has not been observed in all the cases. The combination of *M. incognita* + *F. udum* has been reported to be less pathogenic than *H. cajani* + *F. udum* on variety UPAS 120 (Siddiqui and Mahmood 1996a). Such a synergistic effect of *M. javanica* + *F. udum* was, however, not observed in presence of nickel (Khan and Salam 1990). Inversely proportioned relationship between inoculum densities of *M. incognita* and *F. udum* and plant length, fresh/dry weight of pigeonpea has been reported by Kahkashan *et al.* (1998).

Meloidogyne spp. have been reported to interact with *Rhizobium* also causing reduction in root nodulation in pigeonpea (Salam and Khan 1986). In presence of nickel, *M. javanica* was unable to form galls but it could suppress nodulation significantly (Khan and Salam 1990). The nematode *M. incognita* has been reported to reduce leghaemoglobin content of cowpea root nodules and the reduction was more than that caused by *H. cajani* (Sharma and Sethi 1975).

6.2.6 Host Resistance

Sources of Resistance : Screening of pigeonpea against root knot nematodes has been done mainly in India and few other countries. The sources of resistance so identified are compiled in Table 6.2. It is important that the reaction of a variety may differ greatly due to the existence of several species of nematode and their races pathogenic to pigeonpea. In Nigeria, variety Hope 5989 was found tolerant to *Meloidogyne* spp. (Fennell 1963). In U.S.A., variety Norman was reported as resistant to some species of *Meloidogyne* (Anonymous 1968, Killinger 1968a) but it was seriously attacked by *M. arenaria* in a field having shaded conditions until mid-day (Killinger 1968b). According to Taylor *et al.* (1985) variety Norman was severely infested by *M.*

Table 6.2: Sources of resistance against root knot nematodes of pigeonpea

Nematode species	*No. of entries tested*	*Entries found resistant*	*Reference*
M. incognita	26	PT 8, 12, 15, 16, 17, 21, 22, 26, 27; M 290, C11 (MR to race 3)	Darekar & Jagdale (1989)
	—	ICPL 8, 81, 93, 94, 111, 143, 146, 227, 316, 8324, 8343; ICP 6997, 7025, 7182, 7197, 7234, 7898, 8308, 8662, 10976, 10978, 10979, 10984, 10986, 10991, 10993, 10996, 11049, 11204, 11206, 11207, 11231	Sharma and McDonald (1990)
	69	Forty were immune including NP (WR) 15, Pant A-1, Pant A-2, Pant A-3, Pusa Ageti, T 7, T 17, T 21, UPV 120	Hasan and Khan (1983)
	11	Norman and others	Taylor *et al.* (1985)
	27	All resistant to 4 races except ICP 11292	Sasser & Hartman (1985)
	25	T 66, ICPL 8, 580, 81 and Pant A 10	Bhargava and Pathak (1985)
	47	36 were resistant for 3 races	Ravichander *et al.* (1988)
	—	AGS 522, GAUT 85-25, 89-17; H 83-9, 86-7; ICPL 83015, 86015, 89044, JAS 148-6; KE 1, MTH 15, 23, 26, 28; P 607, MRG 66	Ali (1991)
	10	ICPL 89044	Alam *et al.* (1991)
	43	DA 11, H 86-1, H 87-12, ICPL 87, 227, 371, 88026 88046, 88047, IPH 732, MTH 9, MTH 20, P 606	Ali (1992)
	19	DSRL 95, T 21, Pusa ageti, and P 3789	Imran *et al.* (1992)
	22	AF 239, 276, 284, 293; AL 13-31, 587, 601, MRG 66; P 604, 852, 856; Pant 104, 8507, PPH 4, 19; SPMA 8, T 21	Ali (1994)
	75	AF 239, 286, 293; AL 600, BDN 699, GAUP 9002, 9005, GAUT 88-2, IPA 94-3, 94-5; KM 9, 32; P 862, 605, PBNA 67-2, Pusa 9, 28, SPLA 11	Ali (1995a)
	13	KM 9, AF 239	Anver *et al.* (1997)
M. javanica	11	Norman & 10 others	Taylor *et al.* (1985)
	27	All except ICP 11292, 11295	Sasser & Hartman (1985)
	6	Pusa 33, 85 and 78	Salam and Khan (1986)
	—	ICP 3465, 8864, 9145, 7174 and 11299	Sharma and McDonald (1990)

Table 6.2: *Contd.*

Nematode species	*No. of entries tested*	*Entries found resistant*	*Reference*
	20	PDA 1 and LRG 30	Siddiqui *et al.* (1991)
	43	AK 881, BSMR 203, DA 11, H 82-1, H 86-1, ICPH 8, ICPL 87, 227, 371, 87104, 88026, 88046, IPH 732, MTH 9	Ali (1992)
	22	AF 239, 276, 284, 293, Pant 104, 8507, PPH 4, T 92	Ali (1994)
	75	AF 239, 284, 286, 293; BDN 699, GAUP 9003, 9004; H 86-14, IPA 94-3, 94-5; KM 9, 32, 34; MA 5 P 8621, PBNA 47-1, 47-2, 67-2, Pusa 28, 30 and SPLA 11	Ali (1994)
M.incognita +M. javanica	32	ICP 11295, ICP 234, 2376, 6965, 11287, 11294, 11299, Prabhat and Radhika	Thakar & Patel (1985)
	59	Var 18-1 & 77-1	Patel *et al.* (1987a)
	92	18-1, 77-1, 21-4, 24-4, 49-4, 55-8, 75-1, 99-10; ICPL 93, 111, 143	Anonymous (1990)
M. hapla	27	All were resistant	Sasser and Hartman (1985)
Meloydogyne spp		ICP 8859 TO 8862, 8865, 8866, 11286, 11291, 11299	Anonymous (1985a)
	—	EL 81d, EL 45a, Norman	Reddi & Prine (1981) and Patel *et al.* (1983)
	200	ICP 11289, 11299, ICPL 151	Sharma *et al.* (1992)
	—	P 1148, 1162/1, P 157, P 1169, P 1299, P 2499	Anonymous (1992)
M. arenaria	38	None	Taylor *et al.* (1985)

arenaria race 1 but it was infested least by *M. incognita* race 3 and *M. javanica.* The compiled information indicates that some of the varieties/ lines of pigeonpea are resistance to more than one species of *Meloidogyne.* The variety ICP 11289 was found susceptible by Thakar and Patel (1985) but later, it was reported to be moderately resistant by Patel *et al.* (1987a). Similarly ICP 11295 reported as resistant (Thakar and Patel 1985) was found to be highly susceptible to mixed population of *M. incognita* and *M. javanica* (Patel *et al.* 1987a). So far resistance has not been reported against *M. arenaria* (Taylor *et al.* 1985, Sasser and Hartman 1985).

Technique of Screening: The screening of pigeonpea against root knot nematodes includes growing plants in autoclaved soil in pots, their inoculation at three-leaf stage by pouring suspension of freshly hatched larvae in holes made around plants and covering them with soil (Hasan and Khan 1983). Sandy soil is more suitable for the test. Count of galls and egg masses on roots are taken at 40 to 60 days after inoculation. The larval development within the host can be observed by staining the affected roots in the lactophenol-cotton blue, mashing in a waring blender and then examining under the microscope. Test lines may also be done in microplots having high inoculum pressure (Thakar and Patel 1985, Patel *et al.* 1987a). The roots may be stained by Phloxine B in place of lactophenol-cotton blue (Sasser and Hartman 1985). Number of eggs masses and galls/g of root system are recorded. The eggs can be extracted with 1% sodium hypochlorite as suggested by Taylor and Sassar (1978) and numbers of eggs/g of root mass is counted for assessing the host reaction as per scales used by various workers (Table 6.3).

Table 6.3 : Scales used by various workers for scoring pigeonpea against root knot nematodes (*Meloidogyne* spp.)

Reaction types	*Number of galls/egg masses per plant observed by*			
	Hasan & Khan (1983)	*Hadsoeganda & Sasser (1982)*	*Ali (1992)*	*Ali (1995a)*
Immune	0 gall	0-2 galls	0 gall	0 gall
Highly resistant	—	0-2 galls (1)*	0 gall	0 gall
Very resistant	—	3-10 galls (2)	—	—
Resistant	1-25 galls without egg masses	—	1-2 galls	1-10 galls
Moderately resistant	1-25 galls with egg masses	11-30 galls (3)	3-10 galls	11-30 galls
Susceptible	26-50 galls with egg masses	31-100 galls (4)	11-30 galls	31-100 galls
Highly susceptible	More than 50 galls with egg masses	More than 100 galls (5)	31-100 galls	101 and more

*Figures within the parenthesis are the ratings proposed.

Note : Patel et al. (1987a) considered the reaction on the basis of numerical ratings as 0= Highly resistant, 0.01 to 1.0 = Resistant, 1.01 to 2.0 = Moderately Resistant, 2.01 to 3.0 = Moderately Susceptible,3.01 to 4.0= Susceptible, 4.01 to 5.0 = Highly Susceptible. Similarly Sassar and Hartman (1985) reported scale on the basis of numerical ratings as 0 to 1 = Highly Resistant, 1.1 to 3.0 = Very Resistant, 3.1 to 3.5 = Moderately Resistant, 3.6 to 4.0 = Slightly Resistant, 4.1 to 5.0 = Susceptible, Resistant and Susceptible plants = Variable.

Some workers have used scale as per categories proposed by Patel et al. (1987a) but ratings have been expressed as Root knot Index (Anonymous 1990). The main criteria for categorization is, however, the number of galls or egg masses present in root of a plant.

The gall and egg sac indices are the two important criteria for determining the suitability of host or its variety to *Meloidogyne* spp. However *M. javanica* and *M. incognita* do not produce noticeable galling on pigeonpea roots. Soaking roots in phloxine B for 10-15 minutes stains egg sacs pink but good contrast is not obtained as root tissues are also stained light pink. Staining in 0.25 % trypan blue for 3.5 minutes gives good contrast by staining egg sacs deep blue and no staining of root tissues (Sharma and Mohiuddin 1993). Staining does not affect the viability of eggs adversely.

6.2.7 Control

Chemical: Seed treatment with aldicarb, carbofuran, fensulphothion and phorate @ 1% a.i. W/W have been reported effective in reducing the penetration of pigeonpea roots by larvae of *M. incognita* by 50-80 per cent (Mishra 1985a). Under microplot conditions, seed treatment with aldicarb and carbofuran @ 1 and 2 % W/W while fensulphothion and oxmyl @ 1% W/W using gum arabica reduced the rate of increase of *M. incognita* on pigeonpea by 23.2 to 46.2 % increasing yield, although aldicarb 2% was found phytotoxic (Mishra 1985b). In the same way, seed treatment with furadan 2% and oncol 2% eliminated root galling due to *M. incognita* infesting pigeonpea and also rate of increase of nematodes in soil by 45.2-70.6% (Mishra 1986). Seed treatment of pigeonpea by the aldicarb @ 100 or 1000 ppm controlled *M. incognita* with a significant increase in length and fresh weight of plants (Singh *et al.* 1988). Fensulphothion was better than others (Jaiswal *et al.* 1987).

The plant parasitic nematodes including *M. incognita, M. javanica* and *H. cajani* are controlled by soil fumigation with DD @ 400 ml/ha resulting in better growth and yield of pigeonpea and mungbean (Sethi 1973). Soil application of carbofuran @ 3 kg a.i./ha has been reported to reduce the root knot index and the nematode population by 53.9% and 61.4% respectively (Patel & Patel 1993). In Zimbabwe, use of carbofuran @ 2 kg. a.i./ha each has been recommended to manage *Meloidogyne* spp. (Sharma and McDonald 1990).

Plant Products: In addition to chemicals, certain plant products like aqueous extract of *Azadirachta indica, Brassica rapa, Pongamia glabra,* and *Arachis hypogea* cakes and the leaf extracts of Bhang (*Cannabis sativa*), Bhangra (*Eclipta alba*), Dhatura (*Datura metal*), Katali (*Argemone maxicana*) and Neem (*Azadirachta indica*) have also proved nematocidal reducing juveniles (Majumdar & Mishra 1991).

Out of 23 plant species tested against *M. incognita,* the extracts of fresh leaves, fruits, seeds of *A. indica, Datura fastuosa, Allium cepa, Ricinus communis, Allium sativum* and *Solanum nigrum* at different concentrations reduced hatching of eggs greatly (Upadhyaya *et al.* 1998).

Cultural: Inclusion of non-host crops like Sorghum, pearl millet, *Setaria* spp., maize, paddy etc. in the crop rotation with pigeonpea reduces the density of population of root knot nematodes within 2-3 years. Pigeonpea-wheat cropping system is recommended to control root knot nematodes in Brazil (Sharma and McDonald 1990). Other crops which reduce the root knot population in soil are cabbage, cauliflower, mustard, onion, garlic, cotton, groundnut, etc. Green manure crop *Crotalaria juncea* can also be used. However, selection of crop for rotation/green manure should be done carefully as exceptions are there due to involvement of several species and races of *Meloidogyne* in causing root knot deceased (PANS 1981). Pigeonpea, being a good host of *M. arenaria* is not recommended for incorporation in the crop rotation scheme in south eastern USA (Rodriquez Kabana and Ingram 1978) although, use of resistant pigeonpea varieties EL 81, EL 45a and Norman have been recommended as green manuring for control of root knot nematodes in other crops (Reddy *et al.* 1983). Root exudates may also play important role in disease control. Some plant species like *Tagetes patula* and *Sesamum indicum* produce root exudates toxic to root knot nematodes and may be used for inter-cropping.

A fallow period of 2-3 years can also reduce the nematode population if susceptible weeds are not there in the field. Turning the soil during the fallow gives additional effect. The disease is more severe in sandy light soil than sandy loam.

Biological Control: The second stage juveniles of *M. javanica* are infected with *Pasteuria penetrans* (Anonymous 1988). Eggs of *M. incognita* are parasitized by *Metarhizium anisopliae* and *Beauveria brongniartii* which may be used for managing the root knot nematodes (Vyas *et al.* 1995). The literature on biological control of plant parasitic nematodes has been reviewed by Stirling (1991).

6.3 Dirty Root Disease

The dirty root disease of pigeonpea is caused by *Rotylenchulus reniformis* commonly known as reniform nematode. The association of *Rotylenchulus* spp. with pigeonpea roots was first reported from Puerto Rico (Stener 1960) which later was confirmed as *R. reniformis* (Ayala 1962a). The nematode was found parasitizing the pigeonpea roots in India by Seshadri and Sivakumar (1963). The nematode has been reported to occur on pigeonpea in Australia, Fiji, India, Jamaica, Puerto Rico, Trinidad & Tobago (Nene *et al.* 1996). However, it is reported to be severe in Fiji only where it reduces the pigeonpea production greatly in some areas (Heinlein and Black 1983). In India, the nematode has been found associated with pigeonpea in most of the states specially Andhra Pradesh, Bihar, Gujarat, Haryana, Karnataka, Madhya Pradesh, Maharashtra, Manipur, Rajasthan but it is of economic importance in Gujarat, Maharashtra, Rajasthan and Uttar Pradesh only (Rashid *et al.* 1973, Verma and Prasad 1969, Kaushik and Bajaj 1980, Nath 1986, Ali 1987, 1992, 1995b; Anonymous 1988, Sharma *et al.* 1992b, 1993a, 1996a).

In combination with lance nemadoes, *R. reniformis* may cause 14.5% to 16% avoidable losses to yield of pigeonpea (Ali 1994, 1995a). Under field conditions, a net loss of 19% was worked out due to this nematode (Ali 1996).

6.3.1 Symptoms

The most common below ground symptom is the presence of soil-covered egg masses on roots (Reddy *et al.* 1990). The root development is poor with reduced root masses as compared to healthy plants. The name dirty root is because the infected roots appear dirty due to presence of soil particles which adhere to the mucilaginous egg sacs which are not separated even after shaking the roots (Sharma *et al.* 1992c). Besides poor growth of roots, the nematodes parasitize the root nodules (Ayala 1962b, 1962c).

Above ground symptoms include reduction in plant growth, bulk density of stem parts, number of pods/plant and the chlorophyll contents of leaves (Anver and Alam 1989). Thus the foliage of the infected plant is light green with young leaves becoming yellow. The patches of stunted plants in the field indicate the nematode infection and number of such patches increase under drought conditions (Sharma *et al.* 1992c). The nematode reduces the shoot and root length, number of floral branches, pod setting and the nodulation even at 10 larvae/pot but the fresh weight of root and shoot are reduced significantly at 100 larvae/pot (Mishra and Gaur 1987). On the other hand, some workers have reported this level as 500-1000 nematodes/pot (Mohanty and Pandey 1987, Sharma and Nene 1988). An initial population of 1-2 nematodes/cm^3 of soil could reduce the plant growth significantly in pigeonpea (Sharma 1988).

6.3.2 Causal Nematode

Rotylenchulus reniformis Linford & Oleivera

This species of nematode was first reported infecting pigeonpea in Puerto Rico by Ayala (1962a) and simultaneously in India (Seshadri and Sivakumar 1963). Later, it was found infecting pigeonpea in Trinidad & Tobago (Singh and Farrell 1972), Jamaica (Hammerton 1973), West Indies (Brathwaite 1974) and Fiji (Williams 1980). It is the main species causing dirty root disease in pigeonpea and is described as follows (Ali 1995b):

The juveniles, males as well as young females are vermiform arcuate to spiral upon relaxation.

Females: Young females are vermiform while matured ones are kidney shaped with an irregular, less swollen neck; post-median vulva and short pointed tail. Cuticle annulated; lateral field with 4 incisures, non-aerolated and obliterated. Cephallic region high, continuous. Stylet 2-3 times cephallic width. Orifice of dorsal oesophageal gland usually one stylet length behind the stylet base. Sub-ventral glands in the normal position, dorsal gland shifted laterally to subventrally, former being much longer than the latter. Immature females are vermiform and migratory. Ovaries paired with double flexures. Tail elongate-conoid with prominent, hyaline terminal portion.

Males: Males are vermiform with stylet and oesophagus regressed. Tail similar to that of females; bursa sub-terminal, low, not projecting beyond the tail contour in lateral view. Phasmids located on tail in its anterior region. Spicules slender lacking distal flanges. Gubernaculum fixed, devoid of titillae and telamon. Cloacal lips pointed not forming a tube; hypopygma absent.

Juveniles : They are vermiform with stylet 2-3 times cephalic region width long; Tail more rounded terminally than that of male and with shorter hyaline terminal portion than that of female.

Other species of reniform nematode associated with pigeonpea roots are *Rotylenchulus leptus* and *R. parvus* in Kenya (Sharma *et al.* 1993c) and *R. Parvus* in Australia. However, *R. reniformis* is the important one which is distributed throughout the world and has been studied in detail.

Biology and Disease Cycle: The nematode *R. reniformis* develops to the pre-adult infective stage through a series of three moults without any feeding. It preferably penetrates the root in the zone of elongation and reaches the endodermal layers. Several cells of the pericycle layer surrounding the nematode head form the giant cells (Patel and Patel 1991). The immature female feed semi-endo-parasitically with its anterior 1/3 body inside the root. It establishes its feeding sites in the phloem cells, starts enlarging on the ventral side around the vulval region and finally becoming reniform in shape. The males are found close to females feeding sites. The reinform nematodes are considered bisexual in nature and reproduce by cross fertilization. The female lay eggs in the gelatinous matrix on the host surface (Patel and Patel 1991) and the egg masses contain up to 150 eggs. The time taken for the completion of life cycle is 24-29 days by females and 16-20 days by males (Sivakumar and Seshadri 1971). The thermal limits for the reproduction are 15-36°C with an optimum of 30°C. The nematode is able to survive without host for more than 25 months.

After entry, the nematode causes various cellular modifications which differ with the host and the variety involved with regard to the degree and type. However, in general they cause hypertrophy, hyperplasia, thickening of cell walls, dense granular cytoplasm, enlargement of nucleus giant cell/syncytial formation of feeding peg and feeding tube formation within syncytium etc.

Dasgupta and Seshadri (1971) reported two races of the nematode: race 1 completes its life cycle on castor, cowpea and cotton but race 2 does not complete its life cycle on castor and cotton. In Japan, 3 biological types of *R. reniformis* have been reported (Nakasono 1983).

Pathogenicity and Damaging Levels: No relationship was observed between the number of reniform nematodes in the soil and the number of plants showing symptoms of decline but the plants grew faster and flowered earliest under suppressed nematode population (Hutton and Hammerton 1975). The reduction in plant growth depends on the population densities associated with pigeonpea plants. An initial inoculum level of 4 × 10 larvae/pot could reduce the plant growth significantly (Vilsoni and Heinlein 1984). The inoculum levels for adversely affecting the plant growth have been recorded variably (Mishra and Gaur 1987, Mohanty and Pandey 1987, Sharma 1988 and Sharma and Nene 1988) for pigeonpea. The economic threshold level has been reported to be 100 nematodes/kg of soil by Nath (1986). These levels may also differ from variety to variety due to the extent of their resistance to nematodes. The damaging levels for susceptible and resistant varieties of pigeonpea have been mentioned as 1000 and 10000 larvae/700 g of soil respectively (Thakar and Yadava 1985c). The initial inoculum levels and the final population counts of reniform nematodes have been found correlated negatively (Vilsoni and Heinlein 1984) but such correlation was observed above the inoculum levels of 10 larvae/plant and below this level the correlation was positive (Patel and Patel 1990).

6.3.3 Host Range

The host range of *R. reniformis* has been studied in detail in India. The nematode was first reported on cotton (Siddiqui and Bashir 1957). Later it was found to parasitize pigeonpea, potato (Seshadri and Sivakumar 1963), peas, broadbean, cowpea (Verma and Prasad 1969). Alam *et al* (1979) tested 68 economically important plant species and reported tickseed, rocket, salad, balsam, sesame and marigold as poor hosts; calendula, corn flower and blackgram as moderate and okra, chickpea, cotton, tomato, greengram and egg plant as good hosts while *Cajanus cajan* was a poor host. The nematode was found to occur on some additional hosts also specially sweet potato, cucumbers, potato, ginger, onion, grapes, papaya, citrus, mango, guava, peaches, pears, banana, litchi, jackfruit, beans, castor, groundnut, sunflower, mustard, wheat, rice, maize, sorghum, pearl millet, tea, coffee, tobacco, sugarcane, jasmine, and rose (Sitaramaiah 1984). Sahoo and Padhi (1986) evaluated 21 plant species belonging to 11 families and found soybean, groundnut, pigeonpea, blackgram, and greengram to be susceptible and little millet, kodomillet. common millet, horsegram, jute and niger as the new hosts of reinform nematode. In Puerto Rico, eighty-nine plant species were reported to be the hosts of reniform nematode of which 15 were new to *Rotylenchulus* spp. and 74 were susceptible to *R. reniformis* while pigeonpea was the most susceptible host (Ayala and Ramirej 1964). Marigolds have also been reported to increase the population of this nematodes (Roman 1964).

6.3.4 Relationship With Other Microorganisms

Higher incidence of Fusarium wilt of pigeonpea has been recorded in association with *R. reniformis* (Singh and Jayawant 1985, Anonymous 1987a). It has been reported that the presence of nematode accelerates the wilt in wilt susceptible variety and not in resistant or tolerant ones (Sharma and Nene 1990a). However, in some cases like cultivar ICPL 270, the resistance was affected adversely in presence of nematode (Jain and Sharma 1996). On the other hand, the population of *R. Reniformis* has been found to reduce in presence of *F. udum* (Sharma and Nene 1990a) and *Meloidogyne incognita* (Pathak *et al.* 1985).

The nematode *R. reniformis* and/or *Tylenchorhynchus* spp. have also been suspected to transmit the sterility mosaic of pigeonpea (Narayanaswamy and Ramakrishnan 1965) but it was not confirmed later.

6.3.5 Host Resistance

Screening of pigeonpea for resistance to reniform nematode, *R. reniformis* has been done in India and Fiji where several sources of resistance have been identified (Table 6.4).

Table 6.4 : Sources of resistance against *Rotylenchulus reniformis* in pigeonpea

Country	*No. of entries tested*	*Genotypes identified as resistant*	*Reference*
Fiji	—	QPL 67, 116, 511	Sharma and McDonald (1990)
India	25	UPAS 120 × PL 85, Prabhat, Pant A 10, ICPL 87, 93, 96	Bhargava and Pathak (1985)
	296	Varieties 4658, 2387, 556-1, 4167, 3830-2 and Norman at high inoculum and 2812 and 4217-2 at low inoculum	Thakar and Yadava (1985a, 1987)
	14	Basant and PDM 1	Ali (1987)
	64	ICP 12744, Basant & PDM 1	Patel *et al.* (1987b)
	82	AGS 522, GAUT 82-74, 83-23, and 84-22	Chavda *et al.* (1988)
	414	18-1, 77-1, 21-4, 24-4, 49-4, 55-8, 99-10, 556-1, 2387, 3830-2, 4167, AGS 522, Basant, Gaut 82-74, 83-23, 84-22, ICP 8869, 11291, 12744, ICPL 93, 111, Norman and PDM 1	Anonymous (1990)
	500+40 wild species	*Rhynchosia aurea, R. minima, R. rothii; ICPL 83045, 85024*	Sharma *et al.* (1992)
	—	P1148, P 1162/1, P 157, P 1169, P 1299, P 2499 were resistant to reniform and root knot nematodes and first two to *H.cajani* also	Anonymous (1992)

Sharma and Ashok Kumar (1991) developed a greenhouse method to evaluate the pigeonpea genotypes for resistance to reniform nematodes. The seedlings are grown in the nematode infested soil. The egg sacs are counted at 30-45 days after emergence of seedlings after staining with 0.25% trypan blue for 3 minutes. The exposure of egg sacs to trypan blue enhances the emergence of juveniles from the egg sacs. In this procedure heating is not required and hence, viability of eggs is not affected. The scoring is done on the basis of egg sacs as follows (Anonymous 1990):

Highly Resistant (HR)	: No females/plant
Resistant (R)	: 1-10 females/plant
Moderately Resistant (MR)	: 11-20 females/plant
Susceptible (S)	: 21-30 females/plant
Highly susceptible (HS)	: More than 30 females/plant

The higher levels of phenol in the roots of pigeonpea have been found associated with higher level of resistance to *R. reniformis* (Thakar and Yadava 1985b). The infection by nematode increase the total phenol contents in roots of resistant variety but decreases the same slightly in susceptible ones (Thakar and Yadava 1986). Nematodes at higher inoculum levels are reported to decrease polyphenol oxidase and B-glucosidase activities as well as total phenol contents of pigeonpea roots but peroxidase activity is not altered by nematode infection (Patel and Patel 1990).

6.3.6 Control

Chemical: A good control of reniform nematode in pigeonpea has been reported by seed treatment with fensulphothion, phorate, aldicarb Vyadate, carbofuran or dibromochloropropane @ 1.25 % a.i. W/W followed by granular application of any of these @ 4 kg a.i./ha 4 weeks after sowing (Panda and Seshadri 1979). Similarly seed treatment with 1% aldicarb, fenusulphothion or oxamyl reduced rate of nematode increase by 20-53 per cent with increased yield of pigeonpea (Mishra 1985b). Higher dose of aldicarb (2%) was most effective but showed phytotoxic effect reducing yield. Fensulphothion has been found effective for controlling the reinform nematode in pigeonpea by Jaiswal *et al.* (1987). They also reported gama BHC to possess nematicidal properties better than DBCP. Soil application of aldicarb @ 2.5 kg/ha at sowing and 2.5 kg/ha after sowing has been found highly effective but it induced early senescense (Ali 1996).

In the glass house experiments, a single folliar application of oxamyl (2500 ppm) inhibited the penetration of pigeonpea seedlings by *R. reinformis* in Trinidad (Singh 1975a). Foliar spray of oxamyl @ 3.6 kg a.i./ha in a fallow-planting combination was found effective in Fiji also (Heinlein and Black 1983).

Cultural : In Fiji, Disc fallows for 6 months between the pigeonpea crops was found highly effective in reducing the population of *R. reniformis* (Heinlein and Black 1983). Rotation of pigeonpea with rice or maize has been reported to check the population built up effectively (Sharma *et al.* 1992c). The population of reniform nematode is reduced greatly by growing *Tagetes patula* (Nakasono 1973), *Cynodon dactylon* (Singh 1975c) and pearl millet in rainy season (Singh *et al.* 1994). The population is favoured by sunflower, irrigation and inclusion of cowpea in the cropping system (Singh *et al.* 1994, Sharma *et al.* 1996b) but it is reduced by 80% in fallows from February to June.

The nematodes can be controlled by summer ploughing effectively (Sharma 1991).

Solarization : Pre-sowing solarization of vertisols using transparent polythene tarps during April-May for 8 weeks caused drastic reduction in the population of *R. reinformis* as assessed 58 days after solarization. The population remained low during the crop season up to the maturity of pigeonpea (Sharma and Nene 1985a). The solarization increased the soil temperature by 6-10°C and decreased the population of *Fusarium* and other nematodes also. According to Sharma and Nene (1990b) irrigation followed by solarization was most effective in reducing the juveniles of *R. reniformis* by 100 per cent.

6.4 Lance Nematodes

Lance nematodes include species of the genus *Hoplolaimus*. At least three species of this nematode have been observed occurring on pigeonpea in different countries of which *Hoplolaimus seinhorsti* is wide-spread and is reported from Nigeria (Bridge 1973), Fiji (Williams 1980), India (Sharma *et al.* 1985) and Kenya (Sharma *et al.* 1993c). The species *H. indicus* has been found associated with pigeonpea in India (Rashid *et al.* 1973) while *H. galeatus* occurs in USA only (Ingram and Rodriguez Kabana 1977). The *Hoplolaimus* spp. associated with pigeonpea have been reported from Puerto Rico (Ayala 1962a) and Jamaica also (Hammerton 1973). In India, lance nematode species have been found occurring on pigeonpea in the states of Andhra Pradesh, Karnataka, Uttar Pradesh, Gujarat, Bihar etc.

The lance nematodes are commonly associated with root/rhizosphere soil of pigeonpea and other plants. *H. seinhorsti* reduces the growth of plant which is evident 40-50 days after inoculation. It strongly affects top and root growth (Sharma 1985b), shoot length, fresh weight of root and shoot, leaf area and number of leaflets. Number of nodes are suppressed with increasing level of inoculum (Sharma and Nene 1988).

Lance nematodes are ectoparasites which sometimes feed on a particular site for longer time with nearly half of their body inside the root system and hence, they are considered as sedentary ectoparasites. The juveniles may enter the cortical tissues, become endoparasite causing more injury. The nematode, however, multiplies slowly as compared to other endoparasites. The population has been found more in alfisol than in vertisol and in February than other months. They were confined up to a depth of 30 cm in soil (Sharma 1985b). There is no resistant stage in the life cycle of the nematodes but it could survive for more than 300 days in absence of host (Sharma and Nene 1992). The storage of soil for more than 7 weeks reduced the nematode population. A temperature of 25-30°C has been found more favourable while population decreased at 10°C.

Variability has been observed in genotypes regarding their resistance to nematode. Out of 950 pigeonpea lines tested ICP 290, 554, 715, 830, 933, 1035 and 8077 showed good growth while ICP 1196, 1233, 1336, 7119, 7480, 8852 had good podding in presence of nematodes. The lines ICP 27, 78, 88, 107, 184, 195, 268, 299, 382, 616, 628, 780, 885, 918, 945, 1128, 6630, 8861, 9150, 10977, 10994 and 12734 showed significant plant stunting (Sharma 1985b).

6.5 Root Lesion Nematode

Species of the genus *Pratylenchus* belong to the group of root lesion nematodes. The nematode has been found associated with pigeonpea in Bangladesh, India, Jamaica, Kenya, Nigeria, Philippines, Sudan, Trinidad and Tobago, U.S.A. and Zimbabwe (Nene *et al.* 1996). It has been considered important in Sudan, Brazil, Jamaica, U.S.A., Trinidad and Zimbabwe (Sharma and McDonald 1990). In India, the root lesion nematode has been found occurring on pigeonpea in the state of Andhra Pradesh (Anonymous 1988), Karnataka (Sharma *et al.* 1992b), Uttar Pradesh (Sharma *et al.* 1996a) and Manipur (Ali 1995b).

The root lesion nematodes cause stunting, chlorosis of plants and brownish lesions on the roots of pigeonpea (Sethi 1973). Affected plants show symptoms of malnutrition and poorly developed root system. The feeder roots are damaged considerably as the affected cortical tissues eventually slough off. Careful examination reveal the presence of various stages of nematode.

Several species of *Pratylenchus* have been reported to be associated with pigeonpea in different countries as follows:

Bangladesh	:	*Pratylenchus* spp.
Brazil	:	*P. Brachyurus* (Sharma and McDonald 1990)
Fiji	:	*P. brachyurus, P. zeae* (Williams 1980)
Egypt	:	*P. penetrans*
India	:	*P. coffeae* (Das and Das 1985), *P. delattree, P. zeae* (Sharma *et al.* 1992b), *P. indicus* (Prasad *et al.* 1987)
Jamaica	:	*Pratylenchus* spp. (Hutton and Hammerton 1975)
Kenya	:	*P. neglectus, P. sefaensis, P. sudanensis, P. vulnus, P. zeae* (Sharma *et al.* 1993c)
Sudan	:	*P. scribneri* (Ingram and Rodriguez Kabana 1977), *P. sudanensis* (Sharma and McDonald 1990)
Trinidad	:	*P. zeae* (Sharma and McDonald 1990)
U.S.A.	:	*P. brachyurus* and *P. scribneri* (Ingram and Rodriguez Kabana 1977).

Host range of *P. coffeae* has been studied in India. Out of 63 plant species belonging to 26 families tested, 47 were found susceptible of which blackgram, pigeonpea, groundnut, chrysenthemum and dahlia were categorized as good hosts (Das and Das 1985). The nematode preferred monocot as well as dicot plants; banana being most preferred. Chickpea, Lathyrus, peas and *Dolichos lablab* were fair hosts (Das and Das 1986).

The nematode is controlled by fumigation of soil with DD @ 400 ml/ha resulting in better pigeonpea crop (Sethi 1973). The nematode population has been found to be reduced by tillage (Caveness 1974) and solarization. Due to solarization the nematode population remained low throughout the crop season (Sharma and Nene 1985a) and the reduction was up to 98% (Sharma and Nene 1990b). Inclusion of non-host crops like *Tagetes* spp. in rotation and destruction of weed hosts may be recommended for control of root lesion nematodes.

6.6 Stunt Nematode

The species of *Tylenchorhynchus* are commonly considered as stunt nematode. Several species of *Tylenchorhynchus* have been found associated with pigeonpea from different countries (Table 6.5). In India, stunt nematodes have been reported to occur on pigeonpea in the states of Andhra Pradesh (Sharma *et al.* 1985), Bihar (Anonymous 1987a), Gujarat (Ali 1992b), Haryana (Kaushik and Bajaj 1980), Karnataka (Sharma *et al.* 1992b), Madhya Pradesh (Ali 1987, 1989), Manipur (Ali 1995b) and Uttar Pradesh (Anonymous 1981). *T. brevilineatus, T. brassicae* and *T. vulgaris* occur widely in U.P. (Sharma *et al.* 1996a) while *T. vulgaris* is important in Haryana (Anonymous 1988) and parts of Karnataka (Sharma *et al.* 1992b). For the sake of convenience we may include species of *Bitylenchus, Merlinius* and *Amplimerlinius* under the group of stunt nematodes as all of them previously had been included in *Tylenchorhynchus* group (Ali 1995b).

Table 6.5: Species of stunt nematodes found associated with pigeonpea

Country	*Species reported*
Bangladesh	*Tylenchorhynchus* spp.
India	*Tylenchorhynchus brevilineatus* (Sharma *et al.* 1996a), *T. brassicae* (Alam *et al.* 1979), *T. divittatus, T. goffarti* (Kaushik and Bajaj 1980), *T. indicus* (Ganguli and Khan 1989), *T. mashoodi* (Mahapatra and Das 1979), *T. phaseoli* (Mulk and Jairajpuri 1972), *T. vulgaris* (Upadhyay and Swarup 1972), *Bitylenchus brevilineatus, B. vulgaris* (Ali 1994), *Merlinius* sp. (Ali 1991).
Jamaica	*Tylenchorhynchus* spp. (Nene *et al.* 1996).
Kenya	*T. goffarti* (Nene *et al.* 1996), *T. mashoodi, T. ventrosignatus, Bitylenchus singularis* (Sharma *et al.* 1993c).
Sudan	*Tylenchorhynchus* spp.
Trinidad and Tobago	*Tylenchorhynchus* spp.

The stunt nematodes are obligatory root ectoparasites although, some species are reported as endoparasites. They are economically important. Pigeonpea is the good host of *T. brassicae* supporting free reproduction. The increasing inoculum levels reduce the plant weight, pollen fertility, number of root nodules, water absorption capacity and growth parameter of pigeonpea (Tiyagi and Parveen 1990). They feed on epidermal cells of roots mainly in the region of elongation but occasionally they may be found embeded in host tissues subsequently resulting in severe stunting of plants. The roots of affected plants are seriously reduced.

The inorganic fertilizers increase the nematode population while FYM reduces them greatly (Singh *et al.* 1994). Pre-sowing solarization is reported to reduce the population of stunt nematodes significantly which continued to be lowest during the crop season also (Sharma and Nene 1985a).

6.7 Spiral Nematodes

The typical spiral nematodes include the species of *Helicotylenchus* and *Rotylenchus*. The species of *Scutellonema* have also been considered as spiral nematodes (PANS 1981) although, some workers have mentioned them as closely related to lance nematode (Edward and Mishra 1970). Several species of these genera have been found associated with pigeonpea in different countries as follows (Table 6.6) :

Table 6.6: Species of Spiral nematodes (*Helicotylenchus, Rotylenchus* and *Scutellonema*) found associated with pigeonpea in different countries

Country	*Nematode species reported*
Australia	*Helicotylenchus dihystra.*
Brazil	*H. Dihystra.*
Cuba	*H. dihystra, H. multicinctus.*
Fiji	*H. dihystra, H. indicus, H. microcephalus* (Williams 1980).
India	*H. dihystra* (Muthukrishnan *et al.* 1975), *H. crenacauda, H. abunnamai* (Padhi and Das 1982), *H. elegans* (Das *et al.* 1979), *H. indicus* (Alam *et al.* 1978), *H. retusus* (Sharma 1985a), *Rotylenchus secondus* (Mulk and Jairajpuri 1975), *Scutellonema erectum* (Sivakumar and Khan 1981).
Jamaica	*Helicotylenchus* spp. (Hutton and Hammerton 1975), *Scutellonema* spp., *S. bradys* (Hammerton (1973).
Kenya	*H. dihystra, H. microcephalus, H. paraplatyurus, H. pseudorobustus, Scutellonema anisomeristum, S. brachyurum, S. magniphasmum, S. propelatum,* and *S. unum* (Sharma *et al.* 1993c).
Niger	*Scutellonema clathricaudatum, S. diversicaudatum* (Nene *et al.* 1996).
Tonga	*H. dihystra, H. microcephalus, H. mucronata* (Williams 1980).
Trinidad & Tobago	*H. dihystra, Rotylenchus* spp. (Nene *et. al.* 1996).
U.S.A.	*H. dihystra* (Ingram and Rodriguez Kabana 1977).

Out of these species of spiral nematodes *H. dihystra* is widespread. *Helicotylenchus* spp. are typically ectoparasites and may cause injury effects in the host when present in large numbers by insertion of spear or the head into host tissues. All the stages of the nematode are reported to withstand the adverse soil conditions. *H. retusus* can survive in soil for a longer period even in absence of the host. It could survive for more than 300 days in vertisol and alfisol but was reduced significantly by solarization (Sharma and Nene 1985a). This nematode feeds, on parenchymatous tissues of cortex and after destroying it may penetrate deeper into stelar region.

The *Rotylenchus* spp. are also typical spiral nematodes which are migratory ectoparasites with head inserted in the root tissues. *R. secondus* was found associated with pigeonpea (Mulk and Jairajpuri 1975). It was 0.63-0.77 mm long; lip region faintly striated; spear 24-25 μ; spear knobs anteriorly striated, pointed tail cylindroid and phasmids at anal.

Solarization or fumigation with ethylene dibromide are found to eradicate the spiral nematodes in field.

6.8 Dagger Nematode

The *Xiphinema* spp. are commonly known as Dagger nematode. These nematodes are considerably long measuring up to 5 mm. They are the ectoparasites found deeper in frequently cultivated soil than in undisturbed soil. High population of nematodes cause considerable damage to roots.

Atleast three species of *Xiphinema* have been found associated with pigeonpea. They are *X. americana* and *X. lambertii* reported from India (Bajaj and Jairajpuri 1976), *X. campinense* (= *X. elongatum)* reported from Brazil (Lordello vaj De Ameda 1956), Fiji (Williams 1980) and Kenya. The dagger nematodes have been found associated with the pigeonpea in the states of Delhi (Prasad 1960), Haryana (Bajaj and Jairajpuri 1976), Madhya Pradesh (Ali 1987) and Uttar Pradesh (Ali 1990). The *X. lambertii* is differentiated from *X. americana* in having the smaller body (1.3-1.46 mm) and stylet (odontostyle 55-64 μ) and a larger and differently shaped tail (C = 37-50) as mentioned by Bajaj and Jairajpuri (1976).

Soil fumigation with suitable nematicide can reduce the population effectively.

6.9 Other Nematodes

Large number of nematode species, in addition to described above, have been found associated with the roots of pigeonpea in different pigeonpea growing countries of the world (Table 6.7). They may not be important economically at present but a few of them may cause serious damage to crop under favourable conditions.

Table 6.7 : List of other nematodes found associated with pigeonpea

Name of Species	*Reported from*
Aphasmatylenchus stratulatus	Burkina Faso (Nene *et al.* 1996)
Aphelenchoides sp.	Fiji & Tongo (Williams 1980), India (Sharma *et al.* 1992b), Kenya (Sharma *et al.* 1993c)
A. aligarhiensis	India (Kaushik and Bajaj 1980)
A. bicaudatus	Fiji (Williams 1980), Kenya (Sharma *et al.* 1993c)
Aphelenchus sp.	India (Ali 1992b)
A. radicicolus	India (Kaushik and Bajaj 1980)
Basiria sp.	India (Ali 1991), Kenya (Sharma *et al.* 1993c)
B. graminophila	India (Ali 1995b)
Basirolaimus indicus	India (Ali 1993)
Belanolaimus longicaudatus	U.S.A. (Reddi and Prine 1981)
Boleodorus sp.	India (Ali 1994)
Cephalobus sp.	India (Ali 1995b)
Criconema sp.	India (Prasad *et al.* 1960), Trinidad & Tobago (Nene *et al.* 1996)
Criconemella ornata	India (Das *et al.* 1988)
Criconemoides sp.	Puerto Rico, Trinidad & Tobago (Ayala 1962a), India (Ali 1991), Burkina Faso (Nene *et al.* 1996)
Crossonema spp.	India (Ali 1995b)
Ditylenchus sp.	Fiji (Williams 1980), Sudan (Sharma and McDonald 1990), India (Sharma *et al.* 1992b), Kenya (Sharma *et al.* 1993c)
Dorylaimus sp.	India (Ali 1995b)
Duosullus sp.	Kenya (Sharma *et al.* 1993c)
Filenchus sp.	Kenya (Sharma *et al.* 1993c)
F. filiformis	India (Ali 1995b)
Gracilacus sp.	Kenya (Sharma *et al.* 1993c)
G. peperpotti	Kenya (Sharma *et al.* 1993c)
Hemicriconemoid spp.	India (Prasad *et al.* 1964)
H. cocophillus	Fiji (Williams 1980), India (Kaushik and Bajaj 1980)
Hirschmaniella spp.	India (Prasad *et al.* 1964)
H. mucronata	India (Rashid *et al.* 1973)
H. oryzae	India (Rashid *et al.* 1973), Kenya (Sharma *et al.* 1993c)
Longidorus spp.	India (Prasad *et al.* 1964), Jamaica (Hammerton 1973)
L. siddiqui	India (Kaushik and Bajaj 1980)
Macroposthonia spp.	Trinidad & Tobago, Kenya (Sharma *et al.* 1993c)
M. onensis	Fiji (Williams 1980)
Mulkorhynchus sp.	Kenya (Sharma *et al.* 1993c)
Mylenchulus sp.	India (Ali 1995b)
Neoditylenchus sp.	India (Ali 1992b)
Neoditylenchus gladiolatus	Kenya (Sharma *et al.* 1993c)
Nothotylenchus sp.	India (Ali 1990)
Ottolenchus sp.	Kenya (Sharma *et al.* 1993c)
Paralongidorus sp.	Kenya (Sharma *et al.* 1993c)
Paraphelenchus sp.	Kenya (Sharma *et al.* 1993c)
Paraphylenchus amblyurus	India (Kaushik and Bajaj 1980)

Table 6.7 *contd.*

Name of Species	*Reported from*
Paratrichodorus christiei	USA (Nene *et al.* 1996)
P. minor	Egypt, Kenya (Nene *et al.* 1996)
P.mirzai	India (Kaushik and Bajaj 1980)
Paratylenchus sp.	India (Prasad *et al.* 1964)
P. rotundicephalus	India (Bajaj 1987)
Psilenchus sp.	India (Ali 1990)
Radopholus sp.	Nepal (Nene *et al.* 1996)
R. similis	India (Koshy & Sosamma 1975), Fiji (Sharma & McDonald 1990), Australia and USA (Nene *et al.* 1996)
Sakia sp.	Kenya (Nene *et al.* 1996)
Telotylenchus spp.	India (Prasad *et al.* 1964)
T. lobatus	Kenya (Sharma *et al.* 1993c)
Thornema spp.	India (Ali 1995b)
Trichodorus spp.	Bangladesh (Nene *et al.* 1996)
T. christiei	U.S.A. (Ingram and Rodriguez Kabana1977), Egypt (Nene *et al.* 1996)
T. mirzai	India (Alam *et al.* 1978)
Tylenchus spp.	Trinidad & Tobago, India (Nene *et al.* 1996)
Tylenchus filiformis	India (Alam *et al.* 1978)
Tylenchulus spp.	India (Prasad *et al.* 1964)

REFERENCES

Aboul-Eid, H. Z. and Ghorab, A. I. 1974. Pathological effects of *Heterodera cajani* on cowpea. *Plant Disease Reporter* 58 : 1130-33.

Alam, M.M., Anver, S. and Yadava, A. 1991. Effect of *Meloidogyne incognita* on plant growth and bulk density of plant residues of pigeonpea, *Cajanus cajan*. *Afro-Asian Journal of Nematology* 1 (1): 73-76.

Alam, M.M., Saxena, S. K. and Khan, M. A. 1978. Suitability of crops to certain ectoparasitic nematodes. *Acta Botanica Indica* 6 (Suppl.) : 205-208.

Alam, M.M., Saxena, S. K. and Khan, M. A. 1979. Suitability of crops to the reniform, stunt and root knot nematodes. *Recent Research in Plant Sciences* : 630-634.

Ali, S. S. 1987. Investigations on plant parasitic nematodes associated with pulse crops. *In*: Annual Report 1987. Directorate of Pulses Research Kanpur, India, pp. 127-128.

Ali, S. S. 1989. Occurrence of plant parasitic nematodes associated with pulse crops. Souvenir and Abstract Papers Presented in National Symposium on New Frontiers in Pulses Research and Development. Nov. 10-12, Directorate of Pulses Research, Kanpur, India, p. 28.

Ali, S. S. 1990. Consolidated report on Kharif Pulses 1989-90. Plant Nematology. AICPIP, Kharif Workshop, May 15-18, 1990, Gujarat Agricultural University, Anand, India, pp 25.

Ali, S.S. 1991. Consolidated report on Kharif Pulses, 1990-91. Plant Nematology. AICPIP, Kharif Group Meet, June 4-6, 1991, Banaras Hindu University, Varanasi, India, pp. 40.

Ali, S.S. 1992. Consolidated report on Kharif Pulses, 1991-92. Plant Nematology. AICPIP, Kharif Workshop, 11-13 May, 1992, Rajendra Agricultural University, Pusa, Samastipur, India, pp. 31.

Ali, S. S. 1993. Prevalence of plant parasitic nematodes associated with pigeonpea in Gwalior. *International Pigeonpea Newsletter* 17 : 31.

Ali, S. S. 1994. Consolidated Report on Kharif Pulses, 1993-94. Plant Nematology. AICPIP Kharif Workshop, June 2-4, 1994, Andhra Pradesh Agricultural University, Hyderabad, India, pp. 57.

Ali, S. S. 1995a. Consolidated Report on Kharif Pulses, 1994-95. Plant Nematology. AICPIP Workshop, April 26-29, 1995, JNKVV, Jabalpur, India, pp. 51.

Ali, S. S. 1995b. Nematode problems in chickpea. Indian Institute of Pulses Research, Kanpur, India, pp. 184.

Ali, S. S. 1996. Estimation of yield losses in pigeonpea due to reniform nematode. *Indian Journal of Pulses Research* 9: 209-210.

Ali, S. S. and Sharma, S. B. 1997. Status of nematode problems and research in India. Diagnosis of key nematode pests of chickpea and pigeonpea and their management. Proceeding Patancheru, India, 25-30 November, 1996, pp. 74-82.

Angus, A. 1962. Annotated list of plant pests and diseases in Zambia. Pt. 1. *Plant Pathologists Report*. Chilanga, Zambia : Mt. Makulu Research Station, pp. 21.

Anonymous. 1968. Green manure. *Seed World* 103 : 22.

Anonymous. 1981. All India Coordinated Research Project on Nematode Pests of Crops and Their Control. Proceedings of III Workshop, 10-13 Feb. 1981, TNAU, Coimbatore, India, pp. 65.

Anonymous. 1982. All India Coordinated Research Project on Nematode Pests of Crops and Their Control. Proceedings of Mini Workshop, 27-28 April 1982, IARI, New Delhi, India, pp. 36.

Anonymous. 1985. Annual Report 1984, Biotic Stresses : Nematode, Chickpea/Pigeonpea. ICRISAT, Patancheru, A.P., India, pp. 137-138 and 175-176.

Anonymous. 1987a. All India Coordinated project on Plant Parasitic Nematodes with Integrated Approach for their control. Proceedings of Workshop, 9-12 June 1987, College of Agriculture, Pune, Mahatma Phule Agriculture University, Rahuri, pp. 28.

Anonymous. 1987b. Annual Report (Pigeonpea). ICRISAT, Patancheru, A.P., India, pp. 190-192.

Anonymous. 1988. Annual Report (Pigeonpea). ICRISAT, Patancheru, A.P., India, pp. 91-93.

Anonymous. 1989a. Research Highlights. ICRISAT, Patacheru, A.P., India, pp. 47.

Anonymous. 1989b. Annual Report (Pigeonpea). ICRISAT, Patancheru, A.P., India, pp. 113-115.

Anonymous. 1989c. Annual Report 1988-89 : Nematode Pests. ICAR, New Delhi, India, pp. 75-76.

Anonymous. 1990. Reaction of various crop germplasm to plant parasitic nematodes. Department of Nematology, B. A. College of Agriculture, GAU, Anand. India, pp. 28.

Anonymous. 1992. All India Coordinated Research Project on Nematode Pests of Crops and Their Control. Proceedings of Mini Workshop, 27-28 April 1992, IARI, New Delhi, India, pp. 36.

Anver, S. and Alam, M.M. 1989. Effect of root knot and reniform nematodes on plant growth and bulk density of plant residues of pigeonpea. *Biological Wasts* 30 : 245-250.

Anver, S., Chandel, S. T. and Alam, M. M. 1997. Reaction of pigeonpea accessions to root knot nematode, *Meloidogyne incognita. International Chickpea and Pigeonpea Newsletter* 4: 34-35.

Ayala, A. 1962a. Occurrence of the nematode *Meloidogyne javanica* on pigeonpea roots in Puerto Rico. *Journal of Agriculture of the University of Puerto Rico* 46 : 154-156.

Ayala, A. 1962b. Parasitism of bacterial nodules by the reniform nematode. *Journal of Agriculture of the University of Puerto Rico* 46 : 67-69.

Ayala, A. 1962 c. Pathogenicity of reniform nematode on various hosts. *Journal of Agriculture of the University of Puerto Rico* 46 : 73-82.

Ayala, A. and Ramirez, C. T. 1964. Host range, distribution and bibliography of the reniform nematodes, *Rotylenchulus reinformis*, with special reference to Puerto Rico. *Journal of Agriculture of the University of Puerto Rico* 48: 140-161.

Bajaj, H.K. and Jairajpuri, M. S. 1976. Two new species of *Xiphinema* from India. *Nematol. Medit.* 4: 195-200.

Beeley, F. 1939. A nematode pest of roots of cover plants. *Journal of the Rubber Research Institute of Malaya* 9: 51-58.

Bessey, E.A. 1911. Root knot and its control. *Bulletin, United States, Department of Agriculture* No. 217 : 89 pp.

Bhargava, S. and Pathak, A. K. 1985. Screening of certain varieties of arhar against *Meloidogyne incognita* and *Rotylenchulus reniformis. Indian Journal of Nematology* 15 : 277.

Bhatti, D.S. and Gupta, D.C. 1973. Guar an additional host of *Heterodera cajani. Indian Journal of Nematology* 3 : 160.

Bhatti, D. S. and Walia, R. 1990. Nematode problems of crop plants in Haryana. Pages 543-565, *In*: Progress in Plant Nematology (ed. S. K. Saxena, Wajid Khan, Abdul Rashid M. and R. H. Khan). CBS Publishers and Distributors Pvt. Ltd.

Brathwaite, C.W.D. 1974. Occurrence of plant parasitic nematodes in Monteserrat, West Indies. *FAO Plant Protection Bulletin* 12 : 69-71.

Bridge, J. 1973. *Hoplolaimus seinhorsti*, an endoparasitic nematode of cowpea in Nigeria. *Plant Disease Reporter* 57 : 798-799.

Bridge, J. C. 1981. Nematodes. Pages 111-125, *In* : Pest Control in Tropoical Grain Legumes. Centre for Overseas Pest Research, ODA, London, UK.

Caveness, F. E. 1974. Plant parasitic nematodes population differences under no-tillage and tillage soil regimes in western Nigeria. *Journal of Nematology* 6: 138.

Chauhan, Y. S., Nene, Y. L., Johansen, C., Haware, M.P., Saxena, N.P., Singh, S., Sharma, S. B., Sahrawat, K. L., Burford, J. R., Rupela, O.P., Rao, J.V.D.K.K. and Sithanatham, S. 1988. Effect of soil solarization on pigeonpea and chickpea. Patancheru, A.P., India, ICRISAT, *Research Bulletin*, ICRISAT, pp. 20.

Chavada, J. C., Patel, B. A. and Patel, D. J. 1988. Screening of pigeonpea lines to *Rotylenchulus reniformis*. *International Nematology Network Newsletter* 5 : 28-29.

Collins, J. C. 1938. Nematode investigations. *Rhodesia Agricultural Journal* 35 : 431-438.

Darekar, K. S. and Jagdale, G. B. 1989. Reaction of pigeonpea and greengram varieties/ lines against *Meloidogyne incognita* race 3. *International Nematology Network Newsletter* 6(2) : 12-14.

Darekar, K. S., Mhase, N.L., Soble, A. N. and Azri, D. S. 1985. Occurrence of *Heterodera cajani* in Maharashtra, India. *Current Research Reporter* 1 (2) : 220.

Das, S. and Das, S. N. 1985. Host range of *Pratylenchus coffeae. Indian Journal of Nematology* 15 : 282.

Das, S. and Das, S. N. 1986. Host range of *Pratylenchus coffeae. Indian Journal of Nematology* 16 (2) : 180-184.

Das, S. N., Mishra, C. D. and Mohanty, K. C. 1979. Occurrence and host preference of some plant parasitic nematodes on pulse crops. *Indian Journal of Nematology* 9 (1): 74.

Das, S. N., Mohanty, K. C. and Roy, S. 1988. Population dynamics of *Criconemella ornata* under multiple cropping systems. *International Nematology Network Newsletter* 5(1) : 7-530.

Dasgupta, D. R. and Seshadri, A.R. 1971. Races of reniform nematode, *Rotylenchulus reniformis* Linford and Oliveira, 1940. *Indian Journal of Nematology* 1 : 21-34.

Devi, Sobita L.R. and Gupta, Pramila 1988. Pathogenicity and management of *Heterodera cajani* on some pulse crops. *Indian Phytopathology* 41 : 470-472.

Devi, Sobita and Gupta, P. 1992. Screening of arhar, greengram and urd varieties against cyst nematode, *H. cajani*. First Afro-Asian Nematology Symposium. Afro-Asian Society of Nematologists. Department of Botany, Aligarh Muslim University, Aligarh India, Nov. 29 to Dec. 3, pp. 39.

Devi, Sobita and Gupta, Pramila 1995. Effect of four green manures against *Heterodera cajani* on pigeonpea sown with or without *Rhizobium* seed treatment. *Indian Journal of Mycology and Plant Pathology* 25 : 254-256.

Edward, J. C. and Mishra, S. L. 1968. *Heterodera vigni* n. sp. and second stage larvae of *Heterodera* spp. in Uttar Pradesh, India. *Allahabad Farmer* 43 : 155-159.

Edward, J. C. and Mishra, S.L. 1970. An introduction to Plant Nematology, Central Book Depot, Allahabad, India, pp. 1-82.

Edward, J.C. and Singh, K.P. 1979. Interaction between *Heterodera cajani* and *Fusarium udum* on pigeonpea. *Allahabad Farmer* 50 (1) : 23-24.

Fennell, M.A. 1963. Present status of research on edible legumes in western Nigeria. *Proceeding of the Nigerian Grain Legume Conference* 1 : 16-29.

Ganguli, S. and Khan, E. 1989. Concomitant occurrence of the population of *Heterodera cajani* and *Hoplolaimus indicus* on pulse crops in India. *International Nematology Network Newsletter* 6 (2) : 15-16.

Gaur, H. S., Beane, J. and Perry, R. N. 1996. Effect of storage *in vitro* and in soil on the hatch from the cysts of the pigeonpea cyst nematode, *Hetrodera cajani. Fundamental and Applied Nematology* 19: 537-544.

Gill, J. S. and Singh, R. V. 1990. Nematodes associated with pulse crops and their control. pages 503-514 *In* : Progress in plant Nematology (Eds. S. K. Saxena, Wajid Khan, M. A. Rashid and R. M. Khan). CBS Publishers and Distributors Pvt. Ltd., New Delhi.

Godfrey, G. H. 1928. Legumes as rotation and trap crops for pineapple fields. *Bulletin Hawaiian Pineapple Cannera' Association Experiment Station* No. 10, 21 pp.

Gonzaga, E. and Lordello, L. 1960. Interferences of nematodes in agricultural practices. *Rural Review Society of Rural Brasil* 40: 12-13.

Gunasekaran, C. R., Muthukrishnan, T. S. and Rajendran, G. 1976. Evaluation of Chemicals for control of pigeonpea cyst nematode *Heterodera cajani* in red gram. *Madras Agricultural Journal* 63 : 382-383.

Gupta, P. and Edward, J. C. 1974. Some economically important new hosts of *Heterodera vigni* in Uttar Pradesh, India. *Plant Disease Reporter* 58 : 345-347.

Hadesoeganda, W. W. and Sasser, J. N. 1982. Resistance of tomato, bean, southern pea and garden pea cultivars to root knot nematodes based on host suitability. *Plant Disease* 66 : 145-150.

Hammerton, J. L. 1973. A yellowing and die-back syndrome of pigeonpea, *Cajanus cajan* (L.) Millsp. *Proceedings of the Caribbean Food Crops Society Meeting* 11 : 197-208.

Hasan, A. 1984. Synergism between *Heterodera cajani* and *Fusarium* attacking *Cajanus cajan*. *Nematologica Mediterranea* 12 : 159-162.

Hasan, A. 1989. Efficacy of certain non-fumigating nematicides on the control of pigeonpea wilt involving *Heterodera cajani* and *Fusarium udum. Journal of Phytopathology* 126 (4) : 335-342.

Hasan, Abdul and Khan, Abrar M. 1983. Resistance of some pigeonpea cultivars to root knot nematode. *International Pigeonpea Newsletter* 2: 56.

Heinlein, M. and Black, D. 1983. The use of fallows planting techniques and nematicide application for control of *Rotylenchulus reniformis* in pigeonpea. *Fiji Agricultural Journal* 45 : 35-42.

Hussain, S. I., Siddiqui, Z. A. and Siddiqui, M. R. 1989. Prevalence and geographical distribution of cyst forming nematodes in Uttar Pradesh, India. *Indian Journal of Nematology* 19: 103-104.

Hutton, D. G. and Hammerton, J. L. 1975. Investigating the role of *Rotylenchulus reniformis* in a decline of pigeonpea. *Nematropica* 5: 24.

Imran, M., Fazal, M. and Saxena, S. K. 1992. Morphological response of pigeonpea cultivars to *Meloidogyne incognita*. *Afro-Asian Nematological Network* 1 : 21-24.

Ingram, E. G. and Rodriguez-Kabana, R. 1977. Susceptibility of pigeonpea to plant parasitic nematodes. *Proceedings of the American Phytopathological Society* 4: 177 (Abst.).

Jain, K. C. and Sharma, S. B. 1996. Loss of Fusarium wilt resistance in a pigeonpea line ICPL 270 in reniform nematode infested soil at ICRISAT Asia Centre. *International Chickpea and Pigeonpea Newsletter* 3 : 90.

Jain, S. K., Dave, G. S. and Jain, A. K. 1994. Host range of cyst nematode *Heterodera cajani* in cold weather. *Indian Phytopathology* 47 : 177-178.

Jairajpuri, M. S. 1986. Aligarh Muslim University, Zoology. In : Nematology in India, pp. 51-79.

Jaiswal, B. K., Nath, R.P., Halder, M. G. and Pathak, K. N. 1987. Efficacy of some pesticides on *Meloidogyne incognita* and *Rotylenchulus reniformis* infesting pigeonpea. *Indian Journal of Nematology* 17: 60-61.

Janarthana, R. 1972. Occurrence of the pigeonpea cyst nematode in Tamil Nadu. *Indian Journal of Nematology* 2 : 215.

Kahkashan, Parveen, Haseeb Akhtar and Shukla, P.K. 1998. Influence of root knot nematode and wilt fungus on the growth of pigeonpea. Pages 80-86. *In* Nematology : Challenges and Opportunities in 21st Century. Proceedings of the III International Symposium of Afro-Asian-Society of Nematologists (TISSAN), Sugarcane Breeding Institute, Coimbatore India, April 16-19, 1998 (Eds. Mehta, U.K., Luton, V.K.). Afro-Asian Society of Nematologists.

Kaiser, W. J. 1981. Diseases of chickpea, lentil, pigeonpea and tepary bean in Continental United States and Puerto Rico. *Economic Botany* 35 (3) : 300-320.

Kalha, C. S. and Edward, J. C. 1979. *Heterodera vigni* Edward & Mishra 1968 a synonymy of *Heterodera cajani* Koshy 1967. *Allahabad Farmer* 50 (2) : 143-146.

Kaushik, H. D. and Bajaj, H. K. 1990. Nematodes associated with pulse crops in Haryana. *Indian Journal of Nematology* 20 : 92-96.

Khan, M. W. and Salam, M. A. 1990. Interaction of *Meloidogyne javanica* and *Rhizobium* on pigeonpea in the presence of nickel and cobalt as pollutants. *Annals of Biology* 116 : 549-556.

Killinger, G. B. 1968a. New agronomic crops for Florida. Sunshine State Agricultural Research Report 13 : 3-5.

Killinger, G. B. 1968b. Pigeonpea (*Cajanus cajan* (L.) Druce), a useful crop for Florida. *Proceedings, Soil and Crop Science Society of Florida* 28 : 162-167.

Koshy, P. K. 1967. A new species of *Heterodera* from India. *Indian Phytopathology* 20 : 272-274.

Koshy, P. K. 1968. Studies on the cyst forming nematodes of pigeonpea. Ph.D. Thesis, Indian Agricultural Research Institute, New Delhi, India.

Koshy, P. K. and Sosamma 1975. Host range of the burrowing nematodes *Radopholus similis* (Cobb. 1893) Thorne 1949. *Indian Journal of Nematology* 5: 255-257.

Koshy, P. K. and Swarup, Gopal. 1971. Factors affecting emergence of larvae from cyst of *Heterodera cajani* Koshy. *Indian Journal of Nematology* 1: 209-219.

Koshy, P. K. and Swarup, Gopal. 1971a. Investigations on the life history of pigeonpea cyst nematode *Heterodera cajani*. *Indian Journal of Nematology* 1 : 44-51.

Koshy, P. K. and Swarup, Gopal. 1971b. On the number of generations of *Heterodera cajani*, the pigeonpea cyst nematode in a year. *Indian Journal of Nematology* 1: 88-90.

Koshy, P. K. and Swarup, Gopal. 1971c. Susceptibility of aerial parts of pigeonpea seedlings to *Heterodera cajani* larva. *Indian Journal of Nematology* 1 : 245-246.

Koshy, P. K. and Swarup, Gopal. 1972. Susceptibility of plants to pigeonpea cyst nematode, *Heterodera cajani*. *Indian Journal of Nematology* 2: 1-6.

Koshy, P. K. and Swarup, Gopal. 1979. Histopathology of pigeonpea roots infected with *Heterodera cajani* Koshy 1967. *Indian Journal of Nematology* 9 : 178-179.

Koshy, P. K., Swarup, Gopal and Sethi, C. L. 1970. Further notes on the pigeonpea cyst nematodes *Heterodera cajani*. *Nematologica* 16 : 477-482.

Lordello, L. G. E. and Vaz De Arruda, H. 1956. (Nematodes parasitic on pigeonpea). *Bragantia* 15 : 5-7.

Mahapatra, B. C. and Das, S. N. 1979. Host range and pathogenicity of *Tylenchorhynchus mashoodi* Siddiqui and Bashir 1949 on maize (*Zea mays*). *Indian Journal of Nematology* 9 (1) : 64.

Marley, P. S. and Hillocks, R. J. 1996. Effect of root knot nematode (*Meloidogyne* spp.) on Fusarium wilt in pigeonpea (*Cajanus cajan*). Field Crops Research 46 : 1-3, 15-20.

Mishra, S. D. 1985a. Effect of nematicidal seed treatment on germination, growth and susceptibility to penetration by *Meloidogyne incognita* on pulse crops. *Indian Journal of Nematology* 15:268.

Mishra, S. D. 1985b. Control of nematodes by nematicide seed treatment of pigeonpea. *Indian Journal of Nematology* 15 : 268-69.

Mishra, S. D. 1986. Control of root knot nematode, *Meloidogyne incognita* infesting pigeonpea by nematicidal seed treatment. Pages 34-36. *In* : Proceedings of National Symposium New Dimentions on Parasitology. University of Allahabad 18-19 Jan. 1986.

Mishra, S. D. and Gaur, H. S. 1987. Relation between individual and concomitant population of *Meloidogyne incognita* and *Rotylenchulus reniformis* and the growth of pigeonpea. *Cajanus cajan*. *Indian Journal of Entomology* 49 (1) : 73-75.

Mishra, S. D. and Prasad, D. 1990. Chemotherapeutic management of *Heterodera cajani* in infesting pigeonpea. *In* : Environment Concern and Tissue Injury, *Environment Series* 4: 59-65.

Mohanty, G. B. and Pandey, N. N. 1987. Pathogenic effects of reniform nematode at varying levels of inoculation of pigeonpea. *International Nematology Newsletter* 4 : 15-16.

Mojumdar, V. and Mishra, S. D. 1991. Nematicidal efficacy of some plant products and management of *Meloidogyne incognita* in pulse crops by soaking seed in their aqueous extracts. Current Nematology 2 (1) : 27-32.

Mukiibi, J. 1976. Possible relationship between intercropping and plant disease problems in Uganda. Presented at the Symposium on Intercropping for Semi-arid Areas, 10-12 May 1976. University of Dar-es-Salam, Morogoro, Tanzania.

Mulk, M. M. and Jairajpuri, M. S. 1972. A redescription of *Tylenchorhynchus phaseoli* Sethi and Swarup 1968. *Indian Journal of Nematology* 2: 54-58.

Mulk, M. M. and Jairajpuri, M. S. 1975. Nematodes of leguminous crops in India. IV. Two new species of *Rotylenchus* Filipjeb (Hoplolaimidae). *Indian Journal of Nematology* 5 : 9-14.

Muthukrishnan, T. S., Rajendran and Chandrasekaran, J. 1975. Pathogenicity of *Helicotylenchus dihystra* to chilli (*Capsicum annum*) and its host range. *Indian Journal of Nematology* 5: 180-184.

Nakasono, K. 1973. Relationship between cultivation of *Tagetes* plants and changes in population of the reniform nematode, *Rotylenchulus reniformis*. *Japanese Journal of Nematology* 3 : 38-41.

Nakasono, K. 1983. Plant parasitic nematodes, Problems and Progress. *Journal of Nematology* 12 : 21-25.

Narayanaswamy, P. and Ramakrishnan, K. 1965. Studies on the sterility mosaic disease of pigeonpea. I. Transmission of the disease. *Proceedings Indian Academy of Sciences* Sect. B 62:73-86.

Nath, R.P. 1986. Rajendra Agricultural University Pusa, Samastipur. *In*: Nematology in India, IARI, New Delhi, pp. 149-157.

Nene, Y. L., Sheila, V. K. and Sharma, S. B. 1996. A world list of chickpea and pigeonpea pathogens. Patancheru, A. P., India, ICRISAT, pp. 27.

Padhi, N. N. and Das, S. N. 1982. Host range of the spiral nematode *Helicotylenchus abunamai*. *Indian Journal of Nematology* 12 (1) : 53-59.

Panda, M. and Seshadri, A. R. 1979. Efficacy of few nematicides in controlling the infestations of reniform nematodes in some pulse crops. *Indian Journal of Nematology* 9: 84-85.

PANS 1981. Pest control in tropical grain legumes. Centre for Overseas Pest Research, Overseas Development Administration, London, pp. 206.

Patel, B. A., Chavda, J. C., Patel, S. T. and Patel, D. J. 1987a. Susceptibility of some pigeonpea lines to root knot nematodes *Meloidogyne incognita* and *M. javanica*. *International Pigeonpea Newsletter* 6: 55-57.

Patel, B. A., Chavda, J. C., Patel, S. T. and Patel, D. J. 1987b. Reaction of some pigeonpea lines to reniform nematode, *Rotylenchulus reniformis*. *International Pigeonpea Newsletter* 6: 57-58.

Patel, G.A. and Patel, D.J. 1993. Avoidable yield losses in pigeonpea cultivars Pusa Ageti due to *Meloidogyne javanica*. *International Pigeonpea Newsletter* 17 : 26.

Patel, G. A., Patel, D. J. and Patel, B. A. 1992. Pathogenicity and biochemical changes induced by infection of *Meloidogyne javanica* on pigeonpea. First Afro-Asian Nematology Symposium, Afro-Asian Society of Nematologist. Department of Botany Aligarh Muslim University, Aligarh, India, November 29 to Dec. 3, pp. 39.

Patel, R. G. and Patel, D. J. 1990. Pathogenicity and biochemical changes induced by reniform nematode, *Rotylenchulus reniformis* Linford and Oliveira 1940 in pigeonpea. *Current Nematology* 1(1) : 11-14.

Patel, R. G. and Patel, D. J. 1991. Histopathological changes in pigeonpea infected by reniform nematodes (*Rotylenchulus reniformis*). *Current Nematology* 2(1) : 88.

Pathak, K.N., Nath, R.P. and Haider, M.G. 1985. Effect of initial ioculum levels of *Meloidogyne incognita* and *Rotylenchulus reniformis* on pigeonpea and their interrelationship. *Indian Journal of Nematology* 15 : 177-179.

Prasad, D. 1985. Seed soaking : A prophylactic treatment of pigeonpea against *Heterodera cajani. International Nematology Network Newsletter* 2 (4) : 17-18.

Prasad, J. S., Panwar, M. S. and Rao, Y. S. 1987. The influence of intercropping greengram and red gram with rice on the build up of root lesion nematodes, *Pratylenchus indicus. Biol. Agric. Horticulture* 5 (1) : 61-69.

Prasad, N., Mathur, R. L. and Sehgal, S. P. 1959. Molya disease of wheat and barley in Rajasthan. *Current Science* 28 : 453.

Prasad, S. K. 1960. Plant parasitic nematodes observed at Indian Agricultural Research Institute Farm. *Indian Journal of Entomology* 22 : 127-128.

Prasad, S. K., Dasgupta, D. R. and Mukhopadhyay, M. C. 1964. Nematodes associated with commercial crops in northern India and host range of *Meloidogyne javanica* (Treub 1885) Chitwood 1949. *Indian Journal of Entomology* 26 : 438-446.

Rai, P. K. and Singh, K. P. 1995. Efficacy of certain oilcake amendments on *Heterodera cajani, Fusarium udum* and associated wilt of pigeonpea. *International Journal of Tropical Plant Diseases* 13 (2) : 213-219.

Rai, P. K. and Singh, K. P. 1996. Pathogenicity and histopathology of *Heterodera cajani* and two isolates of *Fusarium udum* on pigeonpea. *National Academy Science Letters* 19 : 1-2, 4-7.

Rajak, R. L., Samathanam, G. T., Khan, M. R., Rao, M. H. and Muthalyan, M. C. 1986. Check list of plant parasitic nematodes. Govt. of India, Ministry of Agriculture and Rural Development, Department of Agriculture and Cooperation, Directorate of Plant Protection, Quarantine and Storage, NH IV. Faridabad, pp. 74.

Rashid, A., Khan, F. A. and Khan, A. M. 1973. Plant parasitic nematodes associated with vegetables, fruits, cereals and other crops in north India. I. Uttar Pradesh. *Indian Journal of Nematology* 3 : 8-23.

Raveendhran, A. and Nadaka, A. M. 1975. An additional list of plants infected by root knot nematode, *Meloidogyne incognita* (Kofoid and White 1919) Chitwood 1949 in Kerala. *Indian Journal of Nematology* 5 : 126-127.

Reddi, K. C. S. and Prine, G. M. 1981. Green manuring of tropical legumes and their effects on soil nitrogen pool and nematode population. *Agronomy Abstract* 1981 : 167.

Reddi, K. C., Soffes, A. R. and Prine, G. M. 1983. Effectiveness of pigeonpea and other tropical legumes in controlling nematodes in following crops. *International Pigeonpea Newsletter* 2:57-59.

Reddy, M. V., Sharma, S. B. and Nene, Y. L. 1990. Pigeonpea : Disease Management. Pages 303-347 *In*: The Pigeonpea (Eds. Y. L. Nene, S. D. Hall and V. K. Sheila). CAB, UK International, ICRISAT.

Rodriguez-Kabana, R. and Ingram, E. G. 1978. Susceptibility of pigeonpea to plant parasitic nematodes in Alabama. *Nematropica* 8 : 32-34.

Roman, J. 1964. Immunity of sugarcane to the reniform nematode. *Journal of Agriculture of the University of Puerto Rico* 48 : 162-163.

Roy, A. K. 1972. Reaction of some plants to the attack of *Meloidogyne incognita* in Assam. *Indian Journal of Nematology* 2: 86-89.

Sahoo, H. and Padhi, M. N. 1986. Susceptibility of plants to the reniform nematodes, *Rotylenchulus reniformis*. *Indian Journal of Nematology* 16 (1): 97-98.

Salam, M. A. and Khan, M. W. 1986. Reaction of some cultivars of pigeonpea against *Fusarium udum* and *Meloidogyne javanica*. *International Nematology Network Newsletter* 3 (4) : 16-17.

Sasser, J. N. 1979. Economic importance of *Meloidogyne* spp. in tropical countries. Pages 359-374 *In*: Root Knot Nematodes (*Meloidogyne* spp.): Systemic Biology and Control (Eds. F. Lamberti and C. E. Taylor). Academic Press, London, UK.

Sasser, J. N. 1989. Plant parasitic nematodes, the farmers hidden enemy. Raleigh, N. C., USA, North Carolina State University.

Sasser, J. N. and Freckman, D. W. 1987. A world perspective on nematology : The role of the society. Pages 7-14 *In*: Vistas on Nematology (Eds. J. A. Veech and D. W. Dickson). Hyattsville, Maryland, U.S.A., Society of Nematologists.

Sasser, J. N. and Hartman, K. M. 1985. Evaluation of some pigeonpea lines for resistance to root knot nematodes *Meloidogyne* spp. *International Pigeonpea Newsletter* 4 : 44-45.

Saxena, K. B., Reddy, M. V., Bhagwat, V. R. and Sharma, S. B. 1996. Preliminary studies on the incidence of major diseases and insects in *Cajanus platycarpus* germplasm at ICRISAT Asia Centre. *International Chickpea and Pigeonpea Newsletter* 3 : 51-52.

Saxena, K. B., Singh, L., Reddy, M. V., Singh, U., Lateef, S. S., Sharma, S. B. and Remanandan, P. 1990. Intra species variation in *Atylosia scarabaeoides* (L.) Benth. A wild relative of pigeonpea. *Euphytica* 49 : 185-191.

Saxena, R. and Reddy, D. D. R. 1987. Crop losses in pigeonpea and mungbean by mungbean cyst nematodes, *Meloidogyne cajani*. *Indian Journal of Nematology* 17 : 91-94.

Seshadri, A. R. and Sivakumar, C. V. 1963. A preliminary note on the occurrence of reniform nematode (*Rotylenchulus reniformis* Linford and Oliviera 1940) on a number of cultivated crops in south India. *Madras Agricultural Journal* 50 : 134-137.

Sethi, C. L. 1973. Nematodes associated with pulses, sugarcane and cotton. Pages 234-235 *In* Pest Management and plant protection training. Directorate of Extension, Ministry of Agriculture and Irrigation, Department of Agriculture, Govt. of India, New Delhi.

Sharma, N. K. and Sethi, C. L. 1975. Leghaemoglobin content of cowpea nodules as influenced by *Meloidogyne incognita* and *Heterodera cajani*. *Indian Journal of Nematology* 45 : 113-114.

Sharma, Renu, and Sharma, S. B. 1989. Sticky swarm disease of *Heterodera cajani* and *Meloidogyne javanica* caused by *Pasteuria penetrans*. *International Pigeonpea Newsletter* 10: 26-27.

Sharma, Renu and Swarup, Gopal. 1988. Pathology of cyst nematodes. Malhotra Publishing House, New Delhi, India, pp. 88.

Sharma, S. B. 1985a. A world list of nematode pathogens associated with chickpea, groundnut, pearl millet, pigeonpea and Sorghum. Pulse Pathology Progress Report-42, Patancheru, ICRISAT, India.

Sharma, S. B. 1985b. Nematode diseases of chickpea and pigeonpea. Pulse Nematology, Progress Report-43, Patancheru, A. P., ICRISAT, India.

Sharma, S. B. 1988. Nematology in the year 2000 AD as I see it in relation to dryland farming. Pages 44-52 *In*: Nematology in 2000 AD, Professor Gopal Swarup Felicitation Committee, ICAR, New Delhi, India.

Sharma, S. B. 1991. Nematode caused problem management in Indian Agriculture. *Everyman's Science*, Feb.-March, 1991 : 3-7.

Sharma, S. B., Ali, S. S., Patel, D. J., Patel, H. V., Patel, B.A. and Patel, S. K. 1993a. Distribution and importance of plant parasitic nematodes associated with pigeonpea in Gujarat state, India. *Afro-Asian Journal of Nematology* 3: 55-59.

Sharma, S. B., Ali, S. S., Upadhyay, K. D. and Ahmed, F. 1996a. Potential nematodes constraints of pigeonpea in Uttar Pradesh in northern India. *Afro-Asian Journal of Nematology* 6:151-155.

Sharma, S. B. and Ashok Kumar, P. 1991. A technique to evaluate pigeonpea for resistance to *Rotylenchulus reniformis*. *Annals of Applied Biology* 119 : 323-330.

Sharma, S. B., Ashok Kumar, P. and McDonald, D. 1991. A greenhouse technique to screen pigeonpea for resistance to *Heterodera cajani*. *Annals of Applied Biology* 118 : 351-356.

Sharma, S. B. and McDonald, D. 1990. Global status of nematode problems of groundnut, pigeonpea, chickpea, sorghum and pearl millet and suggestions for future work. *Crop Protection* 9: 453-458.

Sharma, S. B. and Mohiuddin, M. 1993. Trypan blue strain egg sacs of the root knot nematodes, *Meloidogyne* spp. *International Pigeonpea Newsletter* 17 : 28-29.

Sharma, S. B. and Nene, Y. L. 1985a. Effect of pre-sowing solarization on plant parasitic nematodes in chickpea and pigeonpea fields. *Indian Journal of Nematology* 15 : 277-278.

Sharma, S. B. and Nene, Y. L. 1985b. Additions to host range of pigeonpea cyst nematode *Heterodera cajani*. *International Pigeonpea Newsletter* 4 : 42.

Sharma, S. B. and Nene, Y. L. 1986. Extraction of *Heterodera cajani* cysts using modified sieving technique. *Indian Journal of Nematology* 16 : 123-124.

Sharma, S. B. and Nene, Y. L. 1987. A technique to extract *Heterodera cajani* eggs from egg sacs. *International Pigeonpea Newsletter* 6 : 54-55.

Sharma, S. B. and Nene, Y. L. 1988. Effect of *Heterodera cajani, Rotylenchulus reniformis* and *Hoplolaimus seinhorsti* on pigeonpea biomass. *Indian Journal of Nematology* 18 : 273-278.

Sharma, S. B. and Nene, Y. L. 1989. Interrelationship between *Heterodera cajani* and *Fusarium udum* in pigeonpea. *Nematropica* 19 (1) : 21 -28.

Sharma, S. B. and Nene, Y.L. 1990a. Effect of *Fusarium udum* alone and in combination with *Rotylenchulus reniformis* or *Meloidogyne* spp. on wilt incidence, growth of pigeonpea and multiplication of nematodes. *International Journal of Tropical Plant Disease* 8 : 95-101.

Sharma, S. B. and Nene, Y. L. 1990b. Effect of soil solarization on nematodes parasitic to chickpea and pigeonpea. *Journal of Nematology* 22 (S) : 658-664.

Sharma, S. B. and Nene, Y. L. 1992. Spatial and temporal distribution of plant parasitic nematodes on pigeonpea in Alfisol and Vertisol. *Nematropica* 22 : 13-20.

Sharma, S. B., Nene, Y. L., Reddy, M. V. and McDonald, D. 1993b. Effect of *Heterodera cajani* on biomass and yield of pigeonpea on vertisol. *Plant Pathology* 42 : 163-167.

Sharma, S. B., Patel, H. V., Patel, B. A., Patel, S. K., Ali, S. S. and Patel, D. J. 1992a. First report of *Heterodera cajani* on pigeonpea in Gujarat state in India. *International Pigeonpea Newsletter* 16 : 17.

Sharma, S. B. Reddy, B. M. R. and Krishnappa, K. 1992b. Incidence and importance of plant parasitic nematodes on pigeonpea and groundnut in Karnataka state in southern India. *Afro-Asian Journal of Nematology* 2 : 21-26.

Sharma, S. B., Rego, T. J., Mohiuddin, M. and Nageswara Rao, V. 1996b. Regulation of population densities of *Heterodera cajani* and other plant parasitic nematodes by crop rotations on vertisols in semi-arid tropical production systems in India. *Journal of Nematology* 28 : 244-251.

Sharma, S. B., Saka, V. W. and Nene, Y.L. 1985. Plant parasitic nematodes in pigeonpea fields of ICRISAT Centre. *International Pigeonpea Newsletter* 4 : 41-42.

Sharma, S. B., Siddiqui, M. R.,Omega, P. and Singh, L. 1993c. Distribution and potential importance of plant parasitic nematodes associated with pigeonpea in Kenya. *Afro-Asian Journal of Nematology* 3 : 182-187.

Sharma, S. B., Smith, D. H. and McDonald, D. 1992c. Nematology constraints of chickpea and pigeonpea production in the semi-arid tropics. *Plant Disease* 76 : 868-874.

Sharma, S. B. and Swarup, Gopal. 1984. Cyst Forming Nematodes of India. Cosmo Publications, New Delhi, India, pp. 152.

Siddiqui, M. R. and Basir, M. A. 1987. *In* : Plant Parasitic Nematodes Problems and Progress (Eds. Gopal Swarup, D. R. Dasgupta). Indian Agricultural Research Institute, New Delhi, pp.104-120.

Siddiqui, M. R., Gupta, P. and Ali, Hyder. 1998. Screening of pigeonpea varieties for resistance to the pigeonpea cyst nematode, *Heterodera cajani*. *Annals of Plant Protection Science* 6 : 193-196.

Siddiqui, Z. A., Hussain, S. I. and Fazal, M. 1991. Response of twenty varieties of pigeonpea (*Cajanus cajan* L.) against *Meloidogyne javanica*. *Current Nematology* 2(2) : 139-142.

Siddiqui, Z.A. and Mahmood, I. 1996a. Effect of *Heterodera cajani Meloidogyne* and *Fusarium udum* on the wilt disease complex of pigeonpea. *Indian Journal of Nematology* 26 : 102-104.

Siddiqui, Z. A. and Mahmood, I. 1996b. Biological control of *Heterodera cajani* and *Fusarium udum* on pigeonpea by *Glomus mossae, Trichoderma harzianum* and *Verticillium chlamydosporum*. *Israel Journal of Plant Sciences* 44 : 49-56.

Singh, J. and Rao, A. S. H. 1974. Quantitative estimation of viable *Heterodera* cyst in arhar (*Cajanus cajan*) field at Varanasi. *Indian Journal of Zootomy* 14 (1) : 19-21.

Singh, K. P., Krishna Behari and Singh, U.P. 1989. Effect of culture filtrate of fungi colonizing neem cake on *Heterodera cajani*. *Indian Phytopathology* 42 : 286 (Abst.).

Singh, K. P., Krishna Behari and Singh, V. K. 1991. Effect of cultural filtrates of neem cake on *Heterodera cajani*. *Current Nematology* 2 (1) : 9-14.

Singh, K. P. and Jayawant, Raja. 1985. Association of *Heterodera cajani* and *Rotylenchulus* sp. with wilted arhar plants. *Indian Phytopathology* 38 : 621.

Singh, K. P. and Singh, P. K. 1988a. Effect of different levels of inoculum of *Heterodera cajani* on the manifestating of symptoms in pigeonpea. *Indian Phytopathology* 41 : 279.

Singh, K.P. and Singh, V. K. 1988b. Effect of time of inoculation with standard inoculum of *Heterodera cajani* on the manifestation symptoms in pigeonpea. *Indian Phytopathology* 41 : 279.

Singh, K. P. and Singh, V. K. 1992a. *Terminelia arjuna* leaf powder reduces population density of *Heterodera cajani*. *International Pigeonpea Newsletter* 16: 17-18.

Singh, M. and Sharma, S. B. 1996. Emergence of *Heterodera cajani* juveniles from cysts and egg sacs. *Indian Journal of Plant Protection* 24 : 90-97.

Singh, M., Sharma, S. B. and Anders, M. M. 1994. Plant parasitic nematode densities in cereal and legume based cropping systems on vertisol. *Afro-Asian Journal of Nematology* 4: 44:50.

Singh, N. D. 1975a. Effect of oxamyl applications on eelworm penetration into roots of tomato, lettuce and pigeonpea. *Tropical Agriculture* 52 : 369-373.

Singh, N. D. 1975b. Evaluation of nematode population in pigeonpea. Pages 147-149 *In* : Tropical diseases of legumes (Eds. J. Bird, K. Maramorosch). New York, USA : Academic Press.

Singh, N. D. 1975c. Studies on the selected hosts of *Rotylenchulus reniformis* and its pathogenicity to soybean (*Glycine max*). *Nematropica* 5 : 46-51.

Singh, N. D. and Farrell, K. M. 1972. Occurrence of *Rotylenchulus reniformis* in Trinidad, West Indies. *Plant Disease Reporter* 56 : 551.

Singh, S. K., Ahmad, S., Khan, A. and Mukhtar, J. 1988. Efficacy of aldicarb as seed treatment for the control of root knot nematodes *Meloidogyne incognita* on pigeonpea. *Indian Journal of Applied Pure Biology* 3 (2) : 73-77.

Singh, V. K. and Singh, K.P. 1992b. Effect of some medicinal plants leaves or *Heterodera cajani* and pigeonpea. First Afro-Asian Nematology Symposium, Afro-Asian Society of Nematologists. November 29 to Dec. 3, 1992. Department of Botany, Aligarh Muslim University, Aligarh, India, pp. 39.

Singh, V. K. and Singh, K.P. 1992c. Effect of some granular nematicides on *Heterodera cajani* on pigeonpea. First Afro-Asian Nematology Symposium, Afro-Asian Society of Nematologists. Nov. 29-Dec. 3, 1992. Department of Botany, Aligarh, Muslim University, Aligarh, India, pp. 39.

Singh, V. K. and Singh, K.P. 1995. Development and pathogenicity of *Heterodera cajani* on susceptible and moderately susceptible cultivars of pigeonpea. *International Journal of Tropical Plant Diseases* 13 : 237-244.

Sitaramaiah, K. 1984. Plant Parasitic Nematodes of India. Today and Tomorrows Printers and Publishers, New Delhi, 292 pp.

Sivakumar, C.V. and Khan, E. 1981. Two new species of *Scutellonema* (Nematoda : Tylenchida) from Tamil Nadu, India. *Indian Journal of Nematology* 11 : 47-52.

Sivakumar, C.V. and Seshadri, A.R. 1971. Life history of the reniform nematode *Rotylenchulus reniformis* Linford and Oliveira, 1940. *Indian Journal of Nematology* 1 : 7-20.

Starr, J. L. 1979. Plant parasitic nematodes associated with Sorghum, pearl millet, groundnut, chickpea and pigeonpea of ICRISAT, Hyderabad. *Indian Journal of Nematology* 11 : 314-315.

Steiner, G. 1960. (Three conferences about nematology). Miscellaneous Publication No. 32. Rio Pidras, Puerto Rico : Puerto Rico Agricultural Experiment Station, 41 pp.

Stirling, G. R. 1991. Biological control of plant parasitic nematodes. CAB International, Wallingford, 282 pp.

Subramanyam, P., Reddy, M. V., Likoswe, A. A., Saka, V. W. and Muku, W.A.B. 1995. Diseases of pigeonpea in Malawi. *International Pigeonpea Newsletter* 16 : 75.

Swarup, G. 1983. Plant parasitic nematodes associated with pulse crops. *In*: Pulse Production Constraints and Opportunities. Oxford and IBH Publishing Co. Pvt. Ltd., New Delhi, India.

Swarup, G. and Gokte, N. 1986. Cyst forming nematodes. Pages 172-193 *In*: Plant Parasitic Nematodes of India, Problems and Progress (Eds. G. Swarup and D.R. Dasgupta). IARI, New Delhi.

Swarup, G. and Gokte, N. 1987. Cyst forming nematodes of India. Pages 490-500 *In* : Recent Advances in Entomology (Eds. Y. K. Mathur, A. K. Bhattacharya, N. D. Pandey, K. D. Upadhyay and K. P. Srivastava). Gopal Prakashan, Kanpur, U.P., India.

Swarup, G., Prasad, S. K. and Raski, D. J. 1964. Some *Heterodera* sp. from India. *Plant Disease Reporters* 48 : 235.

Taylor, A. L. and Sasser, J. N. 1978. Biology, identification and control of root knot nematodes (*Meloidogyne* spp.) NCSU and United State Agencies for International Development (USAID) Publication, Ill.

Taylor, S. G., Baltensperger, D.D. and Prine, G. M. 1985. Reaction of pigeonpea lines and five other warm season legumes to root knot nematodes, *Meloidogyne* sp. *International Pigeonpea Newsletter* 4 : 45-47.

Thakar, N. A. and Patel, C.C. 1985. Susceptibility of some pigeonpea varieties to root knot nematodes, *Meloidogyne incognita* and *Meloidogyne javanica. International Pigeonpea Newsletter* 4: 43-44.

Thakar, N. A. and Yadav, B. S. 1985a. Screening pigeonpeas for their resistance to reniform nematodes. *International Pigeonpea Newsletter* 4 : 42-43.

Thakar, N. A. and Yadav, B. S. 1985b. Phenolics in pigeonpea roots confer resistance to reniform nematode. *International Pigeonpea Newsletter* 4 : 47-48.

Thakar, N. A. and Yadav, B. S. 1985c. Comparative pathogenicity of the reniform nematodes, *Rotylenchulus reniformis* on a susceptible and resistant variety of pigeonpea. *Indian Journal of Nematology* 15 : 167-169.

Thakar, N. A. and Yadava, B. S. 1986. Role of total phenols in pigeonpea resistant to reniform nematodes. *Indian Journal of Nematology* 16 : 261-263.

Thakar, N. A. and Yadava, B. S. 1987. Evaluation of pigeonpea varieties/lines for resistance against the reniform nematode. *Indian Journal of Nematology* 17 : 132-133.

Tiwari, S. P. and Sharma, S. B. 1997. Development of Phytonematology in India. pp. 85-86 *In* : Proceedings of Diagnosis of key nematode pests of chickpea and pigeonpea and their management 25-30 November 1996, Patancheru. ICRISAT, Patancheru, India.

Tiyagi, S. A., Anvar, S. and Alam, M.M. 1989. Studies on the pathogenicity of root knot and reniform nematodes on pigeonpea. *International Nematology Network Newsletters* 6 (4): 12-15.

Tiyagi, S. A. and Parveen, M. 1990. Effect of stunt nematode *Tylenchorhynchus brassicae* on pollen fertility, water absorption capacity and plant growth of pigeonpea. *International Pigeonpea Newsletter* 12 : 19-21.

Upadhyaya, K.D., Dwivedi, Kusum and Uttam, S. K. 1998. Effect of some plant products against root knot nematode infesting pigeonpea. Page 81 *In*: Abstracts of National Symposium on Management of Biotic and Abiotic Stresses in Pulse Crops, 26-28 June 1998. ISPRD, Indian Institute of Pulses Research, Kanpur, U.P., India.

Upadhyaya, K. D. and Swarup, G. 1972. Culturing, host range and factors affecting multiplication of *Tylenchorhynchus vulgaris* on maize. *Indian Journal of Nematology* 2: 139-145.

Velayutham, B. 1988a. Screening of some pigeonpea varieties/lines for resistance to cyst nematode, *Heterodera cajani. International Nematology Network Newsletter* 5(1) : 18-19.

Velayutham, B. 1988b. Efficacy of nematicidal seed treatment in the control of pigeonpea cyst nematode, *Heterodera cajani.* Koshy 1967, affecting pigeonpea. *Indian Journal of Nematology* 18(2) : 365-366.

Velayutham, B. 1988c. Intensity of infestation of the cyst nematode, *Heterodera cajani* on pigeonpea in the districts of Tamil Nadu, India. *Indian Journal of Nematology* 18: 383-84.

Verma, S. K. and Prasad, S. K. 1969. The reniform nematode, *Rotylenchulus reniformis* Inford and Oliveira 1940. I. Bioecological studies. *Indian Journal of Nematology* 3 (1) : 36-47.

Verma, A. C. and Yadav, B. S. 1975. Occurrence of *Heterodera cajani* in Rajasthan and susceptibility of certain sesame varieties. *Indian Journal of Nematology* 5 : 235-237.

Vilsoni, F. and Heinlein, M. 1984. Influence of intial inoculum levels of reniform nematodes on the growth of mung, pawpaw, pigeonpea and sweet potato. *Fiji Agricultural Journal* 44: 67-70.

Vyas, R. V., Patel, H. R., Patel, B. A. and Patel, D. J. 1995. Parasitism of muscardine fungi on *Meloidogyne incognita* eggs. *Current Science* 69 : 635-636.

Walia, R. K. 1987. Effect of soil texture on the pathogenicity of pigeonpea, cyst nematodes, *Heterodera cajani*. Koshy 1967 on pigeonpea. *Cajanus cajan*. *Indian Journal of Nematology* 17 (1) : 139-142.

Walia, R. K. and Bajaj, H. K. 1986. Existence of host races of pigeonpea cyst nematodes, *Heterodera cajani* Koshy. *Nematologica* 32 (1) : 117-119.

Walia, R. K. and Bajaj, H. K. 1988. Further studies on the existence of races in pigeonpea cyst nematodes, *Heterodera cajani*. *Indian Journal of Nematology* 18 : 269-272.

Walia, R. K., Bajaj, H. K. and Gupta, D. C. 1985. Prevalence of pigeonpea cyst nematodes, *Heterodera cajani* in Bhiwani district (Haryana) along with a new host record. Haryana Agriculture University. *Journal of Research* 15 (4) : 463-464.

Walia, R. K., Bansal, R. K. and Bhatti, D. S. 1990. A new bacterial parasite (*Pasteuria* sp.) isolated from pigeonpea cyst nematode *Heterodera cajani*. *International Nematology Network Newsletter* 7 (3) : 30-31.

Walia, R. K. and Gupta, D. C. 1986. *In*: Nematodes in India, Haryana Agricultural University, Hissar, India, pp. 99-122.

Williams, K. J. Orton. 1980. Plant parasitic nematodes of the Pacific. Technical Report, Commonwealth Institute of Helminthology, Hertfordshire, England, *Technical Report,* Vol. 8, pp. 1-192.

Yadav, B. S. 1986. Nematode problems of pulse crops. Pages 328-335. *In*: Plant Parasitic Nematodes of India, Problems and Progress (Eds. G. Swarup, D. R. Dasgupta). Indian Agricultural Research Institute, New Delhi, India.

Yadava, U. S. and Walia, R. K. 1988. On the biology of the pigeonpea cyst nematode, *Heterodera cajani* Koshy 1967. *Indian Journal of Nematology* 18 (1) : 35-39.

Zaki, F. A. and Bhatti, D. S. 1986a. Pathogenicity of pigeonpea cyst nematode, *Heterodera cajani*. Koshy 1967 on some pulse crops. *Indian Journal of Nematology* 16 (1) : 30-35.

Zaki, F. A. and Bhatti, D. S. 1986b. Effect of pigeonpea cyst nematode, *Heterodera cajani* Koshy 1967 on macro and micro nutrients of pigeonpea and Moth. *Indian Journal of Nematology* 16(1) : 103-105.

Zaki, F. A. and Bhatti, D. S. 1986c. Control of pigeonpea cyst nematodes *Heterodera cajani* Koshy 1967 by chemical seed treatment. *Indian Journal of Nematology* 16 : 106-108.

Zaki, F. A. and Bhatti, D. S. 1987. Aminoacid composition of *Heterodera cajani* infected pigeonpea plants. *International Pigeonpea Newsletter* 6 : 51-52.

7

Microbes in Ecology of Pigeonpea

7.1 Seed Microflora

Seed may contain large number of microorganisms specially fungi which may deteriorate the quality of seed or cause diseases of the plant created from it. The associated fungus may be pathogenic, parasitic or a saprophyte and may be associated internally, externally or as concomitant contaminant with the seed. In fact, the seed works as a vehicle to carry serious pathogens in new areas. Such pathogens are not detected sometimes by the visual examination of seed and the crop grown from it and even the neighbouring crop may be destroyed. The soil may become contaminated from infected seed and the pathogen may establish there so that subsequent crops suffer from the disease. Seeds of pigeonpea harbour large number of fungi and a few bacteria and viruses. The seed borne pathogens causing diseases are dealt under specific diseases while others are being described in this chapter. The fungi associated with seed have been classified in two groups.

7.1.1 Field Fungi

These are the fungi which invade the seed while in the field. The most common genera are *Alternaria, Drechslera, Fusarium, Diplodia, Chaetomium, Phoma, Colletotrichum, Rhizoctonia* etc. The field fungi may cause discolouration of seed, weakening or death of embryo or may cause diseases of plants at later stages of growth like seed rot, seedling rot, root rot, collar rot, hypocotyl invasion, foliage blight/spoting etc. The fungi infect the seed in the field. In Puerto Rico, Ellis *et al.* (1977b, 1977c) isolated *Phomopsis* sp., *Fusarium semitectum, Botryodiplodia (Lasiodiplodia) theobromae* and *Alternaria tenuissima* from seeds of pigeonpea and reported infection in the field. The pod infection by all the fungi occurred at their green stage. The seed infection was noted after maturity when their colour changed from green to white. The timely harvest escaped the seed from infection while 3 weeks delay in harvesting increased the incidence of *B. theobromae, Fusarium* spp. and other total fungi. According to Maximay *et al.* (1992), the pods are infected first followed by seed. They also recorded high incidence of fungal infection of the ovary in the closed flower stage in the field. The infection was comparatively less in 2 weeks old pods but again increased in 4 weeks old pods. In Nigeria, Bankole *et al.* (1996) also isolated *Alternaria* spp., *B. theobromae, Fusarium* spp. and *Phoma* sp. from the freshly harvested seeds of pigeonpea which disappeared after 5-6 months of storage.

The field fungi are mostly pathogenic causing seed/seedling rot and diseases at later stages of plant growth.

7.1.2 Storage Fungi

These are the fungi which invade the seed making it unsuitable for use as seed and hazardous for the health of human beings and animals due to production of certain toxins. These fungi increase in storage under favourable seed moisture content and temperature of storage. The fungi belonging to this group are mostly molds, specially the species of *Aspergillus, Penicillium, Rhizopus* etc. They replace the field fungi or become predominant over the field fungi during the storage. Hepperly and Rodriguez (1984) reported that after storage the incidence of field fungi, namely *Phomopsis* sp., *Cladosporium* sp. and *B. theobromae* remained 15, 26, 30 and 38 % of their respective pre-storage values while incidence of *Penicillium, Rhizopus* and *Aspergillus* spp. increased during the storage period. In Nigeria, Bankole *et al.* (1996) found that the pigeonpea seed had infection of *Alternaria* spp., *B. theobromae, Fusarium* sp. and *Phoma* sp. which gradually disappeared within 5-6 months of storage and were replaced by the storage fungi like species of *Aspergillus, Rhizopus, Penicillium*. The incidence of the storage fungi increased up to the end of the year.

7.1.3 Fungi Detected on Seed

Large number of field and storage fungi have been found associated with the pigeonpea seed which are listed in Table 7.1. Shariff (1973) studied the seed mycoflora of four crops including pigeonpea in India. In Puerto

Rico, several fungi belonging to genera *Alternaria, Cladosporium, Fusarium, Penicillium* and *Phomopsis* were isolated from the surface sterilized seeds of pigeonpea (Ellis *et al.* 1976). The *Phomopsis* sp. was consistantly associated with non-germinated seeds. Shukla and Bhargava (1976a) detected *A. flavus, A. niger, Fusarium equiseti, M. phaseolina* and *Phyllosticta* sp. from the untreated pigeonpea seed. In the same way, Kamal and Verma (1979) isolated 16 fungi from seeds of pigeonpea variety T 21 of which *A. flavus, A. nidulans, A. niger, Alternaria alternata* and *Trichoderma viride* were predominant. Their cultural filtrates were inhibitory to seed germination. The internally seed borne fungi of pigeonpea detected by Ellis and Paschal (1979) belonged to 7 genera and were located mostly in the seed coat but occasionally to embryo. The varieties of pigeonpea may differ in harbouring the seed borne fungi with regard to their number as well as species (Kannaiyan *et al.* 1980). The abnormally looking, wrinkled and discoloured seeds of pigeonpea showed association of more number of fungi (17) as compared to apparently normal seeds which carried only 11 species (Kumar and Srivastava 1985) of which *Aspergillus candidus, B. cinerea, Cladosporium cladosporioides, Colletotrichum graminicola, Curvularia pallescens, Fusarium semitectum, Penicillium rubrum, Rhizopus arrhizus* and *Rhizopus nigricans* were new records and caused seed rot and seedling mortality in pigeonpea. The pigeonpea seed has been found to be susceptible to at least 52 species of fungi belonging to 35 genera many of which cause economically important diseases (Reddy *et al.* 1989). Pande and Verma (1992a) detected a total of 22 fungi belonging to 12 genera from seeds of 6 pigeonpea varieties in Maharashtra and found *A. alternata, Aspergillus* spp. and *Cladosporium cladosporioides* to be the most frequent. In the same way, Lokesh and Hiremath (1992) isolated 9 fungi from pigeonpea seed of which *A. niger, A. flavus, A. alternata* and *F. moniliforme (Gibberella fujikuroi)* were predominant. In Trinidad, Maximay *et al.* (1992) studied seed borne fungi of pigeonpea and found *Phoma sorghina, F. semitectum, F. avenaceum (Gibberella avenacea), A. flavus, A. niger* and *Phomopsis* sp. to be internally associated with seed. Kasar and Memane (1994a) observed varietal differences in pigeonpea with regard to internally and externally associated fungi of seed. They reported that out of 9 fungi isolated, *A. niger, A. terreus, A. fumigatus, F. oxysporum, F. semitectum* and *A. alternata* were pathogenic. Gill *et al.* (1983) examined seeds of 40 leguminous species including pigeonpea and reported *Aspergillus clavatus, A. flavus, A. fumigatus, A. niger, Aspergillus giganteus* and *A. oryzae* to be the most common.

Table 7.1 : Fungi detected from seeds of pigeonpea and their significance

Fungus	*Significance*	*First reported by*
Alternaria spp.	—	Kannaiyan *et al.* (1980)
Alternaria alternata	ISGV, BC	Kamal and Verma (1979)
A. tenuissima	LS	Kamal and Verma (1979)
Aspergillus awamori	BC	Shukla *et al.* (1988)
A. candidus	SSR	Kumar & Srivastava (1985)
A. clavatus	—	Gill *et al.* (1983)
A. giganteus	—	-do-
A. oryzae	—	-do-
A. flaviceps	—	Kamal and Verma (1979)
A. flavus	ISG, SSR, AF, BC	Shukla and Bhargava (1976a)
A. fumigatus	ISG	Kamal & Verma (1979)
A. nidulans	ISG, BC	-do-
A. niger	ISGV, BC	Shukla and Bhargava (1976a)
A. parasiticus	BC, AF	Singh and Sinha (1985)
A. restrictus	ISG	Pande and Verma (1992a)
A. tamarii	—	Kamal and Verma (1979)
A. terreus	—	-do-
Botrytis cinerea	Mold	Kumar and Srivastava (1985)
Botryodiplodia theobromae	ISG	Ellis *et al.* (1977b)
Chaetomium sp.	—	Arya and Mathew (1991)
C. indicum	—	Kamal and Verma (1979)
Cladosporium sp.	—	Arya and Mathew (1991)
C. cladosporioides	ISG, SSR	*Kumar & Srivastava* (1985)
Colletotrichum cajani	Anthracnose	McRae (1932)
C. capsici	SC	Somani *et al.* (1975)
C. graminicola	SSR	Kumar and Srivastava (1985)
C. truncatum	SA	—
Curvularia sp.	—	Charya and Reddy (1983)
C. lunata	BC	Sinha and Prasad (1979)
C. pallescens	—	Kumar and Srivastava (1985)
Drechslera sp.	—	Charya and Reddy (1983)
D. hawaiiensis	ISG, BC	Sinha and Prasad (1981)
D. tetramera	—	Kamal and Verma (1979)
Fusarium sp.	W	Shukla and Bhargava (1976b)
F. equiseti	SSR	-do-
F. moniliforme	BC	Kamal and Verma (1979)
F. avenaceum	SSR	Maximay *et al.* (1992)
F. oxysporum	—	Kasar and Memane (1994a)
F. semitectum (= *F. pallidoroseum*)	ISG, SSR	Ellis *et al.* (1977b)
F. udum	W, ISG	McRae (1924)
Gibberella avenacea	—	See *F, avenaceum*
G. fujikuroi	—	Lokesh and Hiremath (1992)
Lasidiplodia theobromae	ISG	See *B. theobromae*
Macrophomina phaseolina	SSR, DL	Shukla and Bhargava (1976a)

Table 7.1 *contd.*

Fungus	*Significance*	*First reported by*
Mucor sp.	—	Arya and Mathew (1991)
Nematospora coryli	—	Wallace (1932)
Nigrospora sp.	—	Charya and Reddy (1983)
Penicillium spp.	—	-do-
P. chrysogenum	ISG	Kamal and Verma (1979)
P. funiculsum	—	-do-
P. rubrum	SSR	Kumar and Srivastava (1985)
Phoma sp.	—	Charya and Reddy (1983)
Phoma cajani	SC	—
Phoma sorghina	—	Maximay *et al.* (1992)
Phomopsis sp.	ISG	Ellis *et al.* (1977b)
Phyllosticta sp.	—	Shukla and Bhargava (1976a)
Rhizoctonia sp.	Pathogenic	Charya and Reddy (1983)
R. bataticola	RR	Kannaiyan *et al.* (1980) see *M. phaseolina*
R. solani	RR	Kamal & Verma (1979)
Rhizopus sp.	—	Charya *et al.* (1983)
R. arrhizus	SSR	Kumar & Srivastava (1985)
R.stolonifer	SSR, BC	Kamal and Verma (1979)
Trichoderma sp.	—	Charya and Reddy (1983)
T. viride	ISG, AG	Kamal and Verma (1979)

AF = Aflatoxin production
AG = Antagonistic to fungi
BC = Biochemical changes
DL = Diseases at later stages
ISG = Inhibition of seed germination and vigour
LS = Leaf spots
RR = Root rot
SA = Stem anthracnose
SC = Stem canker
SSR = Seed and seedling rot
W = Wilt

Table 7.2 : Bacteria and viruses associated with pigeonpea seed

Microorganism	Significance	Reported by
Pseudomonas syringe pv. *phaseolicola*	Halo blight	Hayward *et al.* (1983)
Xanthomonas campestris pv. *cajani*	LS, SC	Patel and Jindal (1970)
Tomato black ring virus	—	Kaiser *et al.* (1978)

7.1.4 Significance of Fungi Associated with Seed

Viability and Vigour of Seed: The fungi while growing on seed produce certain metabolites which may prove toxic to seed resulting in its death or loss in vigour. Pathak and Maheswari (1973) studied a sample of pigeonpea seed in which about 60% seeds were distorted and apparently in the form of decay. A number of Aspergilli were associated with such seeds. It has been reported that *A. flavus* causes seed and seedling rot while *Fusarium* spp. are responsible for wilt in pigeonpea (Shukla and Bhargava 1976b, 1978). Reduction in germination of pigeonpea seed has been reported not only by fungus but also by cultural filtrate free from spores, mycelium etc. specially in cases of *A. alternata, Aspergillus flavs, A. fumigatus, A. niger, A. nidulans, A. restrictus, A. terreus, Drechslera hawaiiensis, Cladosporium cladosporioides, Fusarium moniliforme, Penicillium chrysogenum, Rhizopus nigricans, Trichoderma viride* (Kamal and Verma 1979, Pathak *et al.* 1981, Lokesh *et al.* 1987, Arya and Mathew 1991a, Lokesh and Hiremath 1992 and Pande and Verma 1992a). The association of several fungi internally with pigeonpea seed has been reported to be negatively correlated with the germination of seed in laboratory and their emergence in the field. Such fungi are *Phomopsis* sp., *Lasiodiplodia (Botryodiplodia) theobromae, F. semitectum* and *A. tenuissima* (Ellis *et al.* 1977b and 1978, Hepperly and Rodriguez 1984). Not only seed and seedling rots, the fungus associated with seed may cause leaf spots and other diseases at later stages of plant growth (Kumar and Srivastava 1985).

Most of the Aspergilli have been reported to deteriorate the seed and hamper its viability and vigour but a few species have been found to promote the process of seed germination and to increase elongation of radicles and plumules of pigeonpea (Kamal *et al.* 1981).

Mycotoxin Production : Some fungi produce toxins while growing on seed which are highly hazardous for the lives of human beings, birds or animals when consumed. The best known toxin is aflatoxin produced by *Aspergillus flavus* in most of the seeds including pigeonpea. Infection of pigeonpea seed by *A. parasiticus* may cause accumulation of aflatoxin B1 @ 11.44 mg/100g of seed within seven days of incubation (Singh and Sinha 1985). In Nigeria, Bankole *et al.* (1996) reported appearance of storage fungi specially *A. flavus* replacing field fungi within 5-6 months of storage. Accordingly aflatoxin was detected in stored seeds after 3-5 months of storage. The storage fungi as well as aflatoxin contents of seed increased with storage time and faster in seeds stored in jute bags as compared to those in iron seed bins. They evaluated 196 isolates of *A. flavus* of which 48% were found toxigenic.

Nutritive Value of Seed/Biochemcial Changes: The fungi by their biological activities while growing on seed, consume some of the seed contents and produce some of the newer ones altering their food value greatly.

The starch contents of pigeonpea seeds is reduced greatly due to infection by *Curvularia lunata* (Sinha and Prasad 1979), by *Aspergillus flavus, A. niger, Alternaria alternata, Drechslera hawaiiensis, F. moniliforme, R. stolonifer* (Sinha *et al.* 1981), by *Aspergillus parasiticus* (Singh and Sinha 1985). The *A. flavus* and *C. lunata* reduces soluble sugars like sucrose and fructose (Sinha and Prasad 1977 &1979) and total and reducing sugars also (Lokesh and Hiremath 1993).

The protein and total nitrogen of the seed also depletes due to invasion of seed by *A. niger* (Sinha *et al.* 1978), *C. lunata* (Sinha and Prasad 1979), *A. flavus, A. niger, A. awamori* and *A. nidulans* (Shukla *et al.* 1988, Lokesh and Hiremath 1993). The reduction in nitrogen is due to its utilization by the fungus and partly by its conversion into gaseous form. The infection also causes complete loss of some of the aminoacids, some are increased while others like threonine, lysine and arginine appear newly. On the other hand, citric acid, tartaric acid and oxalic acid are increased in quantity (Sinha and Prasad 1977 and 1979).

The seed moisture contents, ambient RH and the temperature in the store influence seed mycoflora quantitatively as well as qualitatively which in turn affect the nutritive value of seeds. The higher seed moisture increases the infestation of *A. flavus* while *A. niger* is favoured at low moisture. The high RH exhibits detrimental effect on the nutritive value but it decreases the incidence of *F. moniliforme* in pigeonpea seeds (Lokesh and Hiremath 1993).

7.1.5 Factors Affecting Seed Infection

The extent of infection of seed in the field as well as in storage depends on several factors which are related to host, environment and the pathogen.

Ellis *et al.* (1977b) reported infection of pigeonpea pods by field fungi at the immature and green stage but seed is not infected till it is matured changing colour from green to white. However, delay in harvest after maturity increased the internally seed-borne fungi decreasing the seed germination *in vitro* and field emergence in pigeonpea (Ellis *et al.* 1979a, Hepperly and Rodriguez 1984). Under such situation, increase in fungal infection of seed was observed in bean, cowpea and soybean also (Ellis *et al.* 1977c). In Trinidad, Maximay *et al.* (1992) observed higher fungal infection of ovaries of pigeonpea in the close flower stage as compared to two week old pods. The infection was again more on 4 week old pods in the field. The variety of the host also plays important role in harbouring the seed fungi. Charya and Reddy (1979) found more fungi associated with seeds of local pigeonpea as compared to three hybrids. According to Kannaiyan *et al.* (1980), the genetic differences rather than weather during the pod maturity or different storage periods seem to influence the intensity of seed-borne mycoflora. The incidence of *B. theobromae* and *Fusarium* sp. have been reported to be higher in the seeds of variety 2B-Bushy which has large, tan coloured seeds but it was much less in segregant of the same having small, flattened, hard and red seeds (Hepperly and Rodriguez 1984).

The seed moisture and the storage temperature are the critical factors in the long term storage of pigeonpea seed. Germination of the seed is reduced by the storage fungi and it could be maintained high (90%) even after 1 year at seed moisture contents of 9-13% at ambient temperature in Puerto Rico but not at 17% moisture even in airtight containers (Ellis *et al.* 1979b). However, in the cold storage at 13°C, germination was maintained high irrespective of the storage containers and seed moisture. The incubation temperature exhibits marked effect on the recovery of seed fungi and germination of seed. The apparant health of the seed of pigeonpea improved significantly in respect of fungal association and *in vitro* germination when incubation temperature was changed from 25°C to 35°C (Ellis and Smith 1978).

The weather conditions of the area also play important role in seed infection by fungi and its quality. In Puerto Rico, Ellis and Paschal (1977) reported lesser seed infection by fungi and greater emergence in case of pigeonpea seeds produced in arid regions as compared to seed produced in regions of the islands receiving higher rainfall. The high RH and rainfall at maturity adversely affect the seed quality and increase the fungal infections.

The virulence of a fungus is also an important factor and it is influenced by its nutritional status. Thus Pande and Verma (1992b) found that *A. alternata* was more virulent to pigeonpea variety BDN 1 when grown on galactose, sucrose or maltose as the carbon sources. The fungus *D. hawaiiensis* was also influenced in similar way.

7.1.6 Methods of Detection

The detection of frequency of a fungus associated with the seed depends on the method used for detection of a particular fungus. The standard blotter paper method has been reported to detect more number of fungi from pigeonpea seed as compared to Agar plate method (Charya and

Reddy 1979, 1983). However, Gill *et al.* (1983), found PDA plating method to be better than blotter method for detection of seed borne fungi of 40 leguminous species including pigeonpea. Similarly, Hepperly and Rodriguez (1984) reported PDA plating method to be superior than the cellulose pad method for detection of *B. theobromae, A. tenuissima* and *Phomopsis* sp. as well as for total fungi associated with seeds of pigeonpea. However, *Cladosporium* spp. were detected best by cellulose pad method. The recovery of *A. alternata* is increased by pre-treating the seed with chlorine (Kumar and Pathak 1985).

The incidence of the storage fungi like *Penicillium, Rhizopus,* and *Aspergillus* spp. increased during the storage. Although, less than 3% *Aspergillus* spp. were detected in the pigeonpea seeds by using cellulose pad assay at 27°C but they increased up to 92% by using pigeonpea seed extract agar and incubating at 35°C (Hepperly and Rodriguez 1984). By this method the losses during the storage were highly correlated with incidence of *Aspergillus* spp. which was in contrast to the results obtained by cellulose pad assay.

7.1.7 Effect of Seed Coat Leachate

During the process of germination, certain chemicals are released through the seed coat which is a site of infection by the seed-borne fungi. The seed leachate so released may be inhibitory to spore germination or growth of seed-borne fungi and hence, the seed invasion by such fungi may be influenced. Pigeonpea seed leachate is reported inhibitory to *Curvularia geniculata, F. oxysporum, D. hawaiiensis, A. flavus, Corynespora cassicola, Drechslera rostrata, Penicillium capsulatum, Phaeotrichoconis crotalarae, R. stolonifer* and *A. alternata.*. The inhibition was maximum (88.6%) in *C. geniculata* and minimum (20.5%) in *A. flavus* (Charya and Reddy 1980). The spore germination of *F. udum* was inhibited by the seed coat leachate of all the pigeonpea cultivars tested (Lokesh *et al.* 1987). However, Reddy *et al.* (1994) reported differential liberation of reducing sugars, proteins and polyphenols from different varieties. These chemicals were less in leachates from the white seeded variety as compared to reddish brown seeded variety. The antifungal properties of leachates from different varieties differ greatly and thus may be correlated with their resistance/susceptibility to a fungus.

While discussing the results, Bhargava and Shukla (1979) mentioned that at one hand seed coat leachate inhibits spore germination while at other, the seed germination itself. Under such type of association, the dominance will be of the party which becomes active first. Not only this, the leachate of a seed and metabolites from the fungus may interact with the seed dressing fungicide and thus influencing the final results.

7.1.8 Control

Chemical Seed Treatment: Treatment of seed by fungicides is the best method for controlling the seed-borne fungi. The organomercurial fungicides like Agrosan GN, Ceresan etc. are the broad spectrum ones and are able to control many of the seed-borne fungal pathogens of pigeonpea (Kamal and Verma 1979, Singh 1981, Gupta *et al.* 1984 and Kumar and Srivastava 1985). However, their use is being discouraged specially in pulses looking to their toxicity to human beings, cattles and *Rhizobium* and their character to enter in the food production chain. The *Rhizobium* is considered as the most important component in the pulse production technology. Other conventional seed dressers which have been reported to be effective and useful in controlling seed-borne fungi of pigeonpea are thiram, captan, mancozeb and difolatan (Ellis *et al.* 1977a, Singh 1981, Gupta *et al.* 1984, Pal and Grewal 1985, Thomas and Vyas 1985, Kumar and Srivastava 1985, Lokesh *et al.* 1987, Solanke *et al.* 1990 and Kasar and Memane 1994b). These fungicides exhibited control of seed-borne fungi and improved the seed germination of pigeonpea to a variable extent. According to Ellis and Poschal (1979), the internally seed-borne fungi in pigeonpea were mostly located in the seed coat and hence, captan and thiram could move up to the seed coat resulting in their control and improvement of germination. The captan was found superior to thiram and even the systemic fungicide benomyl which could penitrate up to the embryo of seed. It was also absorbed by roots of pigeonpea and translocated into leaves (Gadewar and Raut 1976). Seed treatment with Benlate T @ 3g/kg is reported to provide complete control of all the seed-borne fungi of pigeonpea and can be recommended to ensure safe international exchange of seed (Kannaiyan *et al.* 1980). Another systemic fungicide which is highly effective is carbendazim/Bavistin (Kumar and Srivastava 1985, Pande and Verma 1992a and Kasar and Memane 1994b). Use of carbendazim not only controlled seed-borne fungi with improved seed germination but it increased the root nodulation (Thomas and Vyas 1985) as well as the yield of pigeonpea (Pal and Grewal 1985). The root nodulation in pigeonpea is increased by seed treatment with triforine and metalaxyl also (Thomas and Vyas 1985).

The spectrum of efficacy of fungicides may be broadened by using the mixture of fungicides for seed treatment. In this direction, combination of carbendazim + thiram has been reported to be the best for pigeonpea (Solanke *et al.* 1990). It has been reported that the response to seed treatment by fungicides is shown better in case of poor quality seed and not in good quality one (Ellis *et al.* 1979c). It should be kept in mind that best fungicide for seed treatment of pigeonpea should control most of the externally as well as internally seed-borne fungi, should not be phytotoxic and toxic to *Rhizobium*. The fungi produce toxic metabolities which may be controlled considerably by irradiation of seed with NUV (Pathak *et al.* 1981).

Biological Control: Biocontrol of seed-borne fungal pathogens has been dealt in respective chapters for controlling the disease caused by them. Most of the seed-borne pathogens and storage fûngi could be eliminated completely by seed treatment with *Trichoderma viride*.

Fungicidal Spray : The field fungi infect the seed in the field itself and establish internally. Seeds of pigeonpea from field grown plants sprayed with benomyl @ 2.2 kg/ha either twice or 4 times at one week interval had significantly fewer internally seed-borne fungi except *A. tenuissima* and significantly greater *in vitro* germination and field emergence than seeds from the non-sprayed crop (Ellis *et al.* 1977b).

Selection of Area: Selection of area is important for seed production. The seed quality of pigeonpea is reported to be correlated with the site of production. The quality of seed produced at Isabela in Puerto Rico, a high rainfall area, was poor in comparison with seed produced at Fortuna, an arid, low rainfall area (Ellis *et al.* 1978).

Timely Harvesting: The incidence of seed-borne field fungi can be reduced greatly by timely harvest of the crop. In Puerto Rico, delaying the harvest of the seed past maturity resulted in a significant increase in the incidence of *Phomopsis* sp., *A. tenuissima, F. semitectum* and *B. theobromae.* Timely harvest is also desirable to maintain suitable level of the seed moisture (9-13%) which otherwise helps in increasing the storage fungi in seed.

Proper Storage: The storage conditions specially temperature, RH, seed moisture and aeration play important role in development of seed fungi specially the storage fungi and deterioration of the seed in the storage. In Puerto Rico, pigeonpea germination could be maintained high (90%) even after 1 year at seed moisture of 9-13% at the ambient temperature. However, in the cold storage (13°C), germination was maintained high irrespective of the storage conditions and seed moisture

(Ellis *et al.* 1979b). The proper seed moisture can be obtained by timely harvesting the crop and proper seed drying before storage. Early harvesting results in high seed moisture while harvesting delayed after the field maturity reduces seed quality. During the storage, RH controls the seed moisture as the seeds are hygroscopic in nature. Higher temperature accelerates the deterioration of seed by fungi.

The store and seed to be stored should be cleaned well and timely steps should be taken to keep the insects under control. The type of storage containers are also important. The pigeonpea seeds stored in jute bags contain more fungi and deteriorate faster as compared to those stored in iron bins.

Quarantine Regulations: The check on spread of pathogens in new areas through quarantine regulations is important although, these measures have never been considered seriously for pigeonpea. Some diseases like anthracnose, bacterial leaf spot, stem canker, sterility mosaic, yellow mosaic are considered important for quarantine in India (Naidu and Nirula 1979). The pathogen *Colletotrichum cajani* (*Glomerella cingulata*) was intercepted on a flight from the Puerto Rico to U.S.A. (Anonymous 1952).

7.2 Rhizosphere Microflora

The roots of living plants release certain organic substances in the soil in the form of root exudates due to which they create a zone of their own environment around them which is more uniform but different from that of the soil away from it. This zone created around the root is termed as 'rhizosphere'. The substances released by roots differ quantitatively as well as qualitatively in different species and even varieties of plants. Accordingly, microflora developed in the rhizosphere soil of a plant differ greatly from the nearby soil and also from the rhizosphere soil of other species/variety of plants. The rhizosphere microflora may include the pathogen of that plant, the antagonists to the pathogen, stimulator to the pathogen and the non-interfering saprophytes. Thus, their activity in the rhizosphere play important role in the infection by a pathogen and development of the disease caused by root pathogen.

The leguminous plants including pigeonpea have been found to support large bacterial population in their rhizosphere as compared to non-leguminous plants (Agnihothrudu 1953, Bagyaraj and Ramaswami 1965). Sharma (1965) reported more fungi under the cover of pigeonpea as compared to cowpea and suggested that the soil microflora are influenced more by the soil surface cover as compared to edaphic factors although, effect of the rhizosphere is very important. On the other hand, Edward *et al.* (1977) found less number of fungi in rhizosphere of pigeonpea as compared to other legumes which they attributed to rainfed cultivation practices adòpted for pigeonpea which is unfavourable to multiplication of fungi. Large number of fungi have been isolated from the rhizosphere of pigeonpea which include 16 ascomycetes (Agnihothrudu 1958), fifty deuteromycetes (Agnihothrudu 1959) of which *Melanospora brevirostrata, Aspergillus giganteus* and *Oedocephalium coprophilum* were new records for India (Agnihothrudu 1955). Kamal and Verma (1976) isolated several fungal species from pigeonpea field of which 31 were from non-rhizosphere, 23 from rhizosphere and 22 from rhizoplane. But in general, the population is always reported higher in the rhizosphere/rhizoplane than the non-rhizosphere soil (Rao *et al.* 1987). In addition to fungi, bacteria and actinomycetes, and nematodes have also been reported to be influenced by the rhizosphere (Edward *et al.* 1977).

All these microflora, directly or indirectly are influenced in the rhizosphere by several factors relating to host, soil and pathogen itself.

7.2.1 Plant Varieties

The resistance or susceptibility of a variety determines the types of microflora supported by the rhizosphere. Agnihothrudu (1955) isolated *Streptomyces griseolus* and *S. erythrochromogenes* from the rhizosphere of wilt resistant variety of pigeonpea. They were inhibitory to *F. udum* and the inhibitory effect was more when tested on the medium containing exudate from the roots of resistant plant and much less when exudate was used from the susceptible plant. The total population was also larger in rhizosphere of the wilt susceptible than resistant variety of pigeonpea (Agnihothrudu 1957). No potent antagonistic microorganism could be isolated from the rhizosphere of wilt resistant pigeonpea variety C 11-6 (Murthy and Bagyaraj 1978). However, it has been concluded that the pathogen *F. udum* and other *Fusarium* spp. are predominant in the rhizosphere of susceptible variety of pigeonpea while antagonistic fungi like *Trichoderma viride, Aspergillus niger* and certain actinomycetes were isolated from the rhizosphere of resistant variety only (Saik and Nusrath 1987, Rao *et al.* 1987). *T. viride* was found antagonistic to *Fusarium solani* also (Singh and Rai 1983).

7.2.2 Age of the Plant

Age of the plant also influences the activities of the rhizosphere microflora due to change in quality of root exudate. The vegetative growth and sporulation of *F.udum* as well as total fungi in the rhizosphere increased with the increasing age of the plant (Khanna and Singh 1974, Khan and Prakash 1987). According to Rao *et al.* (1987) fungi, bacteria and actinomycetes increase in the rhizosphere of pigeonpea from seedling to pre-flowering but decrease at pod formation stage of plant. In case of the plants inoculated by the wilt pathogen, the parasitic forms increase while saprophytes decrease with the age of plant. On the other hand, Khanna and Singh (1975) found the population of fungi and actinomycetes to be inversely related with the age of plant and the optimum bacterial activity at the stage of maximum plant growth.

7.2.3 Plant Health

In general, the wilt affected plants have shown greater number of fungi than the bacteria in rhizosphere (Agnihothrudu 1957). According to Upadhyay and Rai (1982), the pathogen, *F.udum* was always recorded on the rhizoplane of the wilt affected plants and comprised 90% of the total suppressing the population of actinomycetes. In the early stages, the population of *F.udum* decreased on the decaying roots of the wilted plants but increased on that of the healthy ones. Rhizosphere of healthy Kants had more population of *Aspergillus* and *Penicillium* sp. and bacteria while *F.udum* dominated in rhizosphère of wilt affected plants and non rhizosphere soil (Pandy and Upadhyay 2000). *T. harzianum*, *T. viride* and *Gliocladium virens* were antagonistic to *F.udum* in various ways.

Kàmal *et al.* (1975a) observed differences in the microflora make up in the roots of healthy and arhar mosaic affected plants. The rhizosphere effect was greater in healthy plants than the diseased one. The rhizosphere microflora were reduced in case of infected plant and the reduction was correlated with the severity of infection, although, qualitative change in the microflora was not observed (Kamal *et al.* 1975b).

7.2.4 Crop Rotation

The rhizosphere microflora of pigeonpea was modified when it was grown in the soil previously planted with *Ablemoschus esculentus* and Sorghum (Reddy and Rao 1991).

7.2.5 Soil Amendments

The amendment of soil with oil cakes and the saw dust is reported to enhance the activity of *Fusarium* spp. However, rhizosphere of pigeonpea suppressed the stimulatory effect of amendment and even reversed the low magnitude stimulatory effect into the inhibitory effect (Khanna and Singh 1974). In the another study, the oil cake was found stimulatory while saw dust was inhibitory to microflora. In such case, the pigeonpea rhizosphere reduced the stimulatory effect of oil cake on bacteria and actinomycetes but accentuated the inhibitory effect of saw dust (Khanna and Singh 1975). The wilt pathogen *F.udum* was stimulated in the pigeonpea rhizosphere and also by the root exudate (Kaiser and Sengupta 1978).

7.2.6 Solarization

The solarization increased the soil temperature to 42-46°C after which 6 fungi were recovered from the rhizosphere of resistant variety and 9 from susceptible ones (Arya and Mathew 1993).

7.2.7 Microflora and Soil Fungistasis

The fungal population was maximum at depth of 10 cm along the root of pigeonpea and much less away from the root region (Ghosh and Mukherjee 1969). A close correlation was observed between the soil micropopulation and the fungistasis of the soil (Mishra and Pandey 1975). The fungistasis of the rhizosphere soil of pigeonpea has been found to be more in the month of December-January when the population of microflora was also more. The fungistasis in the soil could be induced by adding fungi like *Alternaria tenuis, Verticillium* spp. and *Fusarium nivale* or their filtrates, the maximum being by *A. tenuis* (Mishra and Pandey 1981).

7.2.8 Activity of Pathogen in the Rhizosphere

The pigeonpea wilt pathogen *F. udum* has been found to possess high survival capacity as it is able to parasitize several fungi in the rhizosphere of pigeonpea. It is reported to produce pectin methyl esterase, polygalacturonase and cellulase and its cultural filtrate when added to the base of 25 days old pigeonpea seedlings, increased the bacterial population in the rhizosphere within 24 h after treatment (Hiremath *et al.* 1973). It could parasitize the mycelium of *Curvularia lunata, Rhizoctonia solani* from the rhizosphere of pigeonpea (Upadhyay and Rai 1983). Similarly, *F. oxysporum* was found parasitic on *Cunninghamella echinulata,* and *Aspergillus luchuensis.* The fungus *Coprinus lagopus* was found frequently associated with *F.udum* in rhizosphere of pigeonpea (Upadhyay and Rai 1979).

7.3 Microflora of the Phyllosphere/Air Over Crop

The air mycoflora over the pigeonpea field included several species of *Aspergillus* (Verma and Kamal 1979). In another studies, *Drechslera* and *Epicoccum* spp. were at maximum concentrations during the winter months with cool and dry environment while *Penicillium* was maximum in the wet and warm seasons (Verma and Kamal 1980). The species of *Curvularia* were the major type followed by *Corynespora, Chaetomium* and *Choanephora* over the pigeonpea field. Out of these, *Chaetomium* was maximum during winter while others during the rainy season (Verma *et al.* 1982). The *Choanephora* is responsible for wet leaf blight disease in pigeonpea while *Corynespora* causes leaf spot/blight in several leguminous plants. The spores of *Cercospora, Diplodia, Drechslera* and *Epicoccum* have also been trapped from the air over the pigeonpea field in the manner which indicates their discontinuous distribution (Verma and Kamal 1982). The *Cercospora* and *Drechslera* were found abundant in the warm wet months while *Diplodia* and *Epicoccum* were favoured by the moderate temperature and low RH. They are considered as the pathogenic genera on leguminous plants and their presence may play significant role in developing epiphytotic of foliar diseases of pigeonpea. The *Choanephora*, a leaf blight pathogen of pigeonpea was caught regularly except November and January peaking in October. They had tendency to occur abundantly in rainy season. It has rapid increase in the catches from morning onwards with the daily peak at noon indicating the existence of a mid-day pattern in the incidence of the conidia which is attributed to increasing temperature and low humidity.

The spores of *Corynespora* appeared with the maximum count in November and September. Its high concentration after the rainy season appears to be related to low humidity and rainfall.

REFERENCES

Agnihothrudu V. 1953. Soil conditions and root disease. Pt 8. Rhizosphere microflora of some of the important corp plants of south India. *Proceedings of the Indian Academy of Sciences,* Sect. B 37 : 1-13.

Agnihothrudu, V. 1955. Incidence of fungistatic organisms in the rhizosphere of pigeonpea (*Cajanus cajan*) in relation to resistance and susceptibility to wilt caused by *Fusarium udum* Butler. *Naturwissenschaften* 42 : 1-2.

Agnihothrudu V. 1957. The density of rhizosphere microflora of pigeonpea (*Cajanus cajan* (L.) Millsp.) in relation to the wilt caused by *Fusarium udum* (*F. merismoides*) Butler. *Naturwissenschaften* 44 : 497.

Agnihothrudu, V. 1958. Fungi isolated from rhizosphere. 4. *Indian Journal of Botanical Society* 37 : 422-431.

Agnihothrudu, V. 1959. Fungi isolated from rhizosphere. 5. *Journal of Madras University* Sect. B 29 (3) : 155-181.

Agnihothrudu, V., Bhuvaneswari, K. and Suryanarayana, S. 1955. Fungi isolated from rhizosphere. 1. *Proceedings, Indian Academy of Science* Sect. B 43 : 98-104.

Anonymous. 1952. List of intercepted plant pests. United States Department of Agriculture 1951. Washington, DC, USA : USDA 61 pp.

Arya, Arun and Mathew, D.S. 1991a. Variation in seed germination of pigeonpea following treatment with fungal metabolites. *Indian Phytopathology* 44 : 392-394.

Arya, Arun and Mathew, D.S. 1991b. Seed mycolfora of pigeonpea. *Acta Botanica Indica* 19: 102-103.

Ayra, Arun and Mathew, D.S. 1993. Studies on rhizosphere microflora of pigeonpea : Qualitative and quantitative incidence of microorganisms after solarization. *Indian Phytopathology* 46 : 151-154.

Bagyaraj, D.J. and Rangaswami, G. 1966. On the variation in the rhizosphere effects of some crop plants. *Current Science* 35:238-239.

Bankole, S.A., Eseigbe, D.A. and Enikuomehion, O.A. 1996. Mycoflora and aflatoxin production in pigeonpea stored in jute sacks and iron bins. *Mycopathologia* 132 (3) : 155-160.

Bhargava, S.N. and Shukla, D.N. 1979. Interrelationship studies on some pulses and oil crop seeds with their seed borne fungi. *Proceedings National Academy of Sciences India* B, 49 : 81-84.

Charya, M.A.S. and Reddy, S.M. 1979. Studies on seed microflora of *Cajanus cajan* Millsp. *Geobios* 6 : 299-301.

Charya, M.A.S. and Reddy, S.M. 1980. Effect of *Cajanus cajan* seed coat leachates on germination of some seed borne fungi. *Indian Phytopathology* 33 : 112-113.

Charya, M.A.S. and Reddy, S.M. 1983. Seed mycoflora of pigeonpea. *International Pigeonpea Newsletter* 2 : 55-56.

Dwivedi, R.S. and Arora, D.K. 1975. Fungal colonization of staled agar discs from rhizosphere soil inocula of pigeonpea. *Proceedings Indian Academy of Sciences* Sect. B 41 : 571-575.

Dwivedi, R.S. and Tandon, R.N. 1976. Studies on some aspects of seed mycoflora of pigeonpea. *Proceedings of Indian Science Congress* 63 : 63-64.

Edward, J.C., Singh, K.P., Tripathi, S.C., Sinha, M.L. and Ranade, K. 1977. Rhizosphere mycoflora and nematode fauna of some field crops and vegetables in Allahabad, India. *Allahabad Farmer* 48 : 131-151.

Ellis, M.A., Foor, S.R. and Melendez, P.L. 1976. Effect of internally seed borne fungi on germination of pigeonpea in Puerto Rico. *Memoria de la Sociedad Puertorriquena de Ciencias Agricolas* 2 : 8-9.

Ellis, M.A., Hepperly, P.R., Foor, S.R. and Paschal, E.H. 1977a. Seed treatment of pigeonpea with fungicides, antibiotics and certain solvents under tropical conditions. *Fungicides and Nematicides Tests* 32 : 177-178.

Ellis, M.A., Minor, H.C., Abrams, R. and Julia, F.J. 1979a. Effect of delayed harvest and fungicide sprays on pigeonpea seed quality in Puerto Rico. *Journal of Agriculture of the University of Puerto Rico* 63 : 428-435.

Ellis, M.A. and Paschal, E.H. II. 1977. Methods of controlling internally seed borne fungi of pigeonpea (*Cajanus cajan*). *Proceedings of the American Phytopathological Society* 4 : 176.

Ellis, M.A. and Paschal, E.H. II. 1979. Effect of fungicide seed treatment on internally seed borne fungi, germination and field emergence of pigeonpea (*Cajanus cajan*). *Seed Science and Technology* 7 : 75-81.

Ellis, M.A., Paschal, E.H. II, and Powell, P. 1977b. The effect of maturity and foliar fungicides on pigeonpea seed quality. *Plant Disease Reporter* 61 : 1006-1009.

Ellis, M.A., Paschal, E.H. II, Rosario, E. 1977c. Similarities in the internally seed borne fungi of four leguminous crops. *Proceedings of the American Phytopathological Society* 4 : 176.

Ellis, M.A., Paschal, E.H. II, Ravalo, E.J. and Rosario, E. 1978. Effect of growing locations on internally seed borne fungi, seed germination and field emergence of pigeonpea in Puerto Rico. *Journal of Agriculture of the University of Puerto Rico 62* : 355-60.

Ellis, M.A., Ravalo, E.J. and Smith, R.S. 1979b. Methods for pigeonpea seed storage in Puerto Rico. *Journal of Agriculture of the University of Puerto Rico 63* : 423-427.

Ellis, M.A. and Smith, R.S. 1978. Effect of incubation temperature on recovery of internally seed borne fungi and germination of pigeonpea seed. *Tropical Grain Legume Bulletin* 13/14 : 22-25.

Ellis, M.A., Smith, R.S. and Sambrano, O. 1979c. Effect of fungicide seed treatment on field emergence of poor and good quality pigeonpea (*Cajanus cajan*). *Journal of Agriculture of the University of Puerto Rico* 63 : 8-12.

Gadewar, A.V. and Raut, N.K. 1976. Translocation of benlate in germinating seeds and seedlings of *Cajanus cajan*. *Indian Journal Mycology and Plant Pathology* 6 : 108-109.

Ghosh, P. and Mukherjee, S. 1969. Preliminary note on the study of microflora from the rhizoshere of *Cajanus cajan* Millsp. *Proceedings of the Indian Science Congress* 56 : 317-318.

Gill, L.S., Obi, J.U. and Husaini, S.W.H. 1983. Mycoflora of some Nigerian leguminous seeds. *Legume Research* 6 : 29-33.

Gupta, R.C., Saxena, A. and Pandey, K.N. 1984. Effect of fungicidal treatment on seed mycoflora of *Cajanus cajan* and *Lens esculenta* grown in Tarai region of Nainital. *Madras Agricultural Journal* 71 : 474-475.

Hayward, A.C., Teakle, D.S., Saxena, K.B., Wallis, E.J. and Moffett, M.L. 1983. Report of halo blight of pigeonpea from Australia. *International Pigeonpea Newsletter* 2 : 54-55.

Hepperly, P.R. and Rodriguez, R. 1984. Mycofloral succession and viability losses in piegeonpea seed in Puerto Rico. *Journal of Agriculture of the University of Puerto Rico* 68 : 19-31.

Hiremath, R.V., Balasubramanyam, R.H. and Puranik, S.B. 1973. Effect of cultural filtrate of *Fusarium udum* Butler on the rhizosphere microflora of *Cajanus cajan* (L.) Millsp. *Indian Journal of Microbiology* 12 : 229-230.

Kaiser, S.A.K.M. and Sen Gupta, P.K. 1978. Population of three formae speciales of *Fusarium oxysporum* in the rhizosphere of host and non-host plants. *Indian Journal of Mycological Research* 16 : 41-46.

Kaiser, W.J., Bock, K.R. Guthrie, E.J. and Meredith, G. 1978. Occurrence of tomato black ring virus in potato cultivar Anett in Kenya. *Plant Disease Reporter* 62 : 1088-1092.

Kamal, Mall, T.P. and Srivastava, R.P. 1975a. Rhizosphere mycoflora of some virus infected cultivars of arhar (*Cajanus cajan* (L.) Millsp.). *Technology* 11 : 234-238.

Kamal, Mall, T.P. and Srivastava, R.P. 1975b. Microfungi at the root-soil interface of arhar (*Cajanus cajan* (L.) Millsp.) infected by pigeonpea sterility mosaic virus. *Technology* 11 : 434-436.

Kamal and Verma, A.K. 1976. Microfungal flora in the root region of arhar (*Cajanus cajan* (L.) Millsp.). *Fertilizer Technology* 13 : 155-157.

Kamal and Verma, A.K. 1979. Seed borne mycoflora of arhar (T 21) effect of culture filtrates of some isolates on seed germination and fungicidal treatment. *Indian Journal of Mycology and Plant Pathology* 9 : 41-45.

Kamal, Verma, A.K. and Verma, R.P. 1981. Effect of culture filtrates of certain Aspergilli on germination of arhar (*Cajanus cajan* (L.) Millsp.) seeds. *Biological Bulletin of India*. 3 : 183-186.

Kannaiyan, J., Nene, Y.L. and Sheila, V.K. 1980. Control of mycoflora associated with pigeonpea seeds. *Indian Journal of Plant Protection* 8 : 93-98.

Kasar, S.R. and Memane, S.A. 1994a. Occurrence of seed borne fungi on red gram. *Indian Phytopathology* 47 : 347.

Kasar, S.R. and Memane, S.A. 1994b. Chemical control of seed borne pathogenic fungi of pigeonpea. *Indian Phytopathology* 47 : 347.

Khan, M.A.A. and Prakash, D. 1987. Rhizosphere and rhizoplane mycoflora of inoculated plant of pigeonpea wilt *Fusarium udum* at varying age. *Fitopatologia Brasileira* 12 (3) : 184-190.

Khanna, R.N. and Singh, R.S. 1974. Rhizosphere population of *Fusarium* species in amended soils. *Indian Phytopathology* 27 : 331-339.

Khanna, R.N. and Singh, R.S. 1975. Microbial population of pigeonpea rhizosphere in amended soils. *Indian Journal of Mycology and Plant Pathology* 5 : 131-138.

Kumar, K. and Patnaik, P. 1985. Seed borne nature of *Alternaria alternata* in pigeonpea, its detection and control. *Indian Journal of Plant Pathology* 3 (1) : 69-73.

Kumar, K. and Srivastava, S.S.L. 1985. Fungi associated with pigeonpea seeds, their effect and control. *Indian Journal of Plant Pathology* 3 (1) : 53-56.

Kumar, Pradeep, Anuja and Kumar, K. 2000. Biocontrol of seed borne fungal pathogens of pigeonpea (*Cajanus cajan* (L.) Millsp.). *Annals of Plant Protecton Sciences* 8 : 30-32.

Lokesh, M.S. and Hiremath, R.V. 1992. Studies on seed mycoflora of red gram (*Cajanus cajan* (L.) Millsp.). *Karnataka Journal of Agricultural Sciences* 5 : 353-356.

Lokesh, M.S. and Hiremath, R.V. 1993. Effect of relative humidity on seed mycoflora and nutritive value of red gram (*Cajanus cajan* (L.) Millsp.). *Mysore Journal of Agricultural Sciences* 27 : 268-71.

Lokesh, M.S., Hiremath, R.V. and Hegde, R.K. 1987. Seed mycoflora of red gram (*Cajanus cajan* (L.) Millsp.). *Plant Pathology Newsletter* 5 (1-2) : 31.

Maximay, S., Duncon, E.J. and Brathwaite, C.W.D. 1992. Internally seed borne fungi of pigeonpea (*Cajanus cajan* (L.) Millsp.) in Trinidad: isolation and occurrence. *Tropical Agriculture* 69 : 260-62.

McRae, W. 1923. Report of the Imperial Mycologist. Scientific reports of the Agricultural Research Institute, Pusa 1922-23. pp. 53-60.

McRae, W. 1924. Report of the Imperial Mycologist. Scientific Reports of the Agricultural Research Institute, Pusa, 1923-24. pp. 41-51.

McRae, W. 1932. Report of the Imperial Mycologist, Scientific Reports of the Imperial Institute of Agricultural Research, Pusa 1930-31 pp. 73-86.

Mishra, R.R. and Pandey, K.K. 1975. Studies on soil fungistasis. Part VII. Studies on colonization of fungi on roots of *Cajanus cajan* in relation to soil fungistasis. *Fertilizer Technology* 12 : 328-330.

Mishra, R.R. and Pandey, K.K. 1981. Studies on soil fungistasis. *Tropical Ecology* 22 : 211-218.

Murthy, G.S. and Bagyaraj, D.J. 1978. Rhizosphere microflora of *Cajanus cajan* in relation to Fusarium wilt resistance. Plant and Soil 50 : 485-487.

Naidu, H.P. and Nirula, K.K. 1979. Quarantine important diseases of sorghum, pearl millet, chickpea, pigeonpea and groundnut. *Indian Journal of Plant Protection* 7 : 175-188.

Nirula, K.K. 1980. Quarantine to the seed exchange at ICRISAT. *Seed Pathology News* 13 : 11-12.

Pal, M. and Grewal, J.S. 1985. Effect of fungicidal seed treatment on emergence and seedling mortality of pigeonpea. *Seed Research* 13 : 204-205.

Patel, P.N. and Jindal, J.K. 1970. Bacterial diseases in seed legumes in 1968 and 1969. Paper presented at the fourth annual workshop conference on pulse crops held at Ludhiana, April, 1970.

Pande, Alka and Varma, K.V.R. 1992a. Seed borne fungi of pigeonpea: their pathogenicity and fungicidal control. *Biovigyanam* 18 : 33-38.

Pande, Alka and Varma, K.V.R. 1992b. Influence of C and N sources on growth and sporulation and aggressiveness of three seed borne fungi in pigeonpea. *Indian Phytopathology* 45 : 213-216.

Pandey, K.K. and Upadhyay, J.P. 2000. Microbial population from rhizosphere and non rhizosphere soil of pigeonpea : Screening for resident antagonist and mode of mycoparasitism. *Journal of Mycology and Plant Pathology* 30 : 7-10.

Pathak, P.D. and Maheshwari, D.K. 1973. Deterioration of seed of *Cajanus cajan* Linn. by *Aspergilli* in storage. *Balwant Vidyapeeth Journal of Agricultural and Scientific Research* 15 : 97-100.

Pathak, P.D., Sharma, O.P. and Sharma, K.D., 1981. Effect of near ultraviolet irrediation on toxin production by certain fungi. *Indian Phytopathology* 34 : 525-527.

Rao, V.K., Ram Chandra Reddy, A.G. and Satyanarayana, K. 1987. Quantitative changes in the rhizosphere microflora of wilt resistant and susceptible varieties of pigeonpea. *Indian Journal of Mycology and Plant Pathology* 17 : 59-61.

Reddy, C.N., Gudige, C.A. and Singh, Rajendra. 1994. Effect of seed coat leachates on seed borne pathogens of pigeonpea. *Indian Journal of Mycology and Plant Pathology* 24 : 128-131.

Reddy, K.S. and Rao, C.G.P. 1991. Studies on the influence of root system of *Ablemoschus esculentus* and *Sorghum vulgare* on the rhizosphere and rhizoplane mycoflora of *Cajanus cajan*. *Journal of Phytological Research* 4 : 41-48.

Reddy, Ravinder, Ch. Ahmad, K.M., Joshi, N.C. and Ratna, A.S. 1989. Health status of seeds of ICRISAT mandate crops in relation to plant quarantine. Pages 210-220 *in* : Proceedings of National Seminar on Advances in Seed Science and Technology, 14-16 Dec. 1989, Department of Studies in Applied Botany, University of Mysore, Mysore, India.

Shaik, Imam and Nusrath, M. 1987. Varietal variation in the rhizosphere and rhizoplane mycoflora of *Cajanus cajan* (L.) Millsp. with special reference to wilt disease. *Indian Journal of Botany* 10 : 126-129.

Shariff, M.H. 1973. Studies on the mycoflora associated with seeds of wheat, paddy, pigeonpea and Bengal gram from three different storage conditions. M.Sc. thesis, University of Allahabad, Allahabad, Uttar Pradesh, India.

Sharma, M.C. 1965. Soil micro-fungi in relation to certain edaphic factors and arhar and cowpea crops. *Proceedings of the Indian Science Congress* 52 : 323.

Shukla, D.N. and Bhargava, S.N. 1976a. Fungi isolated from seeds of pulses. *Proceedings of National Academy of Sciences of India*, Section B 46 : 453-455.

Shukla, D.N. and Bhargava, S.N. 1976b. Some pathogenic fungi from pulses and oil seed crops. *Proceedings of the National Academy of Sciences of India*, Section B 46 : 531-532.

Shukla, D.N. and Bhargava, S.N. 1978. Seed and seeding rot of arhar. *Proceedings of National Academy of Sciences of India*, Section B 48 : 167.

Shukla, H.S., Dube, S. Kum. and Tripathi, S.C. 1988. Changes in protein contents of arhar (*Cajanus cajan*) due to fungal association. *Legume Research* 11 : 85.

Singh, Premlata and Sinha, K.K. 1985. Changes in the seed contents of arhar infected with *Aspergillus parasiticus*. *Indian Phytopathology* 38 : 560-561.

Singh, S. 1981. Control of fungal deterioration of pigeonpea (arhar) seeds during storage. *Seeds and Farms* 7 : 41-42, 46.

Sinha, M.K. and Prasad, T. 1977. Deterioration of "arhar" seeds by *Aspergillus flavus*. *Indian Phytopathology* 30 : 70-72.

Sinha, M.K. and Prasad, T. 1979. Changes in seed contents of "arhar" (*Cajanus cajan* (L.) Millsp.) due to *Curvularia lunata*. *Proceedings of the National Academy of Sciences of India,* Section B 49 : 76-80.

Sinha, M.K., Roy, A.K. and Prasad, T. 1978. Reduction in total N contents of arhar seeds due to storage fungi. *Current Science* 47 : 550-551.

Sinha, M.K., Singh, B.K. and Prasad, T. 1981. Changes in starch content of arhar seeds due to fungi. *Indian Phytopathology* 34 : 269-271.

Solanke, R.B., Choulwar, S.B. and Kore, S.S. 1990. Efficacy of some fungicides on seed mycoflora, seed germination and seedling vigour of pigeonpea. *Research Bulletin Punjab University of Sciences* 41 : 109-111.

Somani, R.B., Wangikar, P.D. and Shukla, V.N. 1975. A new stem canker and die-back disease of pigeonpea. *Indian Phytopathology* 28 : 436-437.

Thomas, M. and Vyas, S.C. 1985. Effect of fungicide seed treatment on pigeonpea nodulation. *International Pigeonpea Newsletter* 4 : 62-63.

Upadhyay, R.S. and Rai, B. 1979. *Coprinus lagopus* as potent saprophytic colonizer of pigeonpea in soil. *Science and Culture* 45 : 171-172.

Upadhyay, R.S. and Rai, B. 1982. Ecology of *Fusarium udum* causing wilt disease of pigeonpea; population dynamics in the root region. *Transaction of British Mycological Society* 78 : 209-220.

Upadhyay, R.S. and Rai, B. 1983. Hyphal interaction and parasitism amongst some rhizosphere fungi of pigeonpea. *Indian Phytopathology* 36 : 302-306.

Verma, A.K. and Kamal 1979. An investigation on mycoflora of air over arhar (*Cajanus cajan* (L.) Millsp.) fields. 1. Aspergilli (*Aspergillus* spp.) over pigeonpea. *National Academy of Sciences Letters* (*India*) 2 : 370-374.

Verma, A.K. and Kamal. 1980. Air-spora studies over arhar (*Cajanus cajan* (L.) Millsp.) field-periodicity in the spores of *Drechslera, Epicoccum* and *Penicillium. National Academy Science Letters* (*India*) 3 : 13-17.

Verma, A.K. and Kamal, 1982. Air-spora studies over an arhar (*Cajanus cajan*) field, the diuranil and seasonal periodicity of certain plant pathogens. *Indian Journal of Mycology and Plant Pathology* 12 : 40-45.

Verma, A.K., Verma, R.P. and Kamal, 1982. Air-spora over arhar field. *Indian Phytopathology* 35 : 126-130.

Wallace, G.B. 1932. Report of the Mycologist. Report Department of Agriculture, Tanganyika, 1930, pp. 53-55.

8

Abiotic Stresses

Several abiotic stresses relating to nutritional deficiencies, micronutrient toxicity, faulty crop production practices, environmental disorders etc. result in typical disease like symptoms in plants. Such disorders of pigeonpea have been described and reviewed in detail (Agarwala and Associates 1973, 1978; Reddy *et al.* 1978, Nichols 1964, 1965; Katyal 1981; Chauhan 1987, Johansen 1990, Sharma 1996 and Kumar Rao *et al.* 1996).

Nutritional Disorders

Pigeonpea requires several macro and micro elements for the growth of plants. These elements are drawn from the soil and their deficiencies may result in abnormal growth and reduced yield.

8.1 Micro-Nutrient Deficiencies

Atleast seven microelements, namely iron (Fe), manganese (Mn), copper (Cu), zinc (Zn), molybdenum (Mo), boron (B) and chlorine (Cl) are required in relatively small quantities but they are essential for proper growth of plants. Their deficiency has been identified as a major constraint in crop production. The reasons responsible for suffering of plants due to micronutrient deficiency may be as follows:

(i) Low contents in soil minerals.
(ii) Adverse physico-chemical conditions of root environment.
(iii) Adverse plant-environment interactions.
(iv) Genotypic inefficiency of their up-take.
(v) Root-shoot transport and their utilization.

The deficiency of a microelement causes typical symptoms on a crop/variety and hence, it comes under the category of non-infectious disease of plant. A good illustrated account of symptoms of micronutrient deficiencies has been given by various workers from time to time (Cook and Miller 1953, Viets *et al.* 1954, Olsen 1958, Wallace 1961, Stiles 1961, Hewitt 1963, Sprague 1964, Chapman 1966, Tanaka and Yoshida 1970, Bergmann and Neubert 1970, Katyal 1981, Bergmann 1992 and Sharma 1996).

In general, deficiency may affect the yield of a crop adversely without exhibiting typical symptoms on plants because symptoms are visible when the deficiency is enough to do so. Such condition is referred as 'Hidden hunger'. The critical concentration of micronutrients in plants is referred to that which distinguishes a nutrient-sufficient-plant from a nutrient-deficient-plant.

8.1.1 Iron Deficiency

Pigeonpea has been reported to be sensitive to iron deficiency (Nichols 1964, Sharma 1966). Since, the iron is immobile in the plant, the youngest leaves show the deficiency symptoms first. The interveinal areas of leaves become pale green. In severe cases, whole of the affected leaf area becomes chlorotic and later, small necrotic patches develop. When the plant is subjected to iron deficiency at 4-5 leaf stage, the young leaves turn chlorotic and gradually entire lamina of these leaves become severely chlorotic. These symptoms further spread systematically to middle and older leaves also. With the advancing deficiency, size of young leaves is reduced, they are bleached, their lamina fails to unfold and shows necrosis and scorching. The apical growth dies prematurely and the plants do not go reproductive phase.

In fact, iron is the constituent of nitrogenase and leghemoglobin but this does not necessarily amounts to dependence of nitrogen fixation on this element. This view has been supported by the work of Nichols (1965) also who demonstrated only marginal effect of iron on nitrogen fixation in pigeonpea. In the solution culture, the pigeonpea plants exhibit iron deficiency symptoms at concentrations of less than 65 ppm of iron.

In the field, high *p*H of soil and high lime contents depress the availability of iron to plants which should be kept in mind for rectifying this disorder in pigeonpea.

8.1.2 Manganese Deficiency

Pigeonpea is sensitive to manganese deficiency, the symptoms of which have been described in detail (Agarwala and Associates 1978, Sharma 1996). The pigeonpea plants grown in sand culture with less than 0.0055 ppm manganese exhibited slight depression in growth after 16 days of sowing while actual visible symptoms appeared in 21 days. The symptoms include fading of the green colour of the lamina of middle leaves. This gradually becomes marked and conspicuous but the veins remain green throughout. Later, small, white and brown spots appear in the chlorotic areas which coalesce forming brown necrotic lesions. The tips and the margins of the middle leaves become necrotic and dry. Middle as well as old leaves appear scorched and shed prematurely but the younger ones remain green. The stem of the affected plant remains week with poor branching and reduced leaf size. Most of the branches remain rudimentary and do not develop normally. The growth of apical shoot is arrested and finally killed under severe cases. The flowering is markedly delayed and severely limited.

Rise in *p*H of the soil adversely affect the uptake of manganese by plants (Dalal and Quilt 1977). The analysis of affected plants have indicated that the manganese is concentrated in the lowest branches.

8.1.3 Copper Deficiency

Symptoms of the copper deficiency in pigeonpea have been described by Sharma (1996). The plant can grow normally up to one month in copper deficient culture but afterward the foliage turns bluish green. The apical part of the leaflet of younger leaves shows chlorosis which spreads gradually from apical to the basal part of the laminae. Afterward, the apical part is bleached severely. The newly emerging leaves remain small and unfolded giving them a boat shaped appearance. In acute cases, the apical growth of primary branches ceases inducing auxiliary branches which in turn remain rudimentary and dry within few days of emergence. In general the young shoots loose turgor. The laminae of matured leaves become thicker than the normal. The copper is distributed evenly in affected plants (Dalal and Quilt 1977).

8.1.4 Zinc Deficiency

Analysis of more than 22000 soil samples collected from Bihar, Andhra

Pradesh, Karnataka and Madhya Pradesh indicated 47% of them being zinc deficient.

Zinc deficiency causes typical symptoms on pigeonpea plants (Agarwala and Associates 1973, Shukla and Associates 1976, Reddy *et al.* 1978, Mehrotra *et al.* 1983 and Sharma 1996). The symptoms start as fading of the green colour of the basal portion of the trifoliates of the middle leaves with inward rolling of their margins. The interveinal chlorosis starts from the tip of the trifoliate leaf on all the three leaflets and spreads to the remaining areas leaving only midrib green. Gradually, irregular interveinal pale/fading of green colour develops followed by appearance of buff areas on both sides of midrib. Subsequently, dark coloured necrotic spots develop in these faded areas. The colour of these necrotic spots differ in different varieties (Mehrotra *et al.* 1983). The leaves show severely scorched appearance and shed prematurely. The size of branches and trifoliates is reduced markedly giving little-leaf syndrome to plant. The lamina of young leaves becomes thicker, brittle and rough to touch. The flowering is delayed and their number is reduced. The fertilization is reduced which results in reduced pod/seed formation under severe deficiency of zinc. The premature buds, flowers and fruits may fall and size of pods and seeds is reduced greatly.

The pigeonpea plants affected by zinc deficiency show decreased contents of zinc which is mainly concentrated in the upper branches (Dalal and Quilt 1977) resulting in decreased shoot : root ratio of zinc. The P : Zn and Mn : Zn ratios on the other hand are increased. In the zinc deficient plants, the activity of catalase is decreased while that of peroxidase, ribonuclease and phosphatase is increased (Mehrotra *et al.*, 1983).

The pigeonpea plants grown in sand culture under zinc deficiency exhibited 30 ppm zinc although, the deficiency symptoms on plants start appearing at less than 15 ppm zinc in soil/sand. The critical limit of DTPA extractable zinc in soil for pigeonpea is however 0.48 ppm which is less than for cereals etc. (Gupta *et al.* 1984). It indicates that the pigeonpea has greater ability to absorb native soil zinc than other crops.

More calcium in soil, high soil *p*H and high phosphorous application reduces the availability of zinc to plants in soil (Dalal and Quilt 1977). Agarwala *et al.* (1973) reported differential response of pigeonpea varieties to zinc. The varieties Pant A3 and Prabhat have been reported to be tolerant than other varieties (Shukla and Associates 1976).

8.1.5 Molybdenum Deficiency

Molybdenum is more important for pigeonpea specially for Rhizobial nodulation. It is required for the key enzyme nitrogenase which is responsible for nitrogen fixation. In fact, the requirement of molybdenum for *Rhizobium* is more than for the host itself.

The symptoms of the molybdenum deficiency in pigeonpea appear as mild interveinal chlorosis of middle leaves which turn yellow and later, brown specks develop on the chlorotic areas (Sharma 1996). These specks coalesce giving rise necrotic patches. At the same time, young leaves also develop chlorosis and yellowing. The lamina is broader than normal. The growth of affected plants is arrested, number of flowers is reduced and podding is limited when the deficiency is acute.

High soil *p*H and presence of calcium in soil enhances the availability of molybdenum to pigeonpea plants while in acid soil, plants do not response even to application of molybdenum (Dalal and Quilt 1977).

8.1.6 Boron Deficiency

The boron contents of soil in arid and semi-arid zones is generally higher than those of humid zones although, it may not insure against boron deficiency because free lime in these soils increases soil *p*H which in turn reduces availability of boron (Katyal 1981). The boron has specific function of cell division and the elongation of the growing points of plant.

The symptoms of boron deficiency in pigeonpea plants includes existance of thick, brittle and dark green leaves (Sharma 1996). The stem is thick and the cotyledonary leaves are thicker and dark green in colour. The youngest leaves remain rudimentary and chlorotic while fully expanded leaves show chlorotic areas. Old leaves show browning in between the veins. Lateral branches develop more than the normal plants. The leaves as well as the stem gradually become necrotic, dried and collapse prematurely. According to Reddy *et al.* (1978), boron deficiency results in die-back, rosetting, multiple branching and ultimately death of plants of pigeonpea.

Spray of boron has been reported to exhibit favourable effect on pigeonpea (Reddy *et al.* 1978).

8.1.7 Potassium Deficiency

Amongst the macro nutrients, pigeonpea has been found to respond marginally to potassium. The potassium deficiency symptoms are less ambiguous to recognize. It includes yellowing followed by marginal chlorosis of older pigeonpea leaves (Nichols 1964). Rao and Rao (1984) recorded typical leaf scorching and decreased chlorophyll contents of older leaves of pigeonpea T 21 seedlings when grown under K deficiency. The foliar application of K was found to increase plant height, dry matter accumulation and reduced flower drop conspicuously ultimately increasing yield (Ravindra Nath *et al.* 1985).

8.1.8 Diagnosis of Nutrient Imbalances

It is very necessary to find out the deficiency of nutrients and ensure their sufficiency for optimizing the yields. This can be done through:

(i) Visible symptoms of the deficiency in plants.
(ii) Plant tissues concentrations of the concerned element.
(iii) Assay of nutrient (microelement) dependent biochemical (enzyme) activity.
(iv) Soil test for available micronutrients.

Out of these methods, diagnosis of nutritional deficiencies on the basis of visible symptoms is simplest. The foliar symptoms give an indication of nutrient imbalances but there are certain limitations. Similar symptoms may appear with some other factors and also they appear only after considerable plant growth inhibition. In fact, the symptom manifestation alone should not form the basis for recommendation but plant growth response in field experiments should also be considered. However, symptoms provide guidelines to designing plant growth tests by suggesting type and severity of nutrient imbalances. Analysis of soil and plant becomes helpful in judging the nature of disorder. The typical diagnostic symptoms due to nutrient deficiencies on pigeonpea have been compiled (Johansen 1990) as follows:

Nitrogen (N) :	Classical yellowing of older leaves as for most legumes.
Phosphorus (P) :	No distinct foliar symptoms, plants stunted. Foliage remain dark green, old leaves eventually shed prematurely.

Potassium (K) :	Yellowing followed by necrosis of outer margins of older leaves.
Calcium (Ca) :	Weekness of stem leading to prostrate growth habit. Random light green patches in marginal interveinal regions of terminal leaves. These patches eventually become necrotic and leaves abscise.
Sulphur (S) :	Even yellowing across lamina of mainly youngest leaves but older leaves also eventually become yellow.
Magnesium (Mg) :	Beginning in oldest leaves, in-rolling of leaf margins, interveinal regions lighter green, mesophyll of interveinal regions become bronzed, eventual necrosis.
Zinc (Zn) :	Yellowish white interveinal chlorosis on youngest leaves, leaflets narrowed, the chlorotic areas become reddish brown and leaves abscise. Plants stunted with shortened internodes.
Iron (Fe) :	Distinct interveinal chlorosis of youngest leaves.
Manganese (Mn) :	Leaf spotting and shedding of younger leaves.
Boron (B) :	Deformed youngest leaves resulting in die-back, rosetting and multiple branching.

8.2 Chemical Toxicity

The agrochemicals used for higher production in the form of plant nutrients/fertilizers, fungicides, insecticides, herbicides etc. as well as the chemical environment developing in the soil or the atmosphere influence the plant growth and yield greatly. Their faulty use and imbalanced presence becomes toxic to plants. Such conditions may develop typical symptoms on plants.

8.2.1 Soil Salinity

The pigeonpea is grown in semi-arid regions that are prone to soil salinity. The soil salinity exerts great influence on the growth parameters and yield of pigeonpea. The salts NaCl and Na_2SO_4 have been reported to adversely affect all the growth and yield parameters in pigeonpea

(Joshi and Nimbalkar 1983). Out of these NaCl has been found to be more deleterious than Na_2SO_4 indicating that in addition to osmotic effect there is also a specific ion effect.

The NaCl salinity increases palisade and spongy parenchyma tissues resulting in increased succulency of pigeonpea leaves (Gururaja and Rao 1982). The salinity damage in pigeonpea is characterized by sudden necrosis of the entire lamina and rapid plant death (Subbarao 1988). At the advanced growth stages, salinity symptoms can also appear as the soil dries out due to the increased salt concentrations in the soil solution. The necrosis of leaf margin is observed primarily of old leaves but also of middle leaves of pigeonpea (Johansen 1990). As stated above, the succulency of leaves is increased and it is associated with reduced dimensions of the vessel lumen, increased thickening of vessel walls, presence of thick cuticle and accumulation of leaf epicuticular waxes. These changes play important role in adaptability of plant to salinity and thus the salt tolerance of a genotype (Gururaja and Rao 1989).

The salinity is reported to reduce as much as 50% dry matter yield of pigeonpea increasing P concentration in leaves (Gupta *et al.* 1985). The sodium chloride and the sodium sulphate have been found to increase sugar, Ca, Mg, Na, Cl and SO_4 contents of pigeonpea leaves but reduce total sugars, starch, P, K and accumulation of proline indicating that there is no regulation of uptake of these elements under saline conditions (Joshi 1984).

Genetic variability to salinity tolerance has been observed in pigeonpea. Three techniques for screening pigeonpea against salinity have been described as: (i) Screening in salinity affected field, (ii) Screening in brick chambers and (iii) Screening in pot cultures (Chauhan 1987). The results of all these techniques are comparable. He has reported varieties C 11 and ICP 3786 to be tolerant to salinity. A substantial sources of salinity tolerance has been reported amongst wild relatives of pigeonpea like *Cajanus platycarpus* and *C. albicans* (Subbarao 1988, Sharma *et al.* 1998). Among the cultivated pigeonpea, ICPL 227 and H 82-52 have been found tolerant to salinity stress (Kuhad and Sheoran 1987). The species *C. albicans* readily crosses with cultivated pigeonpea and the salinity tolerance in it seems to be genetically dominant (Subbarao 1988). On the other hand, the resistance to salt stress in variety ICPL 83024 has been found to be controlled by single recessive gene (Verulkar and Singh 1998).

8.2.2 Effect of Herbicides

Some of the herbicides used for weed control have been found to injure/ damage the pigeonpea crop causing typical disease like symptoms. The important ones are:

Apical Distortion Disease : This disease was noticed at the experimental farm, Faizabad, India on pigeonpea variety T 17 and others by Singh and Singh (1982).

The disease is characterized by symptoms which include twisting of apical tips after a downward bending process followed by a twisting of inwardly rolled leaves. The twisted leaves subsequently dry and shed. New coming leaves also develop similar symptoms and the affected plants fail to flower.

The disease was observed near the wheat field where 2, 4-D was applied. The disease similar to that observed naturally could be produced by application of 2, 4-D to pigeonpea. The chain of symptom production lasted for over 2 months finally resulting in burnt up tips. It was concluded that the disease results from the drift of 2, 4-D to neighbouring pigeonpea fields when applied to wheat crop.

Prometryn Injury : In Puerto Rico, fresh weight of pigeonpea plants was found to be reduced by application of prometryn @ 2.24-3.36 kg/ ha in Mollisol soils specially with increasing irrigation regimes. However, such effect was not observed in Ultisol, Oxisol and Vertisol (Liu 1984).

8.2.3 Sulphur Dioxide

The pigeonpea seedlings exposed to sulphur dioxide (SO_2) were found to exhibit chlorosis, tip-burn and marginal necrosis of leaves. Affected seedlings also showed reduced root growth, root nodulation and dry matter accumulation in all the parts (Satyanarayana *et al.* 1985).

8.3 Water Logging

Pigeonpea is highly sensitive to water logging which is most likely and detrimental during the seedling growth in the clay soils. Such soils crack and the rains lead to short term flooding.

8.3.1 Symptoms

Water logging often results in yellowing of pigeonpea crop followed by mortality of plants if the water logging conditions persist further. According to Chauhan (1987), plants of 40 days age are more susceptible to water logging than those of 60 days. The persistance of water logging for 96 hours could kill 50% plants. The water logging damages the root system through anoxia and possibly the effect of ethylene. The root system is completely rotten and discoloured brown. The seedlings are easily pulled out with discoloured portion of central wood while bark is completely rotten, splitted and mostly remain in the soil. A clear cut brown coloured band can be seen at the base of the stem at the level of water. The foliage of the affected plant show water deficit symptoms (Chauhan 1987). The tolerant genotypes develop a swollen structure at the base of the stem followed by air filled, hypertrophied lenticels and adventitious roots in the submerged zone and just above the water surface (Malima *et al.* 1998).

8.3.2 Cause

Water logging causes extensive rotting of roots of plant which seriously decreases the water uptake by roots. The plant mortality occurs due to water deficit in plant. The transpiration lag due to decreased up take of water by the roots under water logging is one reason for death of plants (Bradford and Young 1981). Under cloudy conditions, even several days of water logging may not cause wilting of plants probably because a transpiration lag does not develop under such conditions. The partial water logging may affect the crop growth rate only and plants may survive.

Several factors are responsible to influence the water logging effect on pigeonpea plants. The effect is more pronounced in hot and clear weather with high ambiant day temperature above 35°C. The amount of decomposable organic matter which acts as a substrate for the ethylene evolution by the microorganisms in waterlogged soil is important for death of plant. In sterilized soil, even prolonged water logging did not cause any appreciable mortality in pigeonpea (Chauhan 1987). The greater mortality occurs in soil rich in organic matter. The pigeonpea planted on flat beds are more prone to waterlogging than ridge planted. The ridge and raised bed sowing of pigeonpea has been found to reduce the incidence of phytophthora blight also appreciably. Pigeonpea genotypes differ in their tolerance to water logging (Dubey and Asthana 1987).

Some of the pigeonpea lines/varieties like BDN 1, ICPL 227, JA 4 have been found tolerant to water logging while Hy 3C was highly susceptible. The techniques for screening pigeonpea in field and in pot culture have been described by Chauhan (1987). The field screening technique has following limitations:

(i) Continuous cropping of pigeonpea in the same field encourages build up of Phytophthora blight.
(ii) The screening depends on the weather conditions like cloudy weather etc.
(iii) Only limited number of lines can be screened.
(iv) Release of water logging may not be uniform in the field.

The pot screening technique is more efficient in summer when the ambiant day temperature rises to 35°C or more in May. The test lines are planted in plastic pots of 18″ diameter. The pots are perforated and lined with muslin cloth at the bottom and filled with black soil. Five seedlings are raised in each pot for 40 days. The pots are then submerged in water filled containers for 5-6 days. The number of dead plants are recorded periodically after relieving the waterlogging. The Phytophthora blight was avoided by using the soil free of inoculum.

8.4 Drought

Pigeonpea is the crop well adopted to drought prone environment. In India, it is grown mainly in rainy season under rainfed conditions depending on the stored soil water. It is thus exposed to periods of transient drought during much of its vegetative stages and then to terminal drought during the reproductive stages. Its production is enhanced greatly if the water deficit is avoided.

The effect of water deficit in pigeonpea has been studied in detail by Teixeira *et al.* (1983). The water deficit reduces the efficiency of interception and efficiency of conversion of PAR to biomass. The efficiency of interception is reduced through reduction in leaf area index due to slower rates of leaf, smaller leaf areas, reduced leaf area duration through faster leaf senescence and decreased K as a consequence of paraheliotropic leaf movement and leaf rolling. The duration and/or reproductive growth is reduced and abscision of pod is excessive. The effect of water deficit on these components depends on timing relative to crop ontogeny duration and intensity. In case water deficit developing gradually, the reduction in the efficiency of interception may be more than in efficiency of conversion. The reverse may be true if the water deficit develops rapidly as in advanced crop with limited soil water reserves. In general, pigeonpea is resistant to water deficit prior to flowering but subsequent to flowering, water deficit may induce abscission of flower-buds and small pods. If it occurs later towards the maturity, causes premature leaf loss reducing seed size. The drought adversely affects the nitrogen fixation. The water deficit reduces the photosynthesis and transpiration rates greatly due to decreased water contents of leaves.

Pre-soaking seeds with sodium benzoate produces plants showing more relative water contents, less water saturation deficit and less saturation deficit in leaves under water deficit conditions. Such hardened plants contained more soluble carbohydrate, free amino acids and proline and gave higher yield (Nilima and Malik 1983).

8.5 Temperature Stress

Pigeonpea is a warm season crop. Its germination is high over a temperature range of 19-43°C but it is rapid at 26-43°C. The optimum range for rate of hypocotyl elongation is 26-36°C and no germination occurs at 7.1°C or 46.5°C (de Jabrun *et al.* 1981). The germination rate is markedly reduced below 19°C. The growth process such as rates of leaf appearance, leaf area per plant and plant height are increased at 20-28°C. The higher day temperature even 35-45°C do not affect growth of pigeonpea seriously if water supply is adequate. However, under controlled conditions, high constant day temperature of 35°C increase floral abortion and decrease pod set (Turnbull 1986).

On the other hand, vegetative growth is slow at 20°C or less and exposure to relatively mild frost may kill leave and meristems. A brief exposure between -2 and -3°C may cause various degree of defoliation but the temperature between -1 and -3°C for 10 hours is lethal (Morton *et al.* 1982). The pod set has been observed to be low in sowings which flowered in periods of low temperature (Akinola and Whiteman 1975). Under low temperature, abscission of floral buds/flowers takes place and pods do not set. However, inherent differences in pigeonpea genotypes with regard to their ability to set pods under cool conditions exists (Saxena *et al.* 1985). The standard varieties like Gwalior 3 and NP (WR) 15 were tolerant.

8.6 Radiation Effect

The pigeonpea is less sensitive to irradiation although, extended periods of clouds during the monsoon and shadding due to companion crop creates conditions of reduced radiation. It is, however, sensitive to low irradiance during the period of pod formation when pod retention depends on current assimilation. If coincides with cloud covers, pod setting is very poor but it recovers on disappearance of such conditions.

In one of the progeny of pigeonpea, development of dark red colour of pods on the side exposed to sun has been reported by Gupta and Saxena (1985). This colour on pods was irreversible. Such a change in colour due to exposure to sun has also been reported in stems of some genotypes of pigeonpea.

8.7 Yellow Ring Disease/Jassid Toximea

The yellow ring disease was observed on several pigeonpea varieties at the research farm Faizabad, India in the month of December by Singh and Singh (1982). As much as 90% plants were observed to show the symptoms in some of the varieties.

8.7.1 Symptoms

The most characteristic symptoms of the disease are formation of red yellow rings throughout the laminae of leaflets. The rings have normal green colour in centre and the number varied 1 to several leaflet. A close examination reveals a minute necrotic speck resulting from an insect feeding puncture in the centre. The rings in some cases may be confined to one side of the midrib. Sometimes rings are oblong or broken. In severe cases, circular, oblong or broken rings may coalesce producing a yellow mosaic effect from a distance. Occasionally ring spots are also observed. In addition to yellow ring symptoms, bright yellowing may be seen around the mid-vein which is more pronounced on one side. Such yellowing normally progresses from the bottom end of the mid-vein towards centre. Sometimes this yellowing is represented by dotting or minute flecking pattern along part or whole of the mid-vein. In later stages, core of the ring or ring spot turns purplish brown in colour.

8.7.2 Cause

The green jassids, *Amaraska kerri* Pruthi could produce the typical symptoms of the disease when fed on healthy plants with or without prior feeding on diseased plants. A proportionate relationship between the number of yellow rings produced and the jassids present on plant was observed. Thus the association of green jassids with the disease is established but possibility of some jassid borne infectious agent involved as its cause cannot be ruled out and need further confirmation. It may be the result of jassid toximea also. Further work on this disease is needed.

8.8 Bracteomania

Some pigeonpea plants of the variety Pusa Ageti were observed with abnormal appearance in the experimental crop in state of Gujarat, India (Desai *et al.* 1981). The abnormality was found to be genetic one and designated as 'bracteomania'.

The affected plants look like if they are affected by some viral disease. Such plants were stunted, greener with fewer branches than normal plants. Instead of normal leaves of three leaflets on a long petiole, only solitary, simple leaves were found attached to the stems, twigs and floral shoots of affected plants. These leaves were with obtuse tips, larger and greener than the normal ones. The axillary floral buds proliferated into abnormal clustered inflorescence. The flowers were bunched and tightly packed giving a knotty appearance. They were sessile buds greatly reduced in size and remained undeveloped with intect bracts and other floral parts remaining green in colour. The flower bud clusters ultimately dried remaining loosely attached to the floral axis. The normal flowers or pods are not formed on affected plants.

8.9 Phyllode

A natural variation was observed in plants of pigeonpea variety Prabhat at Parbhani, India. Some of the plants had green instead of yellow petals. The plants developed pods up to a certain height from the ground level but no seed setting was obtained. Other characters were the same as those of parental (Marekar 1980).

8.10 Allelopathy

The pigeonpea leaf litter is reported to cause root tip necrosis, stunting and reduced germination of several plant species including pigeonpea. Such symptoms were produced by extract of leaf litter with potassium hydroxide and without any pathogen (Hepperly and Mannel 1983).

REFERENCES

Agarwala, S.C. and Associates. 1973. Annual progress Report of ICAR, All India Coordinated Scheme on Micronutrients in Soils and Plants for Lucknow University 1973-74. Lucknow University, Lucknow, Uttar Pradesh, India.

Agarwala, S.C. and Associates. 1978. Annual Progress Report of ICAR, All India Coordinated Scheme of Micronutrients in Soils and Plants for Lucknow University 1978-79. Lucknow University, Lucknow, Uttar Pradesh, India.

Akinola, J.O. and Whiteman, P.C. 1975. Agronomic studies on pigeonpea (*Cajanus cajan* (L.) Millsp.) I. Field responses to sowing times. *Australian Journal of Agricultural Research* 26 : 43-56.

Bergmann, W. 1992, Colour Atlas, Nutritional Disorders of Plants—Visual and Analytical Diagnosis. Gustav Fischer, Jena.

Bergmann, W. and Neubert, P. 1976. Plant diagnosis and Plant analysis. VFb Gustav Fischer, Verlog, Jena.

Bradford, K.J. and Yang, S.F. 1981. Physiological responses of plants to water logging. *Horticultural Science* 16 : 25-30.

Chapman, H.D. 1966. Diagnostic criteria for plant and soil (ed.). University of California, Division of Agricultural Sciences, Berkeley, USA.

Chauhan, Y.S. 1987. Screening for tolerance to salinity and water logging : Case studies with pigeonpea and chickpea pp. 93-103. *In* : Adoption of chickpea and pigeonpea to abiotic stresses. Proceedings of Consultants Workshops, 19-21 Dec. 1984, ICRISAT Centre, Patancheru, India.

Cook, R.L. and Miller, C.E. 1953. Plant nutrient dificiencies. Special Bulletin No. 353. Michigan Agricultural Experiment Station, Michigan State University, East Lansing.

Dalal, R.C. and Quilt, P. 1977. Effect of N.P. liming and Mo on nutrition and grain yield of pigeonpea. *Agronomy Journal* 69 : 854-857.

de Jabrun, P.L.M., Byth, D.E. and Wallis, E.S. 1981. Inhibition by and effects of temperature on germination of mature seed of pigeonpea. pp. 181-187. *In* : Proceedings of the International Workshop on pigeonpea Vol. 2, 15-19 December 1980, ICRISAT Centre, Patancheru, India.

Desai, B.G., Patel, J.C. and Vora, M.S. 1981. Bracteomania : a genetic abnormality giving a virus disease syndrome in pigeonpea. *International Pigeonpea Newsletter* 1 : 20-21.

Dubey, S.D. and Asthana, A.N. 1987. Selection of plant types for resistance to water logging in pigeonpea. page 311 *In* : Food Legume improvement for Asian Farming System (Eds. E.M. Wallis, and D.E. Byth). Proceedings of International Workshop, 1-5th September 1986, Khon Kain, Thailand, ACIAR Proceeding No. 18 ACIAR, Canberra, Australia.

Gupta, S.C. and Saxena, K.B. 1985. Sun red pod colour in pigeonpea. *International Pigeonpea Newsletter* 4 : 28-29.

Gupta, V.K., Hans Raj and Singh, Balwant. 1984. Pigeonpea response to Zn and critical Zn levels. *International Pigeonpea Newsletter* 3 : 32-33.

Gupta, V.K., Yadava, S.S., Potalia, B.S. and Laura, R.D. 1985. Effect of salinity and phosphorus on growth, zinc and P nutrition of pigeonpea (*Cajanus cajan*). *International Journal of Tropical Agriculture* 111 : 95-104.

Gururaja, G. and Rao, R.G. 1982. Anatomical ohanges in the leaves and their role in adoption to salinity in pigeonpea (*Cajanus indicus* Spreg.) and gingelley (*Sesamum indicum* L.). *Proceedings Indian National Science Academy* 48 : 774-778.

Gururaja, G. and Rao, R.G. 1989. Studies on salt tolerance of pigeonpea cultivars, 2. Epicuticular wax and salt tolerance. *Legume Research* 12 : 22-26.

Hepperly, P.R. and Mannel, Diaz 1983. The allelopathic potential of pigeonpea in Puerto Rico. *Journal of Agricultural University Puerto Rico* 67 : 453-463.

Hewitt, E.J. 1963. The essential nutrient elements : Requirements and interactions in plants. pp. 137-360 *In* : Plant Physiology Vol. III (Ed. F.C. Steward). Academic Press, New York.

Johansen, C. 1990. Pigeonpea : Mineral nutrition. Pages 209-231 *In* : The pigeonpea (Eds. Y.L. Nene, Hall, S.D. and V.K. Sheila). C.A.B. International, Wallingford, Oxon, U.K.

Joshi, S.S. 1984. Effect of salinity stress on organic and mineral constituents in the leaves of pigeonpea (*Cajanus cajan* L. var. C 11). *Plant and Soil* 82 : 69-76.

Joshi, S. and Nimbalkar, D. 1983. Effect of salt stress on growth and yield in *Cajanus cajan* L. *Plant and Soil* 74 : 291-294.

Katyal, J.C. 1981. Micronutrient research in pigeonpea. Pages 221-226. *In* : Proceedings of the International Workshop on Pigeonpeas, Vol. 1, 15-19 December 1980, ICRISAT, Patancheru, India.

Kuhad, M.S. and Sheoran, I.S. 1987. Influence of simulated drought and salt stress at iso-osmotic levels on seedlings growth on pigeonpea genotypes. *International Pigeonpea Newsletter* 6 : 48-49.

Kumar Rao, J.V.D., Chauhan, Y.S. and Johansen, C. 1996. Abiotic stresses of extra short duration pigeonpea. pages 80-85 *In* : Prospects of extra short duration pigeonpea in rotation with winter crops. Proceedings of IARI-ICRISAT Workshop and monitoring tour, 16-18 October 1995 (Eds. Laxman Singh, Y.S. Chauhan, C. Johansen and S.P. Singh), New Delhi and Patancheru, India.

Liu Lee-Chyuan 1984. Different irrigation regimes influence phytotoxicity of prometryn to pigeonpeas (*Cajanus cajan* (L.) Millsp) in four soils. *The Journal of Agricultural University Puerto Rico* 48 : 315-321.

Malima, A. Perera, Saxena, K.B., Pooni, H.S. and Chauhan, Y.S. 1998. Genetic control of water logging tolerance in pigeonpea. Pages 154-155 *In* : Abstracts of National Symposium on Biotic and Abiotic Stresses in Pulse Crops, 26th-28th June 1998. IIPR, Kanpur, India.

Mehrotra, N.K., Dube, B.K. and Agarwala, S.C. 1983. Effect of zinc deficiency on uptake of Zn, Mn, P and activity of some enzymes in four pigeonpea genotypes. *Indian Journal of Agricultural Sciences.* 53 : 30-37.

Marekar, R.V. 1980. A case of phyllode in pigeonpea. *Indian Journal of Heridity* 12 (3) : 63.

Morton, J.F., Smith, R.E., Lugo-Lopez, M.A. and Abrams, R. 1982. Pigeonpeas (*Cajanus cajan* (L.) Millsp) : A valuable crop of tropics. Special Publication of

College of Agriculture Sciences, Department of Agronomy and Soils. University of Puerto Rico, Mayguez, Puerto Rico, 123 pp.

Nichols, R. 1964. Studies on the major elements deficiencies of the pigeonpea (*Cajanus cajan*) in sand culture. I. Foliar symptoms of major element deficiencies. *Plant and Soils* 21 : 377-387.

Nichols, R. 1965. Studies on the major elements deficiencies of pigeonpea (*Cajanus cajan*) in sand culture II. The effect of major element deficiencies on nodulation, growth and mineral composition. *Plant and Soils* 22 : 112-126.

Nilima and Malik, C.P. 1983. Physiological and biological changes under water stress in pigeonpea plants grown from seed soaked in water and chemicals. *Indian Journal of Agricultural Sciences* 53 : 550-556.

Rao, V.K. and Rao, M.K.V. 1984. Influence of potassium on chlorophyll content of pigeonpea leaves. *Comparative Physiology and Ecology* 9 : 169-172.

Ravindra Nath, N.N.V.S., Satyanarayana, N.V., Prasad, P. and Rao, K.V.M. 1985. Foliar application of potassium on growth and yield components of pigeonpea (*Cajanus cajan* (L.) Millsp). *Proceedings Indian Academy of Sciences* 94 : 671-676.

Reddy, P.R., Subbarao, I.V. and Madhusudanrao, L. 1978. Nutritional disorders in pigeonpea (*Cajanus cajan* (L.) Millsp) cv. Hy 3c and remedial measures. *Science and Culture* 44 : 36-37.

Satyanarayana, N.V., Prasad, P. and Rao, K.V.M. 1985. Effect of sulphur dioxide on growth and nodulation of pigeonpea. *Proceedings Indian Academy of Sciences* 95 : 199-202.

Saxena, K.B., Gupta, M.D., Chauhan, Y.S. and Faris, D.G. 1985. Low temperature induced floral abscission in pigeonpea. *International Pigeonpea Newsletter* 4 : 27-28.

Sharma, C.P. 1996. Deficiency symptoms and critical concentration of micronutrients in crop plants (ed.). Lucknow University Centre Bulletin No. 1, pp. 1-110.

Sharma, S.K., Dua, R.P. and Singh, D. 1998. Relative performance in sodicity tolerance and genetic variability in wild and cultivated pigeonpea. Pages 164-165 *In* : Abstracts of National Symposium on Management of Biotic and Abiotic Stresses in Pulse Crops, 26-28th June 1998, IIPR, Kanpur, India.

Shukla, U.C. and Associates. 1976. Annual Progress Report of the ICAR, All India Coordinated Scheme of Micronutrients in Soils and Plants for Haryana Agricultural University 1976-77. Haryana Agricultural University, Hisar, Haryana, India.

Singh, R.N. and Singh, H.M. 1982. Apical distortion and yellow ring : two non-infectious diseases of pigeonpea. *Indian Journal of Mycology and Plant Pathology* 12 : 65-67.

Sprague, H.B. (Editor) 1964. Hunger Signes in Crops. A Symposium, 3rd Edition, XXI + 462 pp. London, Longman, New York; David McKay.

Subbarao, G.V. 1988. Salinity tolerance in pigeonpea (*Cajanus cajan* (L.) Millsp.) and its wild relatives. Ph. D. thesis, Indian Institute of Technology, Kharagpur, India, pp. 217.

Teixeira, J.B., Oliva, M.A. and Cambaia, J. 1983. (Efficacy of water use by forage legumes subjected to water deficit). *Revista Ceres* 30 (172) : 463-470.

Turnbull, L.V. 1986. The role of photoperiod and temperature in early vegetative growth and floral development in selected lines of pigeonpea (*Cajanus cajan* (L.) Millsp.). Ph.D. thesis, University of Queensland, Australia, 309 pp.

Verulkar, S.B. and Singh, D.P. 1998. Inheritance of salt tolerance during germination in pigeonpea. pages 163-164 *In* : Abstracts of National Symposium on Biotic and Abiotic Stresses in Pulse Crops 26-28th June 1998, IIPR, Kanpur, India.

Viets, F.G. and Associates. 1954. Zinc contents and deficiency symptoms of 26 crops grown on zinc deficient soils. *Soil Science* 78 : 305-316.

Wallace, T. 1961. The diagnosis of mineral deficiency in plants by visual methods. A colour Atlas and Guide (3rd edition), H.M. Stationery London, U.K.

9

Phanerogamic Parasites

The phanerogamic plant parasites have been reported to attack number of crop plants producing disease like symptoms. These parasites attack roots or stems of the host plant and draw their nutrition causing slow death of host. During this process typical symptoms are produced imparting the plants a diseased appearance. They may be a "Holoparasites" like *Cuscuta* spp. and *Orobanche* spp. which are totally dependent on their host for nutrition while some are "Semiparasites" like *Striga* spp. and *Loranthus* spp. which possess chlorophyll for synthesizing their food but draw water and minerals for their requirement from the host plants. The pigeonpea is reported to be attacked by *Cuscuta* sp. only from India.

Cuscuta spp.

It is also known as dodder, love vine, gold thread, hair weed, devils hair, devils ringlet, pull down, clover silk, and hell bind in English and Amarbel in Hindi. It was reported to attack one of the double cross entry of pigeonpea from ICRISAT severely at the research farm of JNKVV, Jabalpur, India (Kotasthane *et al.* 1980).

The pigeonpea plants attacked by the parasite were underdeveloped with a tendency to dry prematurely. The plants were badly entwined with the slender vines. The transverse section of the host stem exhibited presence of the haustoria of the parasite. The parasite badly infected pigeonpea plants covering all the green parts with coloured stems and branches of inflorescence.

The parasite was identified as *Cuscuta hyalina*. This is a leafless, filiform, branched and orange coloured plant. The flowers of the parasite are minute, in cluster and pale yellow in colour, bracteate with gamopetalous corolla, tetra or pentamerous stamens inserted between the lobes of the corolla. Anthers are yellow in colour, stylet two in numbers, distinct with yellowish capitate stigma. Fruits are capsules with 2-4 seeds, brownish and triangular.

Non-specific control is recommended but use of specific weedicide and the uninfested crop seed is important. They can easily be separated by using 20-22 mesh sieves.

REFERENCE

Kotasthane, S.R., Gupta, Om and Singh, B.R. 1980. A new record of parasitic *Cuscuta* on pigeonpea. *Tropical Grain Legume Bulletin* 19 : 16-18.

10

Integrated Disease Management

Atleast five diseases of pigeonpea, namely wilt, sterility mosaic phytophthora blight, alternaria blight and dry root rot/macrophomina stem canker are of economic importance. More than one of them can occur in the same field/area. For example, in the state of Bihar, Uttar Pradesh, Gujarat and some southern states of India, sterility mosaic and wilt are serious problems while in West Bengal, Madhya Pradesh wilt and phytophthora blight are common. Alternaria blight is serious problem in Bihar while cercospora leaf spot and powdery mildew occur in most of the states to a variable extent. Hence, adoption of control measures with integrated pest management approach for more than one diseases becomes necessary. The IDM system includes the following components:

Resistant Varieties

The pigeonpea germplasm has been found rich for resistance to fusarium wilt, sterility mosaic and alternaria blight but resistance to phytophthora blight and dry root rot is rarely available and not consistant. It is the need of time to develop good varieties of pigeonpea possessing multiple resistance to biotic and abiotic stresses. The intensive work on this aspect has resulted in release and recommendation of some good varieties resistant to more than one diseases. The best examples are ICPL 87119 (Asha), BDN 2, BSMR 736, AL 1, BSMR 175 (All resistant to wilt and sterility mosaic; ICP 8863 (Maruthi) resistant to wilt and early stage seedling mortality etc. Three pigeonpea lines, namely 3D-8111 (UC 5543-1), 3D-8127 (UC 1381-1) and 3D-8104 (UC 5103-1) were developed and released in Ibadan, Nigeria which were claimed to be high yielding early maturing and resistant to most of the diseases (Anonymous 1973). The efforts are being made to combine resistance to insect pests also. The information on multiple resistance in pigeonpea has been reviewed by Onim (1984) and Nene (1988) and the sources of resistance for more than one diseases have been identified (Table 10.1). The first pigeonpea line with multiple resistance seems to be sabour 2E which showed resistance to wilt and sterility (Alam 1931).

Table 10.1 : Sources of multiple disease resistance in pigeonpea

Diseases	*Genotypes found resistant*	*Reference*
Wilt & Sterility mosaic	Purple 1 and 12 others	Venkateswarlu *et al.* (1980, 1981), Venkateswarlu & Singh (1980)
	ICP 3782, 4769, 5097, 6831, 7201, 7273, 7336, 7867, 8861, 8862, 8867, 8869, Purple 1 Sel, Cross No. 74342 and 74363	Reddy *et al.* (1981)
	ICP 7336, 8861, 5133-2-2, 7035, 7217-4-1	Zote *et al.* (1983)
	35 BWSMR series	Zote *et al.* (1987)
	BSMR 65, 242, 243, 270, 294, 493, 511, 519, 528, 539, 540, 544, 697, 736; BWR 97, 153, 159, 175, 177 and 322	Zote and Dandnaik (1987)
	ICP 7198, 8024, 8860 to 8862, 9142, 10960; ICPL 83, 227; PR 5149	Nene (1988)
	AL 1, H 76-51, H 76-65, DA 12, ICPL 267	Reddy *et al.* (1989)
	BWR 23, 369; ICPL 227, 83024	Shirshikar *et al.* (1990)
	ICP 8860, 9174, 11297; BSMR 159, 540, PI 397430, PR 5149 Sel, P7 SMWR 35	Reddy *et al.* (1993)
	ICP 7035, 7336; BDN 2, BWR 22, 23, 24, BSMR 146, 165, 175, 198, 203, 736	Shinde & Zote (1993)
	ICPL 87119	Jain *et al.* (1993)
	BSMR 736 released	Zote *et al.* (1995)
	ICPL 90018, 93179, 93177, 90029, 93175 (Short duration)	Singh *et al.* (1996)
	ICPM 93003 (short genetic male sterile) released 1998.	Saxena *et al.* (1998)
Wilt & Phytophthora	ICP 3753, 7182, 7273	Nene *et al.* (1981)
Blight	No. ICP 7200, 8863, 9080, 80827; KPBR 80-2-2, PI 397430 Sel, PR 5149 Sel.	Prasad & Agrawal (1994)
Wilt, SMD, blight	ICP 7273	Nene *et al.* (1981)
(Phytophthora)	ICP 11302, 11303, 11304, KPBR 80-2	Nene (1988) Anonymous (1990)
Wilt & dry root rot	CO 2	Veeraswamy *et al.* (1975)

Diseases	*Genotypes found resistant*	*Reference*
	CO 3 (S18) a mutant of CO 1	Vidhyasekaran and Arjunan (1976), Sheriff *et al.* (1977a, 1977b)
Wilt, SMD, alternaria blight	ICP 8861, 8862, 10960	Nene (1988)
SMD, Phytophthora blight	ICP 934, 4765, 4866, 5656, 6974, 7185, 7232, 7369, 7273, 7414, 8101, 8127, 8132, 8139, 8147, 8151	Nene *et al.* (1981)
	NPWR 15, 1234, Bahar	Reddy *et al.* (1989)
	ICP 8103, 10958, KPBR 80-2-2	Reddy *et al.* (1993)
Early stage mortality	AGS 522, ICPL 161, 8863, KPBR 80-1, 80-2, 80-3 and T7	Agrawal and Nema (1989)
U. cajani, Phoma, Cercospora and Colletotrichum	64-16A	Rodriguez and Melendez (1984)

For stability of yield and wide adoptability of pigeonpea genotypes, it is essential that cultivars be developed with resistance to important diseases and the races of important pathogens of that area. It would be desirable that breeding programme should involve one parent resistant to wilt and/or SMD and the another be resistant to phytophthora blight (Green *et al.* 1981). Breeding pigeonpea for disease resistance has been reviewed by Reddy and Jain (1992). Saxena *et al.* (1997) developed a male sterile wilt and SMD resistant line by transferring male steile gene (ms 1) from ICPM 93007 through back crossing to the recurring parents ICPL 283 for use in hybrid seed production and released it in 1994.

Tillage Practices

Deep summer ploughing after harvest of the crop exposes the soil borne pathogens to solar heat reducing their quantum specially that of *S. rolfsii, Fusarium* spp., *Rhizoctonia* spp. and nematodes. The efficacy of the solar heat is increased by a technique of 'Solarization' in which the soil is covered with transaparent polythene sheets for 6-8 weeks in April-May. The technique is highly effective if soil is irrigated and treated with carbendazim before covering with polythene. The collar rot pathogen, *S. rolfsii* can also be reduced by removing undecomposed plant debris from the field at the time of field preparation. Removal of pigeonpea diseased plant debris helps in reducing the wilt and phytophthora blight diseases also (Agrawal and Khare 1988).

General sanitation and the tillage methods that burry the crop residues and weeds under the soil are effective against most of the foliar diseases of pigeonpea.

Sowing Time and Methods

Most of the pathogens are restricted in their environmental requirements more as compared to their hosts. An optimum sowing time/season may thus be worked out for growing the crop so that pathogen, although present at the site, is not able to attack the plant. However, optimum sowing time is often locally restricted in its application due to meteorological and biotic factors. The same time or practice may have an entirely different effect under different climatic regions. The pigeonpea wilt is much more less in post-rainy season crop as compared to rainy season crop (Kannaiyan and Nene 1985) while alternaria blight is more serious on post-rainy season pigeonpea. Early sowing of pigeonpea reduces the incidence of sterility mosaic disease. The powdery mildew of pigeonpea is reduced by late sowing and avoiding perennial pigeonpea.

The stem rot of pigeonpea can be reduced greatly by avoiding thick sowing along with seed treatment with captan/thiram. On the other hand less plant spacing 25 × 10 cm has been reported to reduce the incidence of wilt as well as sterility mosaic with increased yield of post rainy season pigeonpea in Mharashtra (Perane *et al.* 1998).

Seed Treatment

The main objective of IPM is to manage the diseases by reducing the use of hazardous chemicals like fungicides so as to avoid the environmental pollution. Seed treatment with fungicides involves much less quantity of chemicals with comparatively high benefits and hence is well included for IPM. Seed treatment with carbendazim + thiram (1 : 2) @ 2.5 to 3.0 g/kg of seed reduces fusarium wilt and alternaria blight greatly. For control of pigeonpea cyst and root knot nematodes, seed soaking with 0.5 to 2% aldicarb for 30-60 minutes is highly effective. Similarly metalaxyl (Apron) as seed treatment @ 6 g/kg has been found effective against phytophthora blight.

Crop Rotation and Intercropping

Crop rotation or intercropping of cereals like Sorghum or tobacco with pigeonpea reduces wilt incidence in pigeonpea. Similarly, use of Sorghum, maize, pearl millet or rice reduces the population of cyst, root knot and reniform nematodes greatly. The crop rotation has been found effective for minimizing certain foliar diseases also. Crop rotation and avoiding bean crop near pigeonpea can reduce the rust of pigeonpea. The crop rotation is effective against foliar anthracnose also. The basic principle of these practices is to make the pathogen devoid of the host so as to reduce its population. The pathogens which can survive for a longer period in absence of the host cannot be controlled by crop rotation or intercropping. However, there are few examples in which pathogen is checked due to the antibiosis.

Nutrient Management

Judicious and balanced use of different plant nutrients is important for getting high yields of pulses. Imbalanced use of the nutrients not only reduces the yields directly but also make the plants prone to attack of various biotic diseases.

Nitrogen is necessary for growth and good yield of crops but its high doses specially with deficiency of other nutrients like P or K make the plant tissues prone to attack by certain pathogens like *Phytophthora drechsleri* f sp. *cajani* on pigeonpea while application of K reduces it regardless of presence or absence of N and P. Not only the quantity but quality of the nitrogen is important. Thus, nitrogen in form of ammonium sulphate reduces the collar rot of pulses caused by *Sclerotium rolfsii.* The pathogenic effects of *S. rolfsii* is reduced by application of calcium also which neutralizes the oxalic acid produced by the pathogen.

Zinc has been reported to retard the colonization of pigeonpea wilt pathogen *F. udum* and hasten its disappearance from the soil. Use of 80 ppm zinc reduces the pigeonpea wilt while urea increases it considerably.

Green manuring with *Crotalaria juncea* reduces the wilt, root rot and the cyst nematodes in pigeonpea.

Water Management

Some of the pigeonpea diseases are influenced by water management practices greatly. The phytophthora blight can be managed well by providing good drainage through sowing crop on ridges or raised beds or by opening dead furrows in the field after every 20 to 30 m. The spread of soil borne pathogens like those of wilt and phytophthora blight diseases can be checked by avoiding flow of water from diseased to healthy fields.

Intercultural Operations

The pathogen *Phytophthora drechsleri* f sp. *cajani* causing blight of pigeonpea is dispersed through water-splashing during rains from soil to stems/branches. Hence, it is reduced in the unweeded areas as compared to weeded one. In place of weeds, fast growing crops like soybean or cowpea may be used as intercrop for this purpose.

The plants are mechanically injured during the weeding which may increase the phytophthora blight and the stem cankers caused by various pathogens specially *Phoma cajani*.

Sanitation

Sanitation practices reduce the inoculum potential of pathogens of most of the diseases in area ultimately resulting in reduction of disease severity. Roguing of diseased plants with roots and their destruction help in minimizing the wilt, root rots, stem cankers, phytophthora blight and several other diseases. Destruction of diseased crop residues is considered as the effective control for phyllosticta leaf spot of pigeonpea.

Timely roguing and destruction of diseased plants also help in minimizing most of the virus diseases due to elimination of source of inoculum.

Harvesting

Delay in harvesting cause yield losses due to shattering and damage by other agencies. In addition it may cause infection of seed by field fungi. Timely harvest helps in reducing most of the seed borne diseases like cercospora leaf spot, alternaria blight and seed and seedling blights caused by several fungi.

Biological control

Several antagonists have been reported against various pathogens of pigeonpea which have been discussed under respective chapters. The most important are *Trichoderma harzianum, T. viride* and *Bacillus subtilis* against *Fusarium udum* (wilt) and *S. rolfsii. T. harzianum* + thiram on seed is reported to control wilt by 68% (Pandey and Upadhyay 1999). *T. harzianum* has been found antagonistic to soil borne pathogens like *R. solani*, and *Pythium* spp. also and is not sensitive to carbendazim, mancozeb, thiram and streptocycline at recommended doses for seed treatment (Mehta *et al.* 1993). Compatibility with *T. harzianum* has been shown by urea, murate of potash, ammonium sulphate while metalaxyl, chlorothalonil, captafol, aldicarb, phorate, carbofuran, ethoprop, sebufos and 2, 4-D were less toxic (Sharma and Mishra 1995). The VAM (*Gigaspora calospora*) has been reported to reduce the incidence of phytophthora blight of pigeonpea. Similarly, *T. harzianum*, a bacterium *Pasteuria penetrans, Gigaspora margarita, Paecilomyces lilacinus* and *Verticillium chlamydosporum* have been reported to control important nematodes specially *Heterodera cajani* and nematode mediated wilt of pigeonpea (Siddiqui and Mahmood 1995). *Glomus mosseae, Paecilomyces liiacinus* and *Pseudomonas fluorescens* alone or in combination controlled *Heterodera cajani* mediated wilt of pigeonpea in spot. They were highly effective in combinaion as compared to used signly (Siddiqui *et al.* 1998).

The soil amendments with Neem, mustard and Mahua cakes are reported to check the nematodes and the nematode mediated wilt of pigeonpea due to increase in population of certain antagonistic fungi in soil.

The method of application and formulations of the antagonist has been a problem in effective biological control of plant diseases. Certain formulations have been made of biofungicides based on *Trichoderma harzianum* (Mehta *et al.* 1995) as follows:

The biomass of the antagonist is produced by solid state fermentation using rice bran and wheat bran. The biomass is dried by pan drying, grinded to reduce the desired particle size, amalgamated with the inert material like lignite and diatomaceous earth and pelleted formulations are made in various concentrations with sodium alginate and inert filler like lignite. This viscous mixture dripped into calcium chloride solution. Beads are then dried for use of storage purpose. Efforts were also made for efficaceous formulations by producing chlamydospores inoculant in molasses corn strip liquor fermentation. After filtering the biomass, pan drying carried out. The dried biomass after grinding is formulated with rice bran in alginate beads for application in soil. While preparing these formulations the factors like easy applications, extended self life, production economics, quality control check, monitoring of product and the nature of the product have also been studied carefully.

Examples of IDM Modules

Several components of the IDM as discussed above have been tested and found effective against various diseases of pigeonpea but these components in combined form have been tested only in few cases. The best example is that of phytophthora blight which is controlled best by integrated treatment involving seed treatment with apron 4 g/kg seed + sowing pigeonpea on ridges or raised beds + sowing of soybean or cowpea as intercrop so as to work as cover crop (Agrawal S.C. and Prasad K.V.V., unpublished data from Sehore Madhya Pradesh, India).

REFERENCES

Agrawal, S.C. and Khare, M.N. 1988. Survival of *Phytophthora drechsleri* f sp. *cajani* causing stem blight of pigeonpea. *Indian Phytopathology* 41 : 250-251.

Agrawal, S.C. and Nema, Sushma, 1989. Multiple disease resistance in pigeonpea (*Cajanus cajan*) genotypes against early plant mortality. *Indian Journal of Agricultural Sciences* 59 : 73.

Alam, M. 1931. Report, Department of Agriculture, Bihar and Orissa 1930-31. pp. 42-65.

Anonymous. 1973. Grain Legume Improvement Programme. In International Institute of Tropical Agriculture Report. Ibadan, Nigeria : IITA. 78 pp.

Green, J.M., Sharma, D., Reddy, L.J., Saxena, K.B., Gupta, S.C., Jain, K.C., Reddy, B.V.S. and Rao, M.R. 1981. Methodology and progress in the ICRISAT pigeonpea breeding programme. pages 437-449 *In* Proceedings, International Workshop on Pigeonpeas, Vol. 1, ICRISAT, 15-19 Dec. 1980, Patancheru, India.

Jain, K.C., Reddy, M.V. and Ariyanayagam, R.P. 1993. Wilt and sterility mosaic resistant pigeonpea variety for central and peninsular India. *International Pigeonpea Newsletter* 17 : 10-12.

Kannaiyan, J. and Nene, Y.L. 1985. Effect of sowing dates on wilt incidence in pigeonpea. *International Pigeonpea Newsletter* 4 : 33-35.

Mehta, R.D., Patel, K.A., Rao, K.K. and Mehta, M.H. 1995. *Trichoderma harzianum* as biocontrol agent in formulated product. *Indian Journal of Mycology and Plant Pathology* 25 : 129 (Abst.).

Mehta, R.D., Shah, R.N., Patel, S.J., Patel, K.A., Rao, K.A. and Mehta, M.H. 1993. *Trichoderma harzianum* : a potential biocontrol agent in the management of soil borne plant pathogens. *Indian Journal of Mycology and Plant Pathology* 23 : 108 (Abst.).

Nene, Y.L. 1988. Multiple disease resistance in grain legumes. *Annual Review of Phytopathology* 26 : 203-217.

Nene, Y.L., Kannaiyan, J. and Reddy, M.V. 1981. Resistance to major diseases of pigeonpea. Pages 121-128 *in* proceedings of the International Workshop on Pigeonpeas, 15-19 Dec. 1980, ICRISAT Centre, India, Vol. 1. Patancheru, India : ICRISAT.

Onim, J.F.M. 1984. Pigeonpea breeding for disease and pest resistance. *F.A.O. Plant Production and Protection Paper No.* 55 : 153-167.

Perane, R.R., Bendre, N.J., Patil, S.D. and Aher, R.P. 1998. Effect of genoypes and spacing on Wilt and sterility mosaic in post rainy season crop of pigeonpea. *Indian Journal of Pulses Research*, 11 : 130-131.

Prasad, K.V.V. and Agrawal, S.C. 1994. Multiple disease resistance in pigeonpea. Abstract No. 19 *in* Group Meeting of Indian Phytopathological Society Central Zone Chapter 3 & 4 Jan. 1994 at JNAU, College of Agriculture Indore, M.P., India.

Reddy, M.V. and Jain, K.C. 1992. Recent advances in breeding for disease resistance in pigeonpea. Pages 77-83 *in* New Frontiers in Pulses Research and Development : Proceedings of National Symposium, 10-12 Nov. 1989. Directorate of Pulses Research, Kanpur, India.

Reddy, M.V., Nene, Y.L. and Kannaiyan, J. 1981. Identification and utilization of multiple disease resistance in pigeonpea. pages 83-85 *in* Proceedings of the EAI Group Discussion on Increasing Pulse and Oilseed Production in India, 4-5 Sept. 1980, New Delhi, India, Fertilizer Association of India.

Reddy, M.V., Nene, Y.L., Raju, T.N., Sheila, V.K., Kannaiyan, J. and Beniwal, S.P.S. 1989. Evaluation of pigeonpea lines for resistance to wilt, sterility mosaic and phytophthora blight. *International Pigeonpea Newsletter* 10 : 22-24.

Reddy, M.V., Raju, T.N., Jain, K.C., Remanandan, P., Ariyanayagam, R.P., Amin, K.S. and Smith, D.H. 1993. Identification of multiple disease resistance in pigeonpea. *Indian Journal of Plant Protection* 21 : 178-182.

Rodriguez, R. and Melendez, P.L. 1984. Field screening of pigeonpea (*Cajanus cajan*) for resistance to foliar diseases in Puerto Rico. *The Journal of Agricultural Research of University of Puerto Rico* 68 : 275-279.

Saxena, K.B., Kumar, R.V., Reddy, M.V. and Singh, L. 1998. Registration of ICPM 93003, a short duration, wilt and SMD resistant genetic male sterile parental line of pigeonpea. *Crop Science* 38 : 577

Sharma, S.D. and Mishra, A. 1995. Tolerance of *Trichoderma harzianum* to agrochemicals. *Indian Journal of Mycology and Plant Pathology* 25 : 129-130.

Sheriff, N.M., Khan, W.M.A. and Annappan, R.S. 1977a. Red gram CO 3—an economic mutant strain for Tamil Nadu. *Madras Agricultural Journal* 64 : 561-564.

Sheriff, N.M., Khan, W.M.A., Iyemperumal, S. 1977b. A note on the study of red gram mutants for resistance to root rot disease under field conditions. *Madras Agricultural Journal.* 64 : 691.

Shinde, V.K. and Zote, K.K. 1993. Management of wilt and sterility mosaic through resistance breeding in pigeonpea (*Cajanus cajam*). *Indian Journal of Pulses Research* 6 : 60-63.

Shirshikar, S.P., Astaputre, J.U., Shinde, V.K. and Deshmukh, R.V. 1990. Screening of pigeonpea entries against wilt and sterility mosaic disease. *Indian Phytopathology* 43 : 307.

Siddiqui, Z.A. and Mahmood, I. 1995. Some observations on the mangement of wilt disease complex of pigeonpea by treatment with a vesicular and arbuscular fungus and biocontrol agents for nematodes. *Bioresource Technology* 54 : 227-230.

Siddiqui, Z.A., Mahmood, I. and Hayat, Shamshul. 1998. Biocontrol of *Heterodera cajani* and *Fusarium udum* on pigeonpea using *Glomus mosseae, Paecilomyces lilacinus* and *Pseudomonas fluorescens. Thai Journal of Agricultural Sciences* 31 : 310-321.

Singh, N.B., Reddy, M.V., Rao, A.N., Raju, T.N., Singh, Laxman and Gupta, S.C. 1996. Newly developed extra short duration and short duration pigeonpea lines with combined resistance to wilt and sterility mosaic, ICRISAT Asia Centre. *International Chickpea and Pigeonpea Newsletter* 3 : 87-88.

Veeraswamy, R., Rangaswamy, P. and Sheriff, N.M. 1975. CO 2—a new strain with early maturity and improved plant type. *Madras Agricultural Journal* 62 : 541-543.

Venkateswarlu, S., Reddy, A.R., Singh, R.M. and Singh, R.B. 1980. Reaction of pigeonpea varieties to wilt and sterility mosaic. *Tropical Grain Legume Bulletin* 17/18 : 25-28.

Venkateswarlu, S., Reddy, A.R., Chauhan, V.B., Singh, O.N., Singh, R.M. and Singh, U.P. 1981. A promising resistant line of pigeonpea (Malviya arhar-1) for wilt and sterility mosaic (virus ?). *Tropical Grain Legume Bulletin* 23 : 27-29.

Venkateswarlu, S. and Singh, R.B. 1980. Pigeonpea improvement at Banaras Hindu University. *Tropical Grain Legume Bulletin* 17/18 : 28-29.

Vidhyasekaran, P. and Arjunan, G. 1976. A new redgram pigeonpea variety resistant to root rot (*Macrophomina phaseolina*). *Madras Agricultural Journal* 63 : 175-176.

Zote, K.K. and Dandnaik, B.P. 1987. Screening of pigeonpea for multiple disease resistance. *Indian Phytopathology* 40 : 59-62.

Zote, K.K., Dandnaik, B.P., Shinde, V.K. and Raut, K.G. 1987. Screening against wilt and sterility mosaic of pigeonpea at Badnapur. *Indian Phytopathology* 40 : 285.

Zote, K.K., Khapre, P.R., Pawar, N.B., Pawar, G.G., Shrirama, M.D., Sable, K.R., Dahiwal, A.L. and Dhutraj, D.N. 1995. High yielding, wilt and sterility mosaic resistant pigeonpea variety released for cultivation in Maharashtra, India. *International Chickpea and Pigeonpea Newsletter* 2 : 54-55.

Zote, K.K., Thombre, P.G., Khalikar, P.V., Dandnaik, B.P., Chavan, G.V. and Olekar, S.S. 1983. Breeding pigeonpea for resistance to wilt and sterility mosaic. *International Pigeonpea Newsletter* 2 : 43-44.

INDEX